BECOMING EAST GERMAN

SPEKTRUM: Publications of the German Studies Association

Series editor: David M. Luebke, University of Oregon

Published under the auspices of the German Studies Association, *Spektrum* offers current perspectives on culture, society, and political life in the German-speaking lands of central Europe—Austria, Switzerland, and the Federal Republic—from the late Middle Ages to the present day. Its titles and themes reflect the composition of the GSA and the work of its members within and across the disciplines to which they belong—literary criticism, history, cultural studies, political science, and anthropology.

Volume 1
The Holy Roman Empire, Reconsidered
Edited by Jason Philip Coy, Benjamin Marschke, and David Warren Sabean

Volume 2
Weimar Publics/Weimar Subjects
Rethinking the Political Culture of Germany in the 1920s
Edited by Kathleen Canning, Kerstin Barndt, and Kristin McGuire

Volume 3
Conversion and the Politics of Religion in Early Modern Germany
Edited by David M. Luebke, Jared Poley, Daniel C. Ryan, and David Warren Sabean

Volume 4
Walls, Borders, Boundaries
Spatial and Cultural Practices in Europe
Edited by Marc Silberman, Karen E. Till, and Janet Ward

Volume 5
After The History of Sexuality
German Genealogies with and Beyond Foucault
Edited by Scott Spector, Helmut Puff, and Dagmar Herzog

Volume 6
Becoming East German
Socialist Structures and Sensibilities after Hitler
Edited by Mary Fulbrook and Andrew I. Port

Volume 7
Beyond Alterity
German Encounters with Modern East Asia
Edited by Qinna Shen and Martin Rosenstock

Volume 8
Mixed Matches
Transgressive Unions in Germany from the Reformation to the Enlightenment
Edited by David Luebke and Mary Lindemann

Volume 9
Kinship, Community, and Self
Essays in Honor of David Warren Sabean
Edited by Jason Coy, Benjamin Marschke, Jared Poley, and Claudia Verhoeven

Volume 10
The Emperor's Old Clothes
Constitutional History and the Symbolic Language of the Holy Roman Empire
Barbara Stollberg-Rilinger
Translated by Thomas Dunlap

Volume 11
The Devil's Riches
A Modern History of Greed
Jared Poley

Becoming East German

Socialist Structures and Sensibilities after Hitler

Edited by

MARY FULBROOK and ANDREW I. PORT

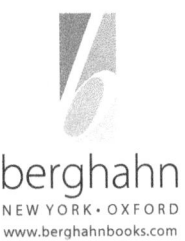

Published in 2013 by

Berghahn Books

www.berghahnbooks.com

© 2013, 2015 Mary Fulbrook and Andrew I. Port
First paperback edition published in 2015

All rights reserved. Except for the quotation of short passages for the purposes of criticism and review, no part of this book may be reproduced in any form or by any means, electronic or mechanical, including photocopying, recording, or any information storage and retrieval system now known or to be invented, without written permission of the publisher.

Library of Congress Cataloging-in-Publication Data

Becoming East German : socialist structures and sensibilities after Hitler / edited by Mary Fulbrook and Andrew I. Port.
  pages cm. — (Specktrum : publications of the German Studies Association ; Volume 6)
  Includes index.
  ISBN 978-0-85745-974-9 (hbk) — ISBN 978-1-78533-027-8 (pbk) — ISBN 978-0-85745-975-6 (ebook)
  1. Germany (East)—Social policy. 2. Germany (East)—Social conditions. 3. Germany (East)—Cultural policy. 4. Socialism—Germany (East) —History. 5. Medical policy—Germany (East) 6. Public health—Germany (East) 7. Socialism and culture—Germany (East) I. Fulbrook, Mary, 1951- author, editor of compilation. II. Port, Andrew I., author, editor of compilation.
  DD283.B427 2013
  943'.10874—dc23

2013005575

British Library Cataloguing in Publication Data

A catalogue record for this book is available from the British Library

ISBN: 978-0-85745-974-9 hardback
ISBN: 978-1-78533-027-8 paperback
ISBN: 978-0-85745-975-6 ebook

❦ CONTENTS ❦

Preface — vii

List of Abbreviations — viii

Introduction. The Banalities of East German Historiography — 1
Andrew I. Port

Part I. Memory and Identity after Nazism

Chapter 1. East Germans in a Post-Nazi State: Communities of Experience, Connection, and Identification — 33
Mary Fulbrook

Chapter 2. Divisive Unity: The Politics of Cultural Nationalism during the First German Writers' Congress of October 1947 — 56
Andreas Agocs

Chapter 3. Communicating History: The Archived Letters of Greta Kuckhoff and Memories of "The Red Orchestra" — 79
Joanne Sayner

Chapter 4. Remembered Change and Changes of Remembrance: East German Narratives of Anti-fascist Conversion — 99
Christiane Wienand

Part II. Health, Food, and Embodied Citizens

Chapter 5. Perceptions of Health after World War II: Heart Disease and Risk Factors in East and West Germany, 1945–75 — 121
Jeannette Madarász-Lebenhagen

Chapter 6. Socialism Fights the Proletarian Disease: East German Efforts to Overcome Tuberculosis in a Cold War Context — 141
Donna Harsch

Chapter 7. The Slim Imperative: Discourses and Cultures of Dieting in the German Democratic Republic, 1949–90 — 158
Neula Kerr-Boyle

Chapter 8. Luxury Dining in the Later Years of the German
   Democratic Republic   179
   Paul Freedman

Part III. Constraints and Conformity: Friends, Foes, and Disciplinary Practices

Chapter 9. Predispositions and the Paradox of Working-Class
   Behavior in Nazi Germany and the German Democratic Republic   201
   Andrew I. Port

Chapter 10. Israel as Friend and Foe: Shaping East German Society
   through *Freund-* and *Feindbilder*   219
   David G. Tompkins

Chapter 11. Humiliation as a Weapon within the Party: Fictional
   and Personal Accounts   237
   Phil Leask

Chapter 12. Playing the Game: Football and Everyday Life in the
   Honecker Era   257
   Alan McDougall

Conclusion. Structures and Subjectivities in GDR History   277
   Mary Fulbrook

Notes on Contributors   291

Index   294

PREFACE

The origins of this book go back to a lively discussion that took place between Andrew Port and Mary Fulbrook when they met for the first time in Germany in October 2009. It was there that the two editors realized that the Atlantic was, despite modern means of electronic communication, still posing a major problem for productive exchanges of ideas about—and the development of innovative approaches to—the history of the German Democratic Republic (GDR). They agreed on the need to foster greater dialogue among scholars trained in Europe and North America who work on the GDR, which ultimately led to the commissioning of the chapters in this volume. These chapters seek to move beyond the tired theoretical debates analyzed in the Introduction and instead develop more fruitful lines of interpretation in light of the new research that has emerged over the past two decades since the dramatic fall of the Berlin Wall. While questions of power can never be absent from discussions of the GDR, there is a shift of focus here to questions of subjectivity and physicality in the historical process of "becoming East German."

The editors would like to thank the two anonymous readers, as well as David Luebke, the editor of the *Spektrum* series, and David Barclay, the executive director of the German Studies Association, for their engagement with and support of this volume. We are also grateful to Marion Berghahn, Ann DeVita, Elizabeth Berg, and the supportive staff at Berghahn Books.

ABBREVIATIONS

BCG	Bacillus Calmette-Guérin
BdM	Bund deutscher Mädel (League of German Girls)
BFC	Berliner Fußballclub Dynamo (Dynamo Berlin Football Club)
BMI	Body Mass Index
BSG	Betriebssportgemeinschaft (Factory Sports Association)
CINDI	Countrywide Integrated Noncommunicable Diseases Intervention
CDU	Christlich Demokratische Union (Christian Democratic Union)
Cominform	Communist Information Bureau
DEFA	Deutsche Film-Aktiengesellschaft (East German Film Studios)
DFV	Deutscher Fußball-Verband der DDR (East German Football Association)
DHMD	Deutsches Hygiene Museum Dresden (German Hygiene Museum)
DSV	Deutscher Schriftsteller-Verband (German Association of Writers)
DTSB	Deutscher Turn- und Sportbund (German Gymnastics and Sports Federation)
FDGB	Freier Deutscher Gewerkschaftsbund (Free German Trade Union Federation)
FDJ	Freie Deutsche Jugend (Free German Youth)
GDR	German Democratic Republic
IM	Inoffizieller Mitarbeiter (unofficial collaborator)
IML	Institut für Marxismus-Leninismus (Institute for Marxism-Leninism)
KPD	Kommunistische Partei Deutschlands (Communist Party of Germany)

LPG	Landwirtschaftliche Produktionsgesellschaft (Agricultural Production Cooperative)
MfS	Ministerium für Staatssicherheit (Ministry for State Security)
MONICA	Multinational MONItoring of trends and determinants in CArdiovascular disease
MRFIT	Multiple Risk Factor Intervention Trial
NATO	North Atlantic Treaty Organization
NDPD	Nationaldemokratische Partei Deutschlands (National Democratic Party of Germany)
NF	Nationale Front (National Front)
NFG	Nationale Forschungs- und Gedenkstatten der klassischen deutschen Literatur (National Research and Memorial Sites of Classical German Literature)
NSDAP	Nationalsozialistische Deutsche Arbeiterpartei (National Socialist German Workers' Party)
NVA	Nationale Volksarmee (National People's Army)
OdF	Opfer des Faschismus (Victims of Fascism)
OMGUS	U.S. Office of the Military Government in Germany
SBZ	Sowjetische Besatzungszone (Soviet Zone of Occupation)
SDA	Schutzverband Deutscher Autoren (Association for the Protection of German Writers)
SDS	Schutzverband Deutscher Schriftsteller (Association for the Protection of German Writers)
SED	Sozialistische Einheitspartei Deutschlands (Socialist Unity Party)
SG	Sportgemeinschaft (sports society)
SMAD	Sowjetische Militäradministration in Deutschland (Soviet Military Administration in Germany)
SPD	Sozialdemokratische Partei Deutschlands (Social Democratic Party of Germany)
SV	Sportvereinigung (sports association)
TB	tuberculosis

USSR	Union of Soviet Socialist Republics
VEB	Volkseigener Betrieb (People's Own Factory)
VVN	Vereinigung der Verfolgten des Naziregimes (Union of those Persecuted by the Nazi Regime)
WHO	World Health Organization
ZIJ	Zentralinstitut für Jugendforschung (Central Institute for Youth Research)
ZK	Zentralkomitee (Central Committee)

INTRODUCTION

The Banalities of East German Historiography

ANDREW I. PORT

For the first decade after the demise of the German Democratic Republic (GDR), professional and popular interest in East German history focused on two broad themes: the forms of power and repression exercised by the ruling elite, and the varieties of dissent and resistance to Communist rule. During this "first wave" of investigation following the opening of the archives, scholarly and public attention fell on spectacular events such as the mass uprising of June 1953 or the construction and fall of the Berlin Wall; the dictatorial, supposedly "totalitarian" nature of the state and its ruling Socialist Unity Party (SED); "high politics" and the significance of Soviet domination, i.e., the formal institutions and structures of power; as well as the threat or use of physical force—symbolized above all by the sinister activities of the State Security Service (Stasi).[1]

Other aspects of life in the GDR were viewed primarily through this lens, with an overwhelming focus on the ways in which people either collaborated with or sought to resist the demands of this highly ideological regime. As a result, interest in the churches or in creative writers and artists, for example, was often limited to their relationships with the regime, their infiltration or cooption by the Stasi, or their contribution to sustaining or undermining the power of the SED. A feverish and often sensational search for former Stasi informers (*Inoffizielle Mitarbeiter*, or IMs)—often with little regard for the exact nature of their collaboration—seemed at times to be a belated attempt to make up for inadequate denazification after 1945.[2]

A gradual move away from this type of top-down, politically inflected, often morally accusatory and triumphalist approach started to emerge in the mid 1990s, as scholars began to broaden their scope and turn to East German society itself as a serious subject of inquiry. These new studies posed the types of questions typically associated with traditional social history, looking at social policies and social developments, as well as at the experiences of social groups such as industrial workers and middle-class professionals, women and youths, writers and artists. Just as this approach began to gather steam and produce substantive results that provided a more nuanced understanding of the relationship between state and society, a "third wave" of studies emerged, influenced by questions associated with the "new cultural history," which relied on the insights of anthropology and linguistic theory. Here the focus of attention was the subjective experiences of "ordinary" East Germans and the possibility of their "agency." It was, above all, scholars working in North America and the United Kingdom who addressed such issues, with an eye to private life and domesticity, material consumption, power in all its guises, perceptions, identities, and discourse.[3]

The boundaries between these "waves" were more porous than this brief, schematic overview suggests; in fact, there was a great deal of overlap among them, both in terms of substance and the actual appearance of individual studies.[4] The general trend has nevertheless been a move away from an almost exclusive focus on high-level "politics" and repression toward one that looks at sociocultural developments at the grassroots level, "everyday history," and questions of agency. This has been accompanied by a broadening of chronological coverage. While many of the initial studies focused on the early decades of the regime under SED leader Walter Ulbricht, more recent ones have looked at its last two decades under Erich Honecker or, in rare cases, the entire forty-year history of the GDR. Some scholars have also adopted a more innovative use of sources, eschewing written documents produced by the regime in favor of a variety of sociocultural artifacts.[5] In short, the historiography of the GDR over the past twenty years has mirrored at breakneck speed the trajectory of postwar historiography more generally, which saw a gradual move away from the "political" to the "social" and then, in turn, to the "cultural."[6]

The Peculiarities of Totalitarian Theory

Out of these various approaches has emerged a major scholarly debate that has come to dominate the field of East German studies—arguably to its detriment. At the heart of the discussion is a deceptively simple question: was the GDR a totalitarian regime in fact as well as in theory? Measured by the various models used to characterize such entities, East Germany—a marginally sovereign state dependent on the USSR for its existence, whose leaders employed Soviet-style methods of rule and provided the mere trappings of democracy in the absence of sustained popular legitimacy—was clearly "totalitarian." Or so it would seem to have been at first glance. Even those who are critical of the concept admit that the regime possessed most, if not all, of the objective traits associated with the term, i.e., rule by a single party or elite that dominated the state machinery; that centrally directed and controlled the economy, mass communication, and all forms of social and cultural organization; that espoused an official, all-encompassing, utopian (or, depending on one's point of view, dystopian) ideology; and that used physical and mental terror and repression to achieve its goals, mobilize the masses, and silence opposition—all of which was made possible by the gradual buildup of a vast state security service.[7] But this was more than a mere dictatorship or run-of-the-mill authoritarian regime relying on single-party rule and repression to do away with genuine political pluralism, guaranteed civil rights, an independent judiciary, and the rule of law. The rulers of totalitarian regimes aspired to complete control of *all* aspects of political, social, economic, and cultural life.

Overviews of the post-Wall historiography routinely claim that "totalitarian theory" enjoyed a renaissance following the demise of state socialism, but this is not accurate. What those who assert this are referring to is the alacrity with which many "first wave" studies referred to East Germany as a totalitarian regime outright—or by employing a variety of euphemisms, all of which suggested that the GDR was a place where "society" had lost all forms of autonomy vis-à-vis the state and thus become a mere reflection of the "political."[8] Yet, the increasing invocation of the term *totalitarian*—or some analogous concept, such as Alf Lüdtke's *durchherrschte Gesellschaft* (thoroughly ruled society)[9]—did not, in itself, constitute a renaissance of this "theory," in the sense of a theory being a set of principles that *explain* a given phenomenon. The term was merely resuscitated, i.e., it once again became a handy label used to describe what was supposedly the essential nature of the GDR. What it—or some variant—helped explain about East Germany remained less clear.

But that is not the main reason why the term *totalitarian* and its use provoked a backlash and came under such vigorous attack by the "sociocultural" historians active during the "second" and "third waves" of GDR-related research. As Peter Grieder argues in a spirited defense of the "theory" as a "tool of historical scholarship," those who reject the term object above all to its politicized nature, moralistic tone, and misuse for conservative political ends; its failure to recognize "agency" or even genuine support on the part of the masses, who are viewed as helpless victims; its static view of developments under such regimes; its uneven focus on the similarities and not differences among various types of "totalitarian" states; its overemphasis on repression as the main stabilizing factor; its neglect of political and social conflicts; and, most important, its tendency to conflate goals with achievements and actual practices.[10] Given the variety of effective limits on official power structures, critics argue, the regime was unable to achieve total control and implement its policies as planned. To cite only one example: the SED may have controlled the media and had a monopoly on the means of communication—a prominent feature of most totalitarian models. But what did that mean in a state where one could, in the privacy of one's home, tune in every evening to West German television and radio?[11] Critics of the term argue, in short, that even as a descriptive label, the "theory" is not useful—or accurate.

These are legitimate objections, but they deserve qualification and further elucidation. It is true, for example, that critics of the term *totalitarian* regard it as a relic of the acerbic ideological Cold War struggles of yore. This makes it politically laden and thus, for some, "academically suspect."[12] Grieder and others have responded to this by pointing out that its pedigree predates the postwar period—but that is beside the point. It is difficult to deny that "totalitarian theory" pinpoints a number of striking similarities between fascism and communism. That, in itself, is not problematic. What is problematic is the subtext of such comparisons—and much of this increasingly tired scholarly controversy revolves around subtexts. In short, the implication is that communism and fascism were cut from the same cloth, that they were two sides of the same coin. That was one point that proponents of the theory were trying to make in a Cold War effort to discredit communism by equating it with fascism—and it is exactly that to which critics of the theory object, namely, its politicized use during the 1950s and 1960s, and then again since 1989–90. (Comparison does not mean equality, Gary Bruce reminds us, but the thrust of *this* comparison seems clear enough.)[13] Critics seem to fear that this not only constitutes an invidious attempt to discredit state socialism for political purposes—but, more important, that it does so by running the risk of relativizing fascist crimes (i.e., genocide) by placing both regimes on an equal plane. In essence, they charge, the theory classifies in order to condemn.

Grieder notes that the misuse of a theory for political purposes does not mean that the theory is incorrect. Again, the similarities between these two types of regimes are undeniable. But what does that mean exactly? What is the heuristic value of this observation? What light does this shed on issues of historical and historiographical significance? As other scholars have pointed out, there is also a great deal of similarity between the bombastic building projects in the 1930s in Moscow under Joseph Stalin and in Washington, D.C. under Franklin Delano Roosevelt.[14] But that is not an argument but rather an observation—and one whose significance is not altogether clear. Besides, the dissimilarities and the significance of those dissimilarities—which totalitarian theorists tend to neglect—are arguably just as important. In the end, what should be determinative when judging the usefulness of a theory or term are their explanatory power and the types of questions they can be used to address and answer. To point out similarities and dissimilarities is not enough.

Other objections to "totalitarian theory" are more weighty, because they call into question the very substance of the claims its proponents make. Grounding their criticism on archivally rich studies that focus on everyday life at the grassroots level, scholars active during the "second" and "third waves" have demonstrated that the intentions and goals of the regime did not automatically translate into practice. There were, in fact, a number of limits that served as an effective check on regime power. They included the weight of past traditions, relatively independent institutions such as the churches, and the overburdening of—and infighting among—party and state officials. But the most forceful criticism of the totalitarian model along these lines points to its failure to take into account the myriad of everyday possibilities for nonconformist, autonomous action and "agency" on the part of "ordinary" East Germans—behavior that not only set distinct limits on the regime's ability to translate its goals into practice, but that could even lead to partial modification of regime policy. Relations between "state" and "society" were asymmetric, in other words, but not entirely one-sided.

Those who discuss such behavior invariably invoke Alf Lüdtke's concept of *Eigensinn*—which, as David Blackbourn once memorably quipped about E.P. Thompson's famous phrase "the enormous condescension of posterity," is a term that seems to have launched a thousand dissertations. But it is also one that remains elusive, which may very well have been the intention of Lüdtke, who himself emphasizes its "ambiguity" (*Vieldeutigkeit*).[15] *Eigensinn* has nevertheless—or perhaps for that very reason—become one of the most popular concepts used to describe a wide range of behavior in East Germany, all of which suggests that the so-called masses were not just passive victims, but that they had "agency."[16] The latter did exist in the GDR, and many people were indeed able to work the system to their own advantage, even if not all of this behavior was necessarily heroic. The larger point is that power relations were far more complex than the simple "state vs. society"—"regime vs. masses"—"rulers vs. ruled" dichotomies have suggested. In fact, the essays in this volume—which look at health and medicine, food and sport, work and leisure, as well as perceptions, memory, ideology, and culture—all serve to help break down those traditional but misleading dichotomies.

Though originally employed by Lüdtke with respect to industrial workers, the term *Eigensinn* has now been applied to almost all social groups in the GDR—and even to entire regions.[17] This inflationary use of the term has not led to greater conceptual clarity. *Eigensinn* refers first and foremost to willful behavior—*Widerborstigkeit, quertreibendes Verhalten*—that allows individuals to demarcate a space of their own.[18] Regardless of its meaning, whenever an author doffs his or her cap to Lüdtke by dropping the word (or some variation thereof) en passant, the reader has some vague and fuzzy feeling of what is meant—or at least thinks that that is the case. According to Lüdtke himself, it is an attempt to go beyond the black-and-white, "either-or" categories of obedience and opposition. Instead, it has become a blanket term used to designate almost any type of resistant or nonconformist behavior in the GDR—becoming in a sense what the problematic term *Resistenz* once was for the Third Reich.[19] In short, it has come to mean everything and, one could argue, nothing at all—beyond the obvious fact that many East Germans had "agency" and that the regime was thus not able to achieve total control.[20]

Rejecting this criticism of totalitarian theory as a straw man, Grieder argues that no one has ever claimed that these regimes were able to achieve complete control. Merle Fainsod, he points out, even spoke of "inefficient" totalitarian rule in his classic study of Soviet rule in Smolensk.[21] That is a fair point. But critics of the theory may be excused for reaching the conclusions that they do about the claims made by the "totalitarian school" given the locution of its practitioners, who favor terms such as *all-powerful* and *all-knowing, omniscient* and *omnipresent*. Writing specifically about East Germany, Klaus Schroeder has unequivocally stated that the regime enjoyed "all-embracing and unlimited, i.e., total, power."[22] This is the type of unrestrained rhetoric to which critics have responded—and that they have rightly rejected.

Faced with an onslaught of criticism over the past decade and a half, some totalitarian theorists have begun to scale back their claims. They now admit, for example, that total control was the aim, not necessarily the reality.[23] In response to criticism about the "static nature" of the theory and its failure to take into account change that took place over the course of these regimes, some have now introduced a series of "hyphenated qualifiers," including ones that try to distinguish among different historical phases, e.g., "late-" or "post-" or "bureaucratic-" totalitarianism.[24] Greater pliability as a descriptive term represents some progress, but one wonders what is left of the "theory" if it is reduced to a model of intentions, and what its purpose and use is if so many variations of the term are not only possible, but now even considered by its own proponents to be necessary. Just as important, it is not clear that this type of revision helps salvage the theory in terms of its explanatory power. Grieder asserts that "it can help *explain* as well as *describe* certain polities," but does not then specify what it is exactly that it explains.[25]

But that is not all: the totalitarian paradigm does not address a whole range of issues that fall beyond its guiding interest in dictatorship and repression. It fails to capture key aspects of everyday life, and gives short shrift to the role played by mentalities and cultural traditions. There was much to life in the GDR that had deeper roots in German history, with echoes and variations in the Federal Republic; at the same time, other major developments there were not unlike those taking place in the other industrial states of postwar Europe—on both sides of the Iron Curtain. Besides failing to tackle the import of this fact, the theory does not explain, or even address, the ways in which East Germans—besides being constrained and formed by the conditions in which they lived—made sense of their own lives, responded to challenges, and adapted to changing conditions. On questions and issues such as these hinge the kinds of interpretation and approach that are adopted—and the totalitarian approach has proven sorely lacking and unfit for the task.

Even if the descriptive and analytical power of totalitarian theory suffers from severe limitations, we should nevertheless be wary of throwing the proverbial baby out with the bathwater. In the first place, the resurgent use of the term, whatever its limitations as a concept and as a descriptive label, has sparked a robust debate about the precise nature of the East German regime. To that extent it has served a useful purpose. But this debate has become sterile, as the same arguments for and against are presented over and over again. Moreover, the discussion itself has become more and more meanspirited, marked by a disturbing tendency to mischaracterize the arguments of one's adversaries, as well as engage in ad hominem attacks and self-righteous moral posturing. This has cut both ways: besides imputing unsavory political motives to those who adopt the term, critics either ignore or deny the more nuanced arguments and valuable observations that the members of the "totalitarian school" make about modern forms of extreme dictatorship. To suggest, for example, that the latter are trying to relativize Nazi crimes by collapsing all distinctions between the two German dictatorships, or that they categorically deny the possibility of agency under such regimes is absurd (though it is true that they do tend to limit their discussion of this to oppositional behavior that is primarily political in character).

Those who brand the GDR a "totalitarian" state make similarly unfair assertions. They suggest that those who call that characterization into question are not only naïve, (n)ostalgic apologists for a monstrous but "ideologically correct" regime, but are also trying to "whitewash" East German history: by trivializing the level and extent of repression, or by "cherry-pick[ing the] attractive aspects of socialism," such as the social welfare benefits, the purported emancipation of women, and the alleged advances made toward the creation of a more egalitarian society. This is a distortion that involves cherry-picking of its own.[26] Such accusations often assume a tone of moral superiority, as if only those who consider the GDR to have been a totalitarian state have realized that it was repressive.

In the end, the main message of the totalitarian school seems to be an obvious one—though no less true for being banal: East Germany was a disagreeable and unpopular dictatorship whose leaders employed repressive methods in order to remain in power. But which scholars have ever denied that? It may be true that many of those who question claims about the totalitarian character of the East German regime, or who focus on the more socially "progressive" aspects of the regime, may still harbor some residual longing for the socialist project. These are often the same scholars who reacted allergically to the crass "triumphalism" in the West that greeted the demise of state socialism in the East.[27] But their view of the GDR as a place that cannot be reduced to the term *totalitarian* does not stem from some misplaced support for the leadership and its ham-fisted methods, but arguably rather from a lingering sympathy with "ordinary" East Germans and a sense of disappointment about the way in which "real existing socialism" really existed.[28] That does not mean that they are apologists for the regime, that they justify or ignore the repressive aspects of the regime, or that they "flirt with exoneration."[29] In fact, no compelling evidence has been offered in support of such claims—which often involve similarly unfounded insinuations about the political motivation and sympathies of those who criticize the totalitarian model. Like most scholars, those on both sides of this debate have political and moral biases that color their views. But what should matter most are the *questions*, and the answers to those questions. It should be possible to discuss these issues without resorting to character attacks.

Whatever its very considerable limitations, and despite its many permutations, totalitarian "theory" can help get at important questions. Because of the way in which it tries to characterize the basic features of modern dictatorships, it can be used as an ideal type with which to compare the empirical evidence, leading to questions about why the regime corresponded—or failed to correspond—to that ideal. In other words, the model can help us to frame important analytical questions about both the nature of state socialism as well as the character of state-society relations in East Germany, such as the extent to which the regime was able to achieve its total claims to reshape society and control the so-called masses.[30]

That is a central question. But it is not the only, or even the most important, question about the history of the GDR. In fact, it is precisely other types of questions that reveal the very serious limitations of totalitarian theory: questions about historical dynamics and change, for example, or ones about individual subjectivities, i.e., about values and norms, and the extent to which and the ways in which the latter became internalized. Getting at motivation, popular opinion, and beliefs is among the most vexing challenges for historians of the GDR, as it is for students of any state that lacks an open public sphere or functioning civil society. It is extremely difficult to measure beliefs and evaluate behavior in a place that has no free elections, uncensored media, or reliable opinion surveys, one permeated by the fear of real or imagined state terror. It is just as difficult to ascertain the motivation of the "true believers" and others who embraced the system. Did they too only go along as part of a "tricky tradeoff" in which loyalty and freedom were given in exchange for social and material security, the motivation often ascribed to the vast majority of East Germans?[31] Or perhaps they were mere dupes who suffered from "false consciousness." That would be something of an irony in a self-styled Marxist regime.[32]

The written sources produced by the regime not only provide a distorted portrait of prevailing opinion (as do any sources), but they also distort the very way in which we write about the GDR, not least concerning questions about motivation and beliefs. Because these reports and analyses tended to highlight critical commentary and "undesirable" behavior—and to allude to popular support in empty-sounding, formulaic phrases that most scholars pass over with a derisory shake of the head—one could gain the impression that the overwhelming majority of East Germans rejected the regime root and branch.[33] The challenge is to get beyond the inexact and impressionistic, to locate the indirect indicators that shine a light on inner values, beliefs, mentalities, and subjectivities, on what East Germans "really" thought, on the extent to which they embraced socialist ideology and values—and then to determine what this tells us, in turn, about larger issues of historiographical significance, such as the reasons for the stability and longevity of state socialism, or about how Germans left their fraught genocidal past behind them and reentered the community of more or less "civilized" and peaceful nations (at least vis-à-vis their neighbors) after 1945.[34]

The written archival record has proven to be more useful in getting at these issues than many researchers had suspected when first entering the former East German archives. "Truth" was not only spoken to power, at least at the grassroots level, but also assiduously recorded in official "public opinion" reports and analyses, petitions, and, most candidly, the minutes of factory, collective farm, and communal meetings—documents that are, in many respects, much richer than the lurid, sensational, and often misleading ones found in the Stasi files that researchers and journalists swooped down upon with alacrity when the archives were first thrown open in 1990. The minutes and petitions are especially valuable because they allow us to hear the voices of ordinary East Germans, and thus help us get at many of the main sources of everyday discontent. What is much harder to ascertain in the archives is, again, "genuine" expressions of loyalty and support, for the stilted phrases (*Floskeln*) used to describe loyalty and support simply do not ring true.[35]

History as Comfort Food

Broad concepts are useful starting points, as long as one remains aware of the potential dangers they pose. The inherent risk of "naming" or "labeling" the GDR totalitarian—or, for that matter, any of the terms used to capture the regime's intrinsically "oxymoronic" character (e.g., "welfare dictatorship," "participatory dictatorship," etc.)—is that the label becomes the content.[36] That is to say, placing it in a fixed category can lead to a static view of something—in this case the GDR—that did indeed change over time. Reification, in other words, runs the risk of impairing our understanding, as well as limiting our ability to recognize nuance and change.

Just as important, no single concept captures the complexity of the GDR. Since 1989, scholars have devised numerous terms to characterize the regime and its defining elements in a pithy, often playful way. Each of these terms—including the ones mentioned in the preceding paragraph—reflects differing methodological and theoretical approaches, as well as contrasting political and even moral agendas. And like the parable of the blind men and the elephant, each only describes a single component or cluster of components and thus misses the larger picture—often by neglecting other important elements that call the characterization at hand into question. Jürgen Kocka, for example, has referred to the GDR as a "modern dictatorship" because of the possibilities for greater social mobility, heightened gender equality, and a decrease in social inequality.[37] Leaving aside the "unmodern" aspects of the regime (which he does not deny), there is a good deal of evidence that calls into question even the "modern" elements identified by Kocka. For example, women were subject to continuing discrimination in terms of earnings and career possibilities and were thus not as "emancipated" or as "equal" to men as official propaganda suggested. In addition, the possibilities for social mobility for both men and women dried up in the 1980s, a development that contributed to the very demise of the GDR by heightening dissatisfaction with the regime.

None of this means that we should abandon the search for useful concepts and labels, but that we must remain aware of the pitfalls they involve and understand that they are only the beginning of a discussion and not the endpoint. In the end, it is perhaps easier to say what the GDR was *not* than to say what it was.

Another question that has attracted a good deal of scholarly attention concerns the extent to which the GDR was a mere "footnote of world history," as the East German author Stefan Heym dismissively commented after the fall of the Berlin Wall. Hans-Ulrich Wehler revived this idea in the final volume of his monumental *Deutsche Gesellschaftsgeschichte*. Claiming that the postwar socialist state was only useful as a foil with which to compare the Federal Republic, Wehler consigned the GDR to the dustbin of history as a "failed" state, a mere "satrapy" of the Soviet Union that had no lasting influence on international developments—or even on German history itself.[38] Scholars have taken issue with Wehler's provocative thesis, arguing that the GDR was historically significant for a number of reasons. According to Donna Harsch, it played an important role in several of the "major stories" of the twentieth century, including the history of Germany itself, the history of communism, and the history of women in the public sphere. Others have suggested different reasons for its importance, e.g., that its very demise demonstrated that Germans too are capable of carrying out a "successful" democratic revolution.[39]

This may all be true, but it seems superfluous to argue about whether the GDR was historically significant—especially if the implication is that only "significant" states and societies are worthy of serious historical analysis. Leaving aside the disturbingly normative aspect of such a question (which is no surprise coming from the leading proponent of the *Sonderweg* [special path] thesis, which essentially asked why modern Germany had not been more like France or Great Britain) and the inherent difficulty in determining what is "significant" (in what respect and for whom? The GDR was certainly significant for millions of Germans): if the "proper" subject of history is the study of past human behavior in all its guises, the "big questions"—such as how and why societies change, or how power is organized and exercised—can fruitfully be asked of *any* historical entity or formation. After all, it is the types of questions one poses, as well as the cogency of the answers that one offers in response, that should count in the end—not the amount of destruction and suffering wrought by a given group or regime, or their "success" or "longevity" (what standard is used to measure or judge such imponderables anyway?). To claim otherwise seems to suggest some sort of unspoken agenda, political or otherwise—and to come perilously close to engaging in a form of history as written by the victors. The Third Reich is not historically more significant than the GDR because it left behind "mountains of dead" and not "mountains of files and dossiers."[40] It is the questions that one is interested in addressing that determine the significance of a regime, event, person, or development. That much would seem obvious.

A different controversy has erupted over the use of the term *normalization* to describe developments in the GDR during the "middle period" of the 1960s and 1970s. In essence, those who have employed the concept are interested in getting at individuals' subjective perceptions of the political, socioeconomic, and cultural circumstances in which they found themselves. More specifically, they are interested in looking at how East Germans "came to terms" with life in the GDR, especially after the construction of the Wall, i.e., the extent to which certain norms, rules, and expectations regarding patterns of behavior became internalized or routinized—and may have come to be seen as somehow "normal" as they became more predictable over time. The "internalization" of norms and values is difficult to measure, of course. But to ask how East Germans came to perceive certain modes of life as "normal" and predictable is not a statement suggesting that life in the GDR was itself "normal." To be clear: no claim is being made about what constitutes a "normal" society. The term is intended to be neutral and does not suggest that East Germans just resigned themselves to their lot, for feelings of distance and alienation no doubt coincided—in greater or smaller measure, depending on the person and the given situation—with a growing sense of what was now "normal."[41]

But what is the heuristic value of such a concept? In the first place, it can help us better understand which factors, besides repression, contributed to the stability of the East German regime—an issue that has attracted a great deal of scholarly attention since the demise of the GDR. At the same time, it suggests one way in which to examine the actual substance of a claim frequently made but rarely demonstrated with evidence: that East Germans chose—or learned—to "accommodate" themselves to the regime after the possibility of escape to the West had more or less disappeared following the construction of the Berlin Wall.[42] Accommodation *with* the regime should not be equated with support *for* the regime. Gauging the latter is, in fact, one of the greatest challenges facing historians of the GDR—not only in terms of ascertaining actual levels of support (for the reasons discussed in the previous section), but also in terms of having to justify why this is a worthy scholarly enterprise without some hidden political agenda. Investigations of popular support for the National Socialist regime have become a staple of the historiography, yet those who examine similar questions about the GDR are, depending on their arguments and findings, subject to accusations of secretly sympathizing with the regime—as if the suggestion that the GDR enjoyed some level of popular support were tantamount to a ringing endorsement of state socialism, the Stasi, and the Berlin Wall.[43]

To investigate or point out those aspects of life in the GDR that enjoyed widespread support is not automatically an attempt to whitewash or relativize the appalling aspects of the regime, though that may be the intention of some scholars. But if one is interested in getting at the central question of, say, regime stability, this is a legitimate and necessary area of inquiry—as long as one avoids clichés. Recent research has shown, for example, that those social benefits that were purportedly most popular—such as low-cost housing, free childcare, and subsidized foodstuffs—were among the most important sources of discontent because of insufficient availability and chronic scarcity, especially during the early decades of the GDR before Erich Honecker decided to place greater emphasis on the satisfaction of material desires and well-being.[44]

With an eye to the latter development, those scholars who have worked on the question of "normality" have made less persuasive claims about a supposed "growth of individualism" during the later decades of the GDR, one that involved "an enhanced focus on the fulfillment of individual goals." According to Mary Fulbrook, the "collective spirit" of the early decades was "displaced in the course of the 1960s and '70s by a retreat into individualistic concerns, with a growing focus on home, family and private gain."[45] It is unclear that such "collective spirit" was really ever as widespread as this suggests—or as official propaganda and rose-colored reminiscences that bathe the early years in a haze of nostalgia about camaraderie, solidarity, and optimism about bright socialist horizons might lead us to believe. In fact, many ordinary East Germans—not least the industrial workers and farmers in whose name the SED claimed to rule—remained doggedly resistant to the blandishments and collectivist propaganda of the regime from the very start. Moreover, if there was indeed creeping "individualism," above all in terms of everyday consumerist and materialist proclivities, its growth was only one of degree: a focus on one's own personal and material interests was very much in evidence from the earliest years of the postwar socialist state—abetted not least by the many economic deficiencies of state socialism itself.[46]

Regardless, the claims about "hidden agendas" are reminiscent of the debate about efforts to "historicize" the Third Reich, which revolved around the question of whether it was legitimate to apply to the history of the Nazi period the same types of questions, dispassionate approach, and methods that historians would apply to any other area of historical inquiry. In many respects, the debate devolved into a *dialogue des sourds* because of the understandable passions it raised. The subtext of the critique voiced by those who objected to this approach seemed to be a fear that a "'normalization' of methodological treatment" (Ian Kershaw) might lead—whatever the intention of those originally calling for this approach—to an insidious relativization of Nazi crimes. The main objection voiced by Saul Friedländer, the most vigorous critic of this approach initially advocated by Martin Broszat, was that the unique genocidal policies of the Nazis made it impossible to approach this period in a "normal" way in any sense of the word. In other words, the enormity and specificity of Nazi crimes placed the period outside the bounds of long-term trends in modern German history; moreover, they forbade an investigation of "normal," everyday life because of the danger that this would lead to misplaced empathy for those who had not suffered themselves under the regime. This was morally questionable, Friedländer argued, given the extreme suffering of those who did.[47]

Similar concerns seem to animate those who object to a historical treatment of "everyday" life or other "normal" developments in the GDR—unless, that is, they have to do with repression, complicity, or active resistance. The message seems to be that it is morally dubious to examine everyday "normality" in a place where life was worse than dismal and often criminally *abnormal* for many others. But if that were the case, it would also mean that one should not be able to write about "everyday" life in, say, the northeast of the United States during the 1950s, given the pervasiveness of Jim Crow in the South at that time. Again, this is not to collapse distinctions: Jim Crow laws and Stasi persecution were not akin to the Holocaust (though the former do invite comparisons to the Nuremberg Laws, as some African Americans in the United States commented themselves at the time).[48] But it seems curious to forbid certain types of questions about, or certain approaches to, certain regimes and certain eras because of certain other developments that took place there—as long as those developments are integrated into any such analyses and not ignored.

At the end of his life, Timothy Mason, the great British historian of Nazi Germany, wistfully regretted that he had failed to realize that race—and not class—was the answer to "the central question of what the Nazi regime was really all about, what its main aims were"—and that this failing had proved to be, in his opinion, an insurmountable shortcoming in his lifelong effort to come to terms with National Socialism.⁴⁹ Those who have tried to move the discussion about the history of the GDR beyond the theme of repression would do well to bear Mason's disheartening realization in mind. Repression did permeate all aspects of life in the GDR. As Gary Bruce has put it, "One can no more place a boundary around the Stasi than one can encircle a scent in a room," and it must be incorporated into any history of East Germany, as Phil Leask explicitly does in this volume in his examination of how humiliation and the arbitrary abuse of power was used to isolate enemies and inculcate discipline, especially among the party loyal.⁵⁰

Documenting the criminality of the regime and its leadership is important and valuable in itself, and it has been the subject of numerous studies. But one must nevertheless ask how that endeavor advances historical debate, and to what questions of scholarly significance it leads. Questions about how repression and terror worked, or failed to work, in practice are important for getting at questions of regime stability, as are questions about why certain people worked for the Stasi, why they reported on family, friends, colleagues, and neighbors, often with enthusiasm. Repression may perhaps be the centerpiece of GDR history—but it is not the end of the story. And it does not explain everything. In fact, what it might explain is sometimes the exact opposite of what one might expect. As Leask paradoxically suggests in his essay, the very policies of repression that the SED used to maintain power may have served, in the end, to undermine its very power.

Was East Germany "totalitarian"? Was it a mere "footnote" of world history? Was it "normal"—or even really "German," given its slavish dependence on Moscow? These questions have become the banalities of East German historiography—history as comfort food for those most interested in moralistic posturing. The *Sonderweg* theory, whatever its shortcomings, tried at least to grapple with a series of important questions about the rise and roots of National Socialism. The historiography of the GDR has, by contrast, tended toward the provincial: as a quick look at the footnotes will reveal, many investigations make little effort to relate their findings to developments outside of East Germany or to issues of greater historical and historiographical importance. This is not surprising, given the rush that greeted the sudden opening of the archives two decades ago, the unprecedented decision to forgo the thirty-year rule that limits access to historical records, as well as the "publish-or-perish" pressures imposed by academe. Graduate students eager to demonstrate their bona fides as historians have produced a flood of often hastily published dissertations that are saturated with archival material, but that, in the words of Sebastian Haffner in a different context, tend to "dump their index cards in the lap of the reader"⁵¹—or that, under the professional pressure of having to demonstrate the utter originality of one's own findings and arguments, fail to give adequate credit to or mischaracterize those of other scholars. This has sometimes been the result of careless or dubious scholarly practices.⁵² But the provincial nature of East German studies has found expression in other ways as well, above all in the general failure of some scholars—especially German-speaking ones—to take into account work on the GDR not produced in their own language.⁵³ This is surprising, given the internationalization of scholarly publications, conferences, and controversies, as well as study in countries other than one's place of birth—a development that casts some doubt on dubious claims about the existence of distinctive "national" perspectives on the GDR, even if there is some variation in emphasis from country to country.⁵⁴

What we need, then, are fresh and innovative approaches, above all to the available source material, both written and nonwritten. As Monica Black has commented:

> Something that has often struck me about East German (and West German, for that matter) historiography is that we have no version of *The Cheese and the Worms* or *The Return of Martin Guerre*. Why this is the case is not obvious, though the simple answer, of course, would be that no one has yet found such a story to write about. I think the issue is different, and lies less with the kinds of sources we have available than with the ways we tend to approach them and the questions we put to them; if we have no work commensurate with that of [Carlo] Ginzburg's or [Natalie Zeman] Davis's, the problem, I think, is not that our sources puzzle us, but that they do not, in fact, puzzle us enough.⁵⁵

In fact, a number of scholars working in North America and the United Kingdom (including Black) have already published rich, archivally based studies that take a more nuanced, less categorical "sociocultural" approach to the history of the GDR, one that has already led to important insights and stimulated novel questions and hypotheses.⁵⁶

All of this has opened new horizons for the study of the GDR, state socialism, and other modern authoritarian regimes—as the essays in this volume demonstrate. Taken together, they demonstrate the fruitfulness of a variety of sociocultural and sociopolitical approaches to the history of East Germany by exploring physical and psychological aspects of life in the GDR, as well as diverse everyday responses at the grassroots level to the well-known political and economic parameters of dictatorship. In so doing, the essays suggest fresh ways of interpreting life behind the Iron Curtain. And, rather than just challenging totalitarian theory on its own ground, or restricting themselves to negative theoretical critiques of that paradigm, they address key issues in East German history from a range of theoretical perspectives, looking at the many ways in which East Germans themselves changed over forty years in negotiating the conditions of life behind the Iron Curtain. The essays in this volume eschew the polarized political and moralistic debates of the past two decades, and instead turn their attention to the ways in which East Germans were themselves both constituted by the physical and cultural, as well as political, parameters of life in the GDR—and, in turn, contributed to the ways in which East German history itself unfolded.

To paraphrase EP Thompson's famous dictum, East Germans were themselves present at the GDR's making.[57] They helped shape the worlds in which they lived, even as they were themselves formed by the circumstances and periods into which they were born. At the risk of stating a truism, how they viewed the regime they helped mold very much depended on their own perspective, perceptions, and sensibilities.

What We Now Know: Fresh Approaches to the History of the GDR

The rich research that has taken place since the fall of the Wall and the subsequent opening of the former East German archives has chipped away at a number of myths about the GDR—tenacious ones that nevertheless still enjoy wide scholarly and popular currency. Where scholars might have expected to find evidence of female emancipation, for example, they instead found continuing sexist discrimination. Where they had expected to discover generous welfare benefits guaranteeing a modicum of social and material security, they often found shortages of housing, childcare, and even the most basic of foodstuffs. Where they had expected to unearth signs of grassroots solidarity, they found social cleavages and divisions.

That was only one side of the coin, however. Where they had assumed they would discover silence and quiescence, they found a surprising and widespread willingness to voice criticism, and a remarkable unwillingness to bow meekly to the many onerous demands of the party and state. There was no deafening silence of the lambs; in fact, many bleated quite vigorously. Where scholars had assumed they would find traces of totalitarian terror, they discovered a repressive apparatus that was not as all-knowing or as effective as once assumed, and a regime that was often weak, incompetent, or overburdened at the grassroots level, one whose representatives were either unable or loath to enforce high-level political and economic directives—and one whose policies aimed at total control in all areas of political, economic, and social life but that produced instead a series of unintended consequences that often had little to do with official intentions. Those unintended consequences not only bore directly on the stability *and* ultimate collapse of the regime, but also suggested the very real limits of the East German dictatorship and of its ability to direct society.[58]

One of the most important insights of the past two decades involves, then, the more nuanced manner in which the complex nature of power and state-society relations in the GDR have come to be characterized. The relationship between the "rulers" and "ruled" was indeed an asymmetrical one, yet the latter were often able to work the system to their own advantage, carving out "spaces for agency and autonomy within a largely paternalistic, coercive, and didactic regime."[59] In their complementary essays in this volume about anti-fascist narratives and memories, Joanne Sayner and Christiane Wienand discuss various ways in which East Germans refused to parrot the official line, but instead advanced their own understanding of anti-fascism and shaped this for their own ends—ones at considerable variance with those of the regime. Andreas Agocs's discussion of the First German Writers' Congress, held in October 1947, similarly looks at the extent to which anti-fascism was more than just a cynical Stalinist tool used by the regime to rally the masses and win support.

Recent research has also led to a partial reconceptualizing of the chronological breaks in East German history, calling into question the extent to which ones traditionally described as major caesura were really as far-reaching as often assumed. Like all states and societies, East Germany changed over time, i.e., it *had* a history. The 1980s were not the same as the Stalinist 1950s—an obvious but essential point often missed by (primarily Western) observers who focus on the contrast between dictatorial and democratic political structures. By the same token, others, in particular younger former East Germans, tend to equate the GDR with its last two decades, i.e., the years of increasing social benefits, of less open and brutal—but therefore more refined—methods of repression and surveillance.

In one way or another, all of the contributions to this volume explore the important ruptures in East German history, looking at when and why they took place, and what their effects were. The extent to which developments in the postwar socialist state represented a dramatic departure from what had come before is another important theme, as is the related issue of continuities across the 1945 divide, i.e., the trends and traditions that survived the war and subsequently shaped the GDR's social, political, and cultural trajectory.[60] While Mary Fulbrook examines "communities of experience, connection, and identification" to get at ways in which "personal legacies of the past" influenced later developments, Donna Harsch and Jeannette Madarász-Lebenhagen address the dynamic mix of tradition and innovation in health-care practices after 1945, looking in particular at East and West German efforts to combat rampant tuberculosis and chronic cardiovascular diseases. In their respective discussions of dieting and luxury dining in the GDR, Neula Kerr-Boyle and Paul Freedman point to East German consumption and behavioral practices that can be traced to the prewar period. Noting striking similarities between slimming aids and advertisements in Weimar, the Third Reich, and the GDR, Kerr-Boyle examines the resurgence of traditional notions of the female body and beauty in the postwar socialist state, as well as the tenacity of traditional dieting and eating habits—including ones frowned on by officials. Along similar lines, Freedman reminds us that the iconic *Spreewaldgurken*—the pickles that have become a major symbol of *Ostalgie* since the popular film *Goodbye, Lenin!*—had a venerable pre-GDR, pan-German history.[61]

The role played by prewar traditions is also a focus of Andreas Agocs's discussion of the acrimonious debate and subsequent split that took place during the First German Writers' Congress in the fall of 1947. These exposed rifts and unresolved conflicts among German intellectuals and within Germany's cultural scene that reached back to at least 1933; they were not, in other words, just the result of escalating Cold War tensions. That said, many of the essays, including Agocs's, do explore the sundry ways in which Germany became a focal point of that conflict—not least as a contest in which the postwar successor states vied with each other to demonstrate the alleged superiority of their own policies and ideologies, as well as the flawed practices of their rival: from the staging of state dinners (Freedman) and the most effective ways of dieting (Kerr-Boyle), to the fight against tuberculosis and heart disease (Harsch and Madarász-Lebenhagen).

Pointing out postwar continuities and placing the postwar period in the context of long-term sociocultural developments is not just about driving another nail in the coffin of the comforting "zero hour" legend.[62] They lay bare the formidable challenges to and limits on the implementation and fulfillment of official policies and desires. The SED did not work in a vacuum, for the long shadow that the past cast on the GDR, as well as the Federal Republic, could not but affect developments in both of them. For example, East German leaders may have hoped to introduce more progressive gender policies and practices—for practical as well as ideological reasons—but, as Kerr-Boyle reminds us, they often ran up against tenacious past practices, prejudices, and expectations.

The year 1945 was not the only major chronological watershed in the history of the eastern half of Germany. Others included 1949, 1953, 1961, 1971, and, of course, 1989, the years in which events regarded as important caesurae took place: the founding of the GDR, the first statewide uprising in the Soviet bloc, the erection of the Berlin Wall, the ascension of Honecker, and the implosion of the regime. Many of the essays in this volume explore the extent to which these were truly turning points, asking implicitly or explicitly whether other types of changes—e.g., social, economic, cultural, generational—corresponded to the well-known *political* caesurae. If they did not fit neatly into the commonly accepted temporal divisions, and if the effects of the political breaks did not always extend beyond the strictly political, there is a need to rethink the traditional periodization of the GDR—a challenge also taken up in this volume. In his discussion of official East German rhetoric about Israel, for example, David Tompkins demonstrates that such shifts were not always related to the well-known caesurae. The gradual darkening of the postwar Jewish state's image from one of "friend" to "foe" began in 1950, intensified later that decade, and then intensified once again in the late 1960s, coinciding with developments not peculiar to the GDR itself, e.g., larger Cold War tensions, anti-Semitic stirrings in the Soviet bloc, and the latter's feverish search for allies in the developing world.

One important reason for reassessing the import and impact of the accepted caesurae is to avoid artificially forcing certain developments into rigid chronological frameworks in a way that does not do justice to the types of changes being discussed or explained. There is a similar need to reexamine some of the blanket statements often made about certain periods, e.g., that the 1960s were a period in which ordinary East Germans came to terms with and accommodated themselves to the regime, that this was a "golden age" in terms of material improvement, that June 1953 represented a turning point in the way officials dealt with workers. It is imperative to ask whether there is actual evidence in support of these assertions; in the absence of evidence they are mere clichés. As I point out in my essay in this volume comparing the behavior of the working classes under the Third Reich and during the GDR, many local officials had been just as solicitous of workers before June 1953, which was one of the underlying reasons that the uprising took place, i.e., as a reaction against efforts to increase worker productivity by raising production quotas.

Whatever chronological reassessments are in order, many changes were indeed linked to the familiar watershed moments. Donna Harsch notes, for instance, that in October 1961, i.e., just two months after the construction of the Berlin Wall, authorities finally introduced obligatory vaccination against tuberculosis despite dogged resistance at the grassroots level—resistance that, incidentally, had its roots in the prewar period.[63] Feeling more confident in the protective shadow of the Wall, they adopted other unpopular policies as well at this time, including compulsory military service and more vigorous campaigns aimed at boosting production levels. But, as Josie McLellan has pointed out, they also introduced more socially permissive policies in an attempt to pacify the population.[64] If the building of the Wall—and this new round of carrots and sticks—did indeed help East Germans, *faute de mieux*, "come to terms" and "make their peace" with the regime, it is important to devise reliable ways in which to measure that process in a meaningful and verifiable way.

Several of the essays identify significant shifts that began in the early 1970s—when Honecker replaced Ulbricht, another transformative moment— and continued into the 1980s. This period, which has received less scholarly attention than the earlier decades of the GDR, is considered to be qualitatively different from what came before, largely because of a vast increase in social benefits, along with a new emphasis on the satisfaction of popular consumer and other material desires. Yet, those were not the only changes. Freedman discusses the introduction of a more "international" dining style at this time, a result of the GDR's increasing openness to the nonsocialist world in the wake of détente, while Kerr-Boyle explores the reasons why official incitement to diet and even popular dieting practices themselves became more pronounced at this time—in the East as well as in the West. In an analysis of everyday sporting practices, Alan McDougall argues that the last two decades of the GDR witnessed growing frustration and disillusionment on the part of those who played amateur soccer, East Germany's most popular mass participatory sport. Though anger and resentment about shoddy facilities and insufficient state support were nothing new, East Germans were now even less willing to put up with longstanding deficiencies. This suggests an important shift in mentality and behavior, suggestive of the type of ferment from below that would usher in the demise of the regime.

Another promising area for future research on the GDR besides questions of continuities and ruptures is a more systematically comparative approach to its history—a recurrent theme in the essays in this volume. While my own piece compares the behavior of workers under the Nazis and the SED, others focus on the similarities and differences between the GDR and Federal Republic: from the commemoration and memory of the National Socialist past, to health-care, culinary, and dieting practices, to the types of pressure placed on women on both sides of the Wall. What is interesting in this respect, as Harsch and Madarász-Lebenhagen show in their work on disease prevention, is that similar developments and outcomes sometimes came about in the two postwar states—but sometimes for vastly different reasons.[65]

Comparisons between the GDR and the Federal Republic are fruitful and revealing for another reason: with regional variations, they shared similar pre-1945 political, socioeconomic, and cultural traditions. This makes them a valuable case study—or "laboratory"—for examining in a comparative manner the ways in which the capitalist West and Communist East faced challenges common to all modern, industrialized (or industrializing) societies. This was a flawed "experiment," however, because the two states were not kept in strict isolation—no matter how hard the East German leadership may have tried! As several of the essays suggest, policies in one state often had a direct or indirect influence on those adopted on the other side of the Elbe.[66]

Comparisons of the GDR with the Third Reich and the Federal Republic already exist, of course.[67] After all, the main thrust of totalitarian theory has been to compare communism and state socialism to fascism. Even if "comparing does not mean equalizing" but rather searching for similarities *and* differences, this comparison in particular has tended toward the former, both before and after 1989—even if the more obvious differences between the GDR and the Third Reich are always acknowledged as part of an obligatory nod toward nuance: East Germany did not unleash a world war or commit genocide, it did not have a charismatic leader or enjoy the same type of popularity as the Third Reich, it did not have the same type of impact on gender relations, it did not come about or even end in the same manner. Yet, the similarities remain obvious enough. Both were one-party dictatorships that used various forms of pressure and propaganda, as well as repression and social goodies—from the plump to the more subtle—to mobilize the masses and keep them in check; both pursued social engineering and reconstruction informed by an official hegemonic ideology; both engaged in "social scapegoating" to rally support for the regime. Similar comparisons have also been made between the GDR and the Federal Republic, but with the emphasis falling in that case on the obvious and essential differences between the two. In brief, the East German dictatorship lacked all of the things that characterized West Germany, as well as other liberal-democratic states and pluralistic societies in the West: due process and a functioning constitution; party competition, democratic elections, and a largely unfettered market economy; an independent judiciary, an uncensored media, and guarantees of basic civil rights.[68]

These are the obvious points of comparison in both cases. But it is also worth asking about the neglected or unexpected similarities and differences. By way of example, let us pose a rhetorical question that is sure to raise some hackles: was the GDR truly more repressive than the Federal Republic—or other Western states, for that matter? To many, the question will seem absurd, if not downright offensive. But it is not difficult to draw up a lengthy list of politically repressive measures that Western states have employed against their own citizens since 1945—from the House Un-American Activities Committee (HUAC), the Internal Security Act of 1950, and the Counter Intelligence Program (COINTELPRO) in the United States, for instance, to Article 21 of the Basic Law and the 1972 Anti-Radical Decree in the Federal Republic, to the more recent anti-terrorism laws.[69] It will be objected that the comparison is unfair because there are "obvious differences." Such repression was much more widespread and violent east of the Elbe, where the possibilities for redress and reform were also much less limited.

The last two points are essential ones, and the difference may be an important one of degree, in the end. After all, it was not the Federal Republic that saw itself forced to build a concrete wall to keep its citizens from fleeing. But that is little solace to those in the West who have themselves suffered from oppression.[70] Along Foucauldian lines, one might even counter that repression in the West was even more invidious for being more subtle and refined.[71] But one does not have to appeal to Michel Foucault and the disciplining effect of discourse to get at the invidious nature of repression on *both* sides of the Elbe, as those who were members of "out-groups" knew and experienced all too well. Dolores Augustine reminds us that there were distinct limits to East Germany's "progressive" sexual policies—especially when it came to homosexuals, who suffered from "rampant homophobia" and (like other so-called "asocials") repression in the GDR.[72] These and other limits as well affected certain groups, the members of which were considered social outcasts for political, religious, cultural, and other reasons.

The West had pariahs of its own, of course. Surveying the past century, one thinks, for instance, of the Jim Crow laws and other forms of racial discrimination in the United States, as well as the treatment there of Communists, homosexuals, Jews, and other minorities. It is not surprising that some American blacks remarked at the time that the Nuremberg racial laws of 1935 sounded "suspiciously like Miami."[73] It is also worth recalling in this context the Tuskegee Syphilis Study, which began a year before Adolf Hitler came to power and lasted until the year the Munich Olympics were held forty years later. This was a shameful episode in U.S. history—but one should not collapse all distinctions: its exposure did lead to the creation of the federal Office for Human Research Protections.[74]

The GDR does not appear to have been similarly "adaptive," in light of its ultimate demise. Yet, one wonders whether it might at least have had the potential to be. Some scholars have (longingly) interpreted the Ulbricht reform era as a "missed opportunity" to carry out salutary modifications that might have salvaged the Socialist project—not unlike the musings in American popular culture about how things might have turned out had John F. Kennedy not been assassinated.[75] But in the end, the GDR proved stubbornly resistant to fundamental reform because it did not have the appropriate channels or possibilities for unfettered communication and public debate—or, for that matter, any willingness on the part of its leadership to relinquish even partial control (until it was too late). Sigrid Meuschel has argued that this is why the postwar Socialist state could in the last resort only end in revolution and dissolution.[76]

There are good reasons for posing such questions and making such observations—despite the obvious differences between these rival political and socioeconomic systems. It is not merely to turn totalitarian theory on its head, create false equivalencies, and apply a moralistic *tu quoque* argument in order to condemn the West by comparing it to the East. Pointing to parallels such as the existence of denunciatory acts, police brutality, and a socioeconomic underclass, as well as the disciplining power of moral strictures under both systems, does have heuristic value. Like totalitarian theory, this exercise can help us frame important questions—for example, ones about stability, longevity, and ultimate collapse. In fact, the foregoing discussion raises a series of essential questions related to these very issues: why did Western states enjoy so much more popular legitimacy and support than those in the East? Why, in other words, were the GDR and the other states in the Soviet bloc unable to win the "hearts and minds" of the masses? And why was the capitalist West able to do so? Was it because of the intrinsic appeal of democracy and "basic freedoms"? As Eric Hobsbawm muses, "Just how and why capitalism after the Second World War found itself, to everyone's surprise including its own, surging forward into the unprecedented and possibly anomalous Golden Age of 1945–73, is perhaps the major question which faces historians of the twentieth century."[77]

It is worth recalling that most East Germans (and other eastern Europeans) had had no, very little, or a decidedly poor experience with and memory of democracy. After all, formal democratic institutions had only existed on what would become East German territory for slightly more than a decade in the 1920s—and they had not been an unmitigated success, to say the least. The reputation of the democratic states in the West was not overwhelmingly positive either in places like Czechoslovakia, for example, which had been abandoned by the Western powers in the late 1930s. Last but not least, the Great Depression had not provided incontrovertible evidence of capitalism's superiority as an economic system.[78] How so many East Germans and their neighbors in eastern Europe came to be so enamored of democracy—not only in the 1980s but also, as recent research about "popular opinion" has found, much earlier—is thus an intriguing question.[79]

An equally intriguing question is why this changes after 1945, i.e., why the West comes to be seen as "superior" in normative as well as functionalist terms[80]—even on the part of those who benefitted least, and suffered most, under prevailing conditions of socioeconomic inequality and, in some countries, institutionalized racism and sexism. One possible reason is that it proved much better able to deliver both necessary and desired material goods—especially to those who "mattered" most in shaping public opinion and the "discourse" of civil society (for is it not true, to paraphrase Judith Butler, that some lives "matter" more than others?).[81] There are other possible reasons. Historical prejudices against the "Russians" and the Soviet Union—fueled for over a decade by Nazi propaganda—may have doomed the Socialist project from the very start in Eastern Europe and the GDR, tarnished precisely for being imposed from without. It could also be that the West simply conveyed a more effective message.

In the United States, even the most downtrodden have learned that they live in "the greatest country in the world"—a place where everyone is "born equal" and has "equal opportunity" in a land of "unlimited opportunities." They are aware of injustices, of course, but they also imbibe from a young age the hegemonic idea (à la Max Weber) that a failure to "succeed" is somehow a personal failing. This idea becomes hardwired and is perhaps *the* most important factor underlying domestic peace and stability. Was the GDR—to put it crudely—a "worse" place than the United States? One wonders how an African American youth from Detroit, where infant mortality, crime, and poverty rates rival those of many developing countries, might answer this question. But in the end, he or she would most likely not exchange "freedom" and the possibility of "making it big one day" for more modest material "security." It could be that totalitarian systems "go against the grain of human nature," as Grieder contends—or because some forms of propaganda have been more effective than others.[82] It is difficult to demonstrate the validity of either proposition. But if it is indeed the latter, why might that be the case? An answer to that question sheds light on subjectivities, values, beliefs, and mentalities—the subjects of this volume. And an understanding of those intangibles can help us better understand, in turn, why one system proved more tenacious and more resilient than the other. That is indeed a question of central historical significance.

Suggested Readings

Bruce, Gary. *The Firm: The Inside Story of the Stasi*. Oxford, 2010.
Eppelmann, Rainer, Bernd Faulenbach, and Ulrich Mählert, eds. *Bilanz und Perspektiven der DDR-Forschung*. Paderborn, 2003.
Fulbrook, Mary. "The State of GDR History." *Francia. Forschungen zur westeuropäischen Geschichte* 38 (2011): 259–70.
———. *The People's State: East German Society from Hitler to Honecker*. New Haven, C.T., 2005.
———, ed. *Power and Society in the GDR, 1961-79*. New York, 2009.
Grieder, Peter. "In Defence of Totalitarianism Theory as a Tool of Historical Scholarship." *Totalitarian Movements and Political Religions* 8/3–4 (2007): 563–89.
Jarausch, Konrad, ed. *Dictatorship as Experience: Towards a Socio-Cultural History of the GDR*. New York, 1999.
Jesse, Eckhard. "War die DDR totalitär?" *Aus Politik und Zeitgeschichte* B40 (1994): 12–23.
Jessen, Ralph. "DDR-Geschichte und Totalitarismustheorie." *Berliner Debatte INITIAL* 4/5 (1995): 17–24.
Kaeble, Hartmut, Jürgen Kocka, and Hartmut Zwahr, eds. *Sozialgeschichte der DDR*. Stuttgart, 1994.
Kocka, Jürgen. *Civil Society & Dictatorship in Modern German History*. Hanover, N.H., 2010.
Lindenberger, Thomas, ed. *Herrschaft und Eigen-Sinn in der Diktatur. Studien zur Gesellschaftsgeschichte der DDR*. Cologne, 1999.
Lüdtke, Alf. *Eigen-Sinn. Fabrikalltag, Arbeitererfahrungen und Politik vom Kaiserreich bis in den Faschismus*. Hamburg, 1993.
Pence, Katherine and Paul Betts, eds. *Socialist Modern: East German Everyday Culture and Politics*. Ann Arbor, M.I., 2008.
Port, Andrew I. *Conflict and Stability in the German Democratic Republic*. New York, 2007.
Ross, Corey. *The East German Dictatorship: Problems and Perspectives in the Interpretation of the GDR*. London, 2002.

Notes

1. The preeminent example of this approach remains Armin Mitter and Stefan Wolle, *Untergang auf Raten: Unbekannte Kapitel der DDR — Geschichte* (Munich, 1993).

2. For a more recent specimen, see Hubertus Knabe, *Die Täter sind unter uns. Über das Schönreden der SED-Diktatur* (Berlin, 2007).
 3. This was the subject of an innovative series of papers presented at the conference "Writing East German History: What Difference Does the Cultural Turn Make?" University of Michigan, Ann Arbor, M.I., 5–7 December 2008.
 4. For example, one of the earliest and most important contributions to the post-Wall social history of the GDR appeared less than half a decade following unification: Hartmut Kaeble, Jürgen Kocka, and Hartmut Zwahr, eds., *Sozialgeschichte der DDR* (Stuttgart, 1994).
 5. Despite a general neglect of what is described here as the "third wave," useful overviews of the historiography include Rainer Eppelmann, Bernd Faulenbach, and Ulrich Mählert, eds., *Bilanz und Perspektiven der DDR-Forschung* (Paderborn, 2003); Corey Ross, *The East German Dictatorship: Problems and Perspectives in the Interpretation of the GDR* (London, 2002); Beate Ihme-Tuchel, *Die DDR* (Darmstadt, 2002); Arnd Bauerkämper, *Die Sozialgeschichte der DDR* (Munich, 2005); Günter Heydemann, *Die Innenpolitik der DDR* (Munich, 2003); Jens Gieseke and Hermann Wentker, eds., *Die Geschichte der SED. Eine Bestandsaufnahme* (Berlin, 2011).
 6. For an accessible overview of the postwar historiography, see Geoff Eley, *A Crooked Line: From Cultural History to the History of Society* (Ann Arbor, M.I., 2006).
 7. Early contributions to the emerging debate include Eckhard Jesse, "War die DDR totalitär?" *Aus Politik und Zeitgeschichte* B40 (1994): 12–23; Mary Fulbrook, "The Limits of Totalitarianism: God, State and Society in the GDR," *Transactions of the Royal Historical Society* 7 (1997): 25–52. Also see Eckhard Jesse, ed., *Totalitarismus im 20. Jahrhundert. Eine Bilanz der internationalen Forschung* (Bonn, 1996); Achim Siegel, ed., *Totalitarismustheorien nach dem Ende des Kommunismus* (Cologne, 1998); Wolfgang Wippermann, *Totalitarismustheorien. Die Entwicklung der Diskussion von den Anfängen bis heute* (Darmstadt, 1997).
 8. See Jürgen Kocka, *Civil Society & Dictatorship in Modern German History* (Hanover, N.H., 2010), 37.
 9. Alf Lüdtke, "'Helden der Arbeit'—Mühen beim Arbeiten. Zur mißmutigen Loyalität von Industriearbeitern in der DDR," in Kaelble, Kocka, and Zwahr, *Sozialgeschichte*, 188.
10. Peter Grieder, "In Defence of Totalitarianism Theory as a Tool of Historical Scholarship," *Totalitarian Movements and Political Religions* 8/3–4 (2007): 563–89.
11. Ralph Jessen, "DDR-Geschichte und Totalitarismustheorie," *Berliner Debatte INITIAL* 4/5 (1995).
12. Grieder, "In Defence," 565.
13. See Gary Bruce, *The Firm: The Inside Story of the Stasi* (Oxford, 2010), 7. Two classic accounts of totalitarian theory are Carl J. Friedrich and Zbigniew Brzezinski, *Totalitarian Dictatorship and Autocracy*, 2nd ed., rev. (New York, 1966); Hannah Arendt, *The Origins of Totalitarianism* (New York, 1951).
14. See, e.g., Karl Schlögel, *Terror and Traum. Moskau, 1937* (Munich, 2008), 304–27. Also see the essays in Boris Groys and Max Hollein, eds., *Dream Factory Communism: The Visual Culture of the Stalin Period* (Ostfildern, 2003).
15. Alf Lüdtke, "Geschichte und Eigensinn," in Berliner Geschichtswerkstatt, ed., *Alltagskultur, Subjektivität und Geschichte. Zur Theorie und Praxis von Alltagsgeschichte* (Munster, 1994), 19; David Blackbourn, *A Sense of Place: New Directions in German History* (London, 1999).

16. That is especially the case since the publication of Thomas Lindenberger, ed., *Herrschaft und Eigen-Sinn in der Diktatur. Studien zur Gesellschaftsgeschichte der DDR* (Cologne, 1999).
17. See the perceptive discussion of this term in Christoph Vietzke, *Konfrontation und Kooperation. Funktionäre und Arbeiter in Großbetrieben der DDR vor und nach dem Mauerbau* (Essen, 2008), 26–29.
18. See Alf Lüdtke, *Eigen-Sinn. Fabrikalltag, Arbeitererfahrungen und Politik vom Kaiserreich bis in den Faschismus* (Hamburg, 1993), 10–12, 136–43.
19. See Martin Broszat, "Resistenz und Widerstand. Eine Zwischenbilanz des Forschungsprojektes," in Martin Broszat, Elke Fröhlich, and Anton Grossmann, eds., *Bayern in der NS-Zeit. Herrschaft und Gesellschaft im Konflikt*, vol. 4 (Munich, 1981), 691–709; Klaus-Michael Mallmann and Gerhard Paul, "Resistenz oder loyale Widerwilligkeit? Anmerkungen zu einem umstrittenen Begriff," *Zeitschrift für Geschichtswissenschaft* 2 (1993): 99–116.
20. Similar arguments are made in Andrew I. Port, "The Dark Side of Eigensinn: East German Workers and Destructive Shop-floor Practices," in *Falling Behind or Catching Up? The East German Economy, 1945-2010*, ed. Hartmut Berghoff and Uta Balbier (New York, 2013), 111–28.
21. See Merle Fainsod, *Smolensk under Soviet Rule* (Boston, 1989), 449–50; Grieder, "In Defence," 570–72.
22. Klaus Schroeder, *Der SED-Staat. Geschichte und Strukturen der DDR* (Munich, 1998), 633.
23. Bruce, *Firm*, 8. Also see Ilko-Sascha Kowalczuk, *Stasi konkret. Überwachung und Repression in der DDR* (Munich, 2013).
24. Mary Fulbrook, "The State of GDR History," *Francia. Forschungen zur westeuropäischen Geschichte* 38 (2011): 264.
25. Grieder, "In Defence," 565.
26. For claims about "whitewashing" (*Weichspülung, Weichzeichnung*) see Klaus Schroeder's review of Mary Fulbrook, *Ein ganz normales Leben. Alltag und Gesellschaft in der DDR* (Darmstadt, 2008) in *Zeitschrift des Forschungsverbundes SED-Staat* 26 (2009), 178; also see Ilko-Sascha Kowlczuk's review of Mary Fulbrook, ed., *Power and Society in the GDR, 1961-79* (New York, 2009) in *Historische Zeitschrift* 291 (2010): 279. These are cited in Fulbrook, "State of GDR History," 267. The quote about "cherry-picking" comes from a contribution made by Dolores Augustine on H-German in October 2007 during an online discussion sparked by Gary Bruce's review of Andrew I. Port, *Conflict and Stability in the German Democratic Republic* (New York, 2007) (http://h-net.msu.edu/cgi bin/logbrowse.pl?trx=vx&list=H-German&month=0710&week=d&msg=ric35JS88CzrSyQG83Y3nA&user=&pw=).
27. The classic example of such "triumphalism" remains Francis Fukuyama, *The End of History and the Last Man* (New York, 1992). Also see Ellen Schrecker, *Cold War Triumphalism: The Misuse of History after the Fall of Communism* (New York, 2006).
28. It is true that many of those who deny the totalitarian character of the regime became interested in the GDR for personal reasons: they had traveled to the East before 1989 and often had friends there. If their sympathies lay anywhere, it was undoubtedly with ordinary East Germans and not the leadership and its policies.
29. Gary Bruce made this claim in the review referred to in note 26. The irony is that Bruce comes close to exoneration in his own work when he approvingly cites a claim reminiscent of Hannah Arendt's "banality of evil" thesis: that those who served such

repressive regimes were not "sadists," "fanatics," or "even evil" does not make such people themselves "more sinister, but rather the state that [they] wanted to serve so unconditionally." This focus on the character of the state runs the risk of downplaying personal responsibility for individual actions—reminiscent of the way in which Daniel Goldhagen inadvertently let individuals (as well as Adolf Hitler) "off the hook" in his controversial study of the Holocaust. That is, after all, the implication of Goldhagen's claim that the attempted extermination of European Jewry was the result of some virulent strain of "eliminationist antisemitism" lying dormant since the Middle Ages. See Bruce, *Firm*, 182–83; Daniel J. Goldhagen, *Hitler's Willing Executioners: Ordinary Germans and the Holocaust* (New York, 1996); Hannah Arendt, *Eichmann in Jerusalem: A Report on the Banality of Evil* (New York, 1963).

30. These arguments are made in Port, *Conflict and Stability*, 281–82.
31. Dolores L. Augustine, "The Power Question in GDR History," *German Studies Review* 34/3 (2011): 10.
32. Fulbrook, "State of GDR History," 265.
33. Port, *Conflict and Stability*, 274–75.
34. This last issue is the driving question behind Konrad H. Jarausch, *After Hitler: Recivilizing Germans, 1945-1995* (Oxford, 2006). Gary Bruce opines, not very persuasively, that the "question of responsibility for crimes … remains the single most important question of twentieth-century Germany history." See Bruce, *Firm*, 2. See my contribution in this volume on the question of indirect indicators (pp. 202–3).
35. Port, *Conflict and Stability*, 274. For a discussion of the special language and phraseology used by East German functionaries, also see Matthias Judt, "'Nur für den Dienstgebrauch'—Arbeiten mit Texten einer deutschen Diktatur," and Ralph Jessen, "Diktatorische Herrschaft als kommunikative Praxis. Überlegungen zum Zusammenhang von 'Bürokratie' and Sprachnormierung in der DDR-Geschichte," in *Akten. Eingaben. Schaufenster. Die DDR und ihre Texte. Erkundungen zu Herrschaft und Alltag*, ed. Alf Lüdtke and Peter Becker (Berlin, 1997), 29–38, 58–75.
36. For a useful overview of some of the more popular terms that have been used, see Torsten Diedrich and Hans Ehlert, "'Moderne Diktatur'—'Erziehungsdiktatur'—'Fürsorgediktatur' oder was sonst? Das Herrschaftssystem der DDR und der Versuch seiner Definition," *Potsdamer Bulletin für Zeithistorische Studien* 12 (1998): 17–25; Fulbrook, "State of GDR History," 260.
37. Jürgen Kocka, "The GDR: A Special Kind of Modern Dictatorship," in *Dictatorship as Experience: Towards a Socio-Cultural History of the GDR*, ed. Konrad Jarausch (New York, 1999), 47–69.
38. See Hans-Ulrich Wehler, *Deutsche Gesellschaftsgeschichte, 1949-1990* (Munich, 2008), 361, 424–25.
39. Or as Lutz Niethammer retorted in response to Heym's comment: "even so: [a footnote] of world history" (*immerhin: der Weltgeschichte*). See Donna Harsch, "Footnote or Footprint? The German Democratic Republic in History," and Thomas Lindenberger, "What's in this Footnote? World History!" in *Bulletin of the German Historical Institute* 46 (Spring 2010): 9–31; Lutz Niethammer, "Erfahrungen und Strukturen. Prologomena zu einer Geschichte der Gesellschaft der DDR," in Kaeble, Kocka, and Zwahr, *Sozialgeschichte*, 96. Also see the contributions to the online forum (*Lesesaal*) about Wehler's claims, sponsored in August 2008 by the *Frankfurter Allgemeine Zeitung* (http://lesesaal.faz.net/wehler/exp_forum.php?rid=12).
40. Quotes from Kocka, *Civil Society & Dictatorship*, 35.

41. See Fulbrook, *Power and Society*, especially pp. 1–30. Also see the following exchange: Thomas Lindenberger, "Normality, Utopia, Memory, and Beyond: Reassembling East German Society," and Mary Fulbrook, "Response to Thomas Lindenberger," *German Historical Institute London Bulletin* 33/1 (May 2011): 67–98.
42. For a study that calls into question claims about popular resignation and quiescence following the construction of the Wall, see Elke Stadelmann-Wenz, *Widerständiges Verhalten und Herrschaftspraxis in der DDR. Vom Mauerbau bis zum Ende der Ulbricht-Ära* (Paderborn, 2009).
43. See Mary Fulbrook's contribution to the online H-German discussion cited in note 26.
44. See Port, *Conflict and Stability*.
45. Mary Fulbrook, *The People's State: East German Society from Hitler to Honecker* (New Haven, C.T., 2005), 9, 15, 59.
46. See Port, *Conflict and Stability*.
47. The exchange between Friedländer and Broszat is reprinted in Peter Baldwin, ed., *Reworking the Past: Hitler, the Holocaust, and the Historians' Debate* (Boston, 1990), 102–32. Also see Ian Kershaw, *The Nazi Dictatorship: Problems and Perspectives of Interpretation*, 2nd ed. (London, 1989), 150–67 (quote on p. 153); Charles S. Maier, *The Unmasterable Past: History, Holocaust, and German National Identity* (Cambridge, M.A., 1988), 90–94.
48. See Jonathan Rosenberg, *How Far the Promised Land? World Affairs and the American Civil Rights Movement from the First World War to Vietnam* (Princeton, 2005), 101–28. Also see Maria Höhn and Martin Klimke, *A Breath of Freedom: The Civil Rights Struggle, African American GIs, and Germany* (New York, 2010).
49. Tim Mason, *Social Policy in the Third Reich: The Working Class and the "National Community,"* ed. Jane Kaplan, trans. John Broadwin (Oxford, 1993), 278.
50. Bruce, *Firm*, 12.
51. Sebastian Haffner, *Zur Zeitgeschichte. 36 Essays* (Munich, 1982), 9.
52. See Port, *Conflict and Stability*, xiii n. 1.
53. A glaring example is Eppelmann, Faulenbach, and Mählert, *Bilanz und Perspektiven*. Only a handful of the more than 2,000 books and articles listed in the bibliography appeared in languages other than German.
54. This claim was one focus of the conference "Writing East German History" mentioned in note 3. For a similar point about this misleading claim, see Fulbrook, "State of GDR History," 261.
55. Monica Black, "Death and the History of East German Sensibilities," paper presented at the conference "Writing East German History" (see note 3).
56. Monica Black, *Death in Berlin: From Weimar to Divided Germany* (New York, 2010). Also see, e.g., Eli Rubin, *Synthetic Socialism: Plastics and Dictatorship in the German Democratic Republic* (Chapel Hill, N.C., 2008).
57. EP Thompson, *The Making of the English Working Class* (New York, 1966), 9.
58. Andrew I. Port, "The Silence of the Lambs, and Other Myths about the German Democratic Republic," paper presented at "Past and Future: East Germany before and after 1989," Munk Centre of International Relations, University of Toronto, 30–31 March 2007.
59. Katherine Pence and Paul Betts, eds., *Socialist Modern: East German Everyday Culture and Politics* (Ann Arbor, M.I., 2008), 23.
60. The essays in Pence and Betts, *Socialist Modern*, similarly attempt to place the GDR within the longer sweep of German history by emphasizing the supposedly "modern"

aspects of the DDR. To that end, they emphasize the interplay of tradition and innovation and claim that what came after 1945 was an amalgam of the old and new.
61. See, e.g., Seán Allan, "Good Bye, Lenin! Ostalgie und Identität im wieder vereinigten Deutschland," GFL German as a foreign language 1 (2006): 46–59.
62. For an assessment of 1945 as a major caesura, see the essays in Hans-Erich Volkmann, ed., Ende des Dritten Reiches—Ende des Zweiten Weltkrieges. Eine perspektivische Rückschau (Munich, 1995). For a more sympathetic view of the term "zero hour," see Richard Bessel, Germany 1945: From War to Peace (New York, 2009), 395–96.
63. In 1929, as Harsch discusses in her contribution to this volume, the city of Lübeck administered batches of the vaccine contaminated by a virulent strain of the bovine bacillus. This led to the death of seventy-two infants, effectively ending such vaccination in Germany until after 1945. Such resistance nevertheless had a long tradition in Germany. See, e.g., Claudia Huerkamp, "The History of Smallpox Vaccination in Germany: A First Step in the Medicalization of the General Public," Journal of Contemporary History 20/4 (1985): 617–35.
64. See Josie McLellan, "State Socialist Bodies: East German Nudism from Ban to Boom," Journal of Modern History 79 (2007): 74.
65. Developments in the primary sector, especially flight from the countryside to the city by East and West German youths, provide another example of this phenomenon. See Andrew I. Port, "Democracy and Dictatorship in the Cold War: The Two Germanies, 1949-1961," in The Oxford Handbook of Modern German History, ed. Helmut Smith (Oxford, 2011), 634–35.
66. Also see Udo Wengst and Hermann Wentker, eds., Das doppelte Deutschland. 40 Jahre Systemkonkurrenz (Berlin, 2008).
67. See, e.g., Günter Heydemann and Heinrich Oberreuter, eds., Diktaturen in Deutschland—Vergleichsaspekte. Strukturen, Institutionen und Verhaltensweisen (Bonn, 2003); Peter Bender, Deutschlands Wiederkehr. Eine ungeteilte Nachkriegsgeschichte 1945-1990 (Stuttgart, 2007); Port, "Democracy and Dictatorship."
68. This is usefully summarized in Kocka, Civil Society & Dictatorship, 39, 40, 57; also see Pence and Betts, Socialist Modern, 8; Augustine, "Power Question," 13.
69. These are only some of the more prominent examples. See, e.g., Shane Harris, The Watchers: The Rise of America's Surveillance State (London, 2010); Tim Weiner, Enemies: A History of the FBI (New York, 2012); Ellen Schrecker, Many Are the Crimes: McCarthyism in America (Boston, 1998); Gary Marx, Undercover: Police Surveillance in America (Berkeley, 1988); Brian Glick, War at Home: Covert Action against U.S. Activists and What We Can Do About It (Boston, 1989); Karrin Hanshew, Terror and Democracy in West Germany (New York, 2012); Josef Foschepoth, Überwachtes Deutschland. Post- und Telefonüberwachung in der alten Bundesrepublik (Göttingen, 2012); Stefanie Waske, Nach Lektüre vernichten! Der geheime Nachrichtendienst von CDU und CSU im Kalten Krieg (Munich, 2013). A major conference organized by the German Institute for Contemporary History also explored this theme: "Staat gegen Terrorismus. Demokratie und Sicherheit in Westeuropa 1979-1990," Institut für Zeitgeschichte, Munich, 8–9 November 2012.
70. As Michael Hunt has written, "Americans went crusading in foreign lands in the name of freedom even as those freedoms significantly narrowed at home. That those who fell victim to McCarthyism lost their jobs and reputations and not their lives and that their numbers were far fewer than those exiled to Soviet labor camps or executed serves to qualify, not invalidate, the comparison and to extenuate, not excuse, the betrayal of

fundamental American political values." Michael Hunt, *The World Transformed: 1945 to the Present* (Boston, 2004), 72.
71. See Michel Foucault, *Discipline and Punish: The Birth of the Prison* (New York, 1977).
72. Augustine, "Power Question," 6. Also see Sven Korzilius, *"Asoziale" und "Parasiten" im Recht der SBZ/DDR. Randgruppen im Sozialismus zwischen Repression und Ausgrenzung* (Cologne, 2005); Andrew I. Port, "When Workers Rumbled: The Wismut Upheaval of August 1951 in East Germany," *Social History* 22/2 (1997): 168–71.
73. See note 48.
74. See Susan Reverby, *Examining Tuskegee: The Infamous Syphilis Study and Its Legacy* (Chapel Hill, N.C., 2009).
75. See, e.g., Herbert Wolf, *Hatte die DDR je eine Chance?* (Hamburg, 1991); Jörg Roesler, *Zwischen Plan und Markt. Die Wirtschaftsreform 1963-1970 in der DDR* (Berlin, 1990); Monika Kaiser, "Die Reformversuche der sechziger Jahre im Kontext der innerparteilichen Richtungskämpfe," in *Pankower Vorträge* 23/2 (2000): 53–65. For a more realistic assessment, see André Steiner, *Die DDR-Wirtschaftsreform der sechziger Jahre. Konflikte zwischen Effizienz- und Machtkalkül* (Berlin, 1999).
76. Sigrid Meuschel, *Legitimation und Parteiherrschaft in der DDR. Zum Paradox von Stabilität und Revolution in der DDR, 1945–1989* (Frankfurt am Main, 1992).
77. Eric Hobsbawm, *The Age of Extremes: A History of the World, 1914-1991* (New York, 1994), 8. For a similar warning against the assumption that liberal democracy was "destined" to emerge victorious after 1945, see Mark Mazower, *Dark Continent: Europe's Twentieth Century* (New York, 2000), 3–6.
78. For such sentiments, see the important memoir by the disillusioned wife of a Czech Communist functionary "purged" and executed following the 1952 Slánský Trial: Heda Margolius Kovály, *Under a Cruel Star: A Life in Prague 1941-1968* (New York, 1997).
79. Equally intriguing is the question of why there has been such "nostalgia," or *Ostalgie,* for what had been, while it still existed, an extremely unpopular regime—whereas earlier Germans had been able to distance themselves so quickly from another regime that had, in its time, enjoyed much greater support, namely, the Third Reich. Some obvious answers include the difference in the magnitude of the crimes committed by the two regimes, how they initially came about and how they ultimately met their demise, and what came afterward. See my own essay in this volume and, on the topic of *Ostalgie,* Katja Neller, *DDR-Nostalgie. Dimensionen der Orientierung der Ostdeutschen gegenüber der ehemaligen DDR, ihre Ursachen und politische Konnotationen* (Wiesbaden, 2006). On popular support for the Nazi regime, see Robert Gellately, *Backing Hitler: Consent and Coercion in Nazi Germany* (Oxford, 2001); Götz Aly, *Hitlers Volksstaat. Raub, Rassenkrieg und nationaler Sozialismus* (Frankfurt am Main, 2005).
80. Kocka, *Civil Society & Dictatorship,* 60.
81. Judith Butler, *Bodies That Matter: On the Discursive Limits of "Sex"* (New York, 1993).
82. Grieder, "In Defence," 584.

PART I

Memory and Identity after Nazism

CHAPTER 1

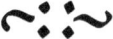

East Germans in a Post-Nazi State
*Communities of Experience,
Connection, and Identification*

MARY FULBROOK

The pre-1945 dimension to the German Democratic Republic (GDR) is central to understanding its history. Yet, the implications at a personal, subjective level of the radical historical rupture of 1945 still remain relatively unexplored and undertheorized. The continuing legacies of a still salient past have often been subsumed under a now inflated notion of "collective memory."[1] Historians have tended to focus on public practices of remembrance, memorialization, and representation, often following Pierre Nora's conception of "sites of memory" that stand for and may displace "real memories."[2] Historians have less frequently engaged with the collective construction of accounts of the past among the kinds of small communities, families, and informal groups discussed by Maurice Halbwachs and which are of interest to social psychologists; or with the lingering individual legacies and representations of trauma with which literary scholars and psychotherapists have been particularly concerned.[3] These wider theoretical emphases and omissions appear magnified when considering the historiography of the GDR. While historians looking at the legacies of the Holocaust and the relations between trauma and memory have largely focused on Western societies, historians of "collective memory" in the GDR have focused almost exclusively on state-sponsored and official representations of the GDR as the "anti-fascist state."

The purpose of this essay is to suggest ways of connecting the familiar narrative of public practices of remembrance in the GDR with personal legacies of the past, by focusing on what may be termed communities of experience, connection, and identification. What follows is intended merely to give a preliminary indication of the complexity of the ways in which the significance of the Nazi past was transformed in the GDR. It is also intended to suggest a more differentiated way of exploring significations of past and present than is offered by approaches focusing on "collective memory" understood primarily in terms of cultural and political representations and dominant narratives.[4]

Communities of Experience, Connection, and Identification

There is a tendency in dichotomous approaches to the GDR to consider "state" and "society" as relatively static, all-encompassing categories, juxtaposing public and private as though collective actors remained the same over time. But East German society was no more homogeneous with respect to personal legacies of the Nazi past across generations than it was in any other respect. In exploring relationships with a specific past, it is helpful to distinguish between what may be called communities of experience, connection, and identification. These are conceptual categories developed for purposes of analysis: theoretical terms, not concepts that people themselves would have necessarily recognized or accepted—although they do often map onto substantive concepts current either at the time or later, such as "victims of fascism," "second generation," and "war children." What, then, is signified by each of these conceptual terms?

The term "community of experience" designates those who personally lived through a particularly significant historical event or period and shared certain experiences—even if what they shared were common challenges rather than individual responses, as they faced divergent twists and turns of fate. "Communities of connection" are made up of those people who did not themselves consciously experience this "salient past," but who nevertheless, and not necessarily by choice, were in some way linked with the people who did: the children and grandchildren of Nazi perpetrators or Holocaust victims and survivors, for example, but also friends, relatives, and other members of society who were emotionally or practically affected in some way. Hence this is not a purely generational or familial term; nor do all relatives necessarily have any sense of "connection"; nor do those who are affected necessarily have to be aware of the consequences of the past for their own lives. Choice is, however, a greater component of the final category—though with qualifications, since the availability and desirability of particular forms of identification depend on the social, political, and cultural context of "choosing." "Communities of identification" are those who, by identifying or empathizing with the fates of others, find a particular past to be one of heightened personal significance. Patterns of identification are likely to be more variable than the legacies of the past among the directly affected communities of experience. But the extent to which such variations are primarily bounded by national public representations, or vary with, for example, personal experiences, family backgrounds, social networks, or transnational cultural developments, is an empirical question requiring further exploration.[5]

A particular past may not be of persisting relevance to everyone in any specific area at any given time. But these categories may provide a useful way in which to understand the undulating and shifting landscapes of confrontations with the past, as the remembering agents who endow it with significance change over time. This people-centered approach allows us to look at the changing interrelations between "public" and "private," between dominant, prevalent, and marginalized narratives, between cultural representations, socially current interpretations, and personal significations of a salient past in later circumstances. It also allows us, in principle, to make comparisons, exploring the ways in which the "same" past can have different significance under later circumstances. This essay focuses on just a few examples, but the theoretical approach is designed specifically to allow for broader comparisons across a far broader geographical and temporal range.

Structural Filters among Communities of Experience

Experiences of Nazism and war entailed seismic shifts in identity—both self-chosen and externally attributed, even forcibly imposed—during the 1930s and early 1940s. There were, correspondingly, many differing communities of experience across Europe, where people had experienced Nazism, Stalinism, and the violent upheavals of war in a variety of ways: "victimhood," "resistance," or "collaboration," for example, could mean quite different things depending on context—both at the time of the experiences and in later reinterpretations.[6]

Postwar circumstances both filtered and reshaped how key "defining experiences" were perceived and how people felt they could or should express themselves about their past, partially deflecting the political and "racial" fault lines of the Nazi period. Among those who had, to some degree, supported and gone along with Nazism, earlier faith in Adolf Hitler and pride in being German, while now publicly rejected, could nevertheless continue in new ways in face of unpopular denazification policies, while other experiences evoked a new "community of fate." Memories of wartime air raids were augmented and complicated by postwar experiences of flight and expulsion, of rape and robbery at the hands of Soviet soldiers, of personal bereavement and worry about missing friends and family members. Survivors of "racial" persecution often faced further experiences of rejection, as in the case of Polish Jews who were widely met with hostility upon seeking their former homes in Poland. Identities continued to be reconsidered and reconfigured in the maelstrom of postwar population movements and migrations. In short, narratives of the past were crucially affected not only by experiences under Nazism, but also by rapidly changing postwar contexts.

Personal narratives were shaped in the context of emergent wider, prevalent, and dominant discourses about the past. Considerations about the "politics of the past" varied according to political circumstances, with key differences between dictatorial and democratic conditions. In Konrad Adenauer's West Germany, the desire to appeal to a wide constituency meant not only public acknowledgment of historical responsibility—in which many prominent West Germans later took an almost perverse pride—but also, paradoxically, the practical, material, and symbolic inclusion of former Nazis and beneficiaries of Nazism. The dominant narrative was thus one of acknowledging collective responsibility without any concession of guilt, while looking after those who had actively sustained the Nazi racial community. Thus there was relatively little incongruity between official proclamations and private narratives in the first decade or so of West Germany's existence.[7]

In the Soviet Zone of Occupation (SBZ) and subsequently the GDR, the dominant public narrative was that of active "anti-fascist" resistance.[8] The regime developed shrines to Communist martyrs such as Ernst Thälmann; it designated and orchestrated visits to "national" sites of memory such as Buchenwald, Sachsenhausen, and other quasi-sacred places; and it sought to influence younger generations.[9] The ruling Socialist Unity Party (SED) also went to considerable lengths—through, for example, the activities of the National Front (NF) and the German National Democratic Party (NDPD)—to attempt to win over and "convert," or at least neutralize and contain, those former "nominal" Nazis deemed capable of redemption. The official conception of an "anti-fascist state" was intrinsically distorted and never entirely successful: the emphasis on liberation at the hands of the Soviets was at odds with private memories of defeat; denazification could be critiqued as serving Communist political and socioeconomic goals; the official line was partially undercut by family narratives; it was progressively overlaid by Cold War rhetoric and instrumentalized for political purposes. That the SED based much of the GDR's claim to legitimacy on being *the* "anti-fascist state" is nevertheless significant: it served to filter and color public expressions of private memories, and to exclude certain areas almost entirely from the consciousness of later generations.

This is evident even when we ask about private narratives of the past among victims of persecution on "racial" grounds. With respect to Western Europe and North America, the "myth of silence," or the notion that Holocaust survivors "did not talk" about their experiences in the early postwar years, has been radically revised.[10] Yet this is an area that has only recently been addressed with respect to the GDR. This question is one with many aspects. Holocaust scholars have begun to focus on discussing the ways in which the character of such accounts changed, with differences between accounts produced close to the experiences of persecution and those produced years later. "Bearing witness" could mean very different things for diarists in the ghetto, for witnesses at later war-crimes trials, for writers of memoirs at different stages of life, and for oral history interviewees half a century after the war's end.[11]

Clearly there are varying personal reasons why some survivors prioritized putting what energy they had into making a new life and tried not to burden the next generation, allowing their own wounds to form scar tissue. It was often only later in life, when personal losses were partially overlaid by the intervening years and the mission for the future was not so much to protect as to educate the next generation, that some started to speak openly and in public. These personal concerns were as relevant to survivors in the GDR as elsewhere. But the political and social context mattered alongside the individual dynamics of adjustment and strategies for personal and family survival. The question is not always or only that of "who talked," but rather "to whom" they talked, who was prepared to listen, and what effect this had on the character of their accounts. In many Western states the problem was not so much that survivors "did not talk," but rather that dominant communities were only selectively prepared to listen, and that "talking" did not readily translate into "voice" on the public stage. Communities "talked past" each other: suppressing uncomfortable aspects of their respective narratives in public; selectively recounting or silencing the past within distinctive community or private settings—but not communicating across the boundaries of different communities of experience. In the early postwar period, unlike later in the twentieth century, audiences for accounts of the suffering of others were relatively lacking. When such narratives were heard in the public sphere, they inevitably bore traces of what was both acceptable and desirable—from a number of perspectives—to say.

Accounts in the GDR were constrained and shaped by the emergent Communist-dominated organizational and narrative framework. The Union of those Persecuted by the Nazi Regime (*Vereinigung der Verfolgten des Naziregimes*, VVN) was formed to unite a variety of victims' groups that had sprung up after the war in both the Western and Eastern zones, and a branch was founded in the Soviet zone in 1947. This was dissolved without discussion in 1953, when the SED-controlled Committee of Antifascist Resistance Fighters (*Komitee der antifaschistischen Widerstandskämpfer*) took over. Those designated "victims of fascism" (*Opfer des Faschismus*, OdF) eventually received certain privileges, such as higher pensions and regular health checks, but were from the start seen as less worthy than active "fighters against fascism." Thus distinctions emerged between the racially persecuted and the political opponents of the Nazi regime, with the former deemed less important than the latter—a situation not radically dissimilar, incidentally, to that of Jews returning to France, where, in different political colors, the patriotic myth of French resistance tended to take precedence over Jewish victimhood.

Those involved in the VVN were explicitly conscious of the fact that they constituted an "imagined community," linked by common experiences of the past and related later goals. They referred to each other as "comrades"; they cooperated in attempts to bring former perpetrators to trial; there was considerable activity both by official representatives and individuals.[12] There was a sense of community persisting through time: each action, each case of bringing a former perpetrator to trial, was seen as achieving something on behalf of the millions who had suffered and died at the hands of the Nazis. The sense of community not only registered a sense of having something in common with other survivors, but also with the dead, and indeed the dead of many nations (now in some contrast to the French case, where patriotism remained dominant). Moreover, it implied that those who died were *Opfer* (victims) in the dual sense possible in German: they died not merely as "victims" but also as a "sacrifice" for a larger, still enduring cause that was wider and greater than any individual life. This was accompanied by the sense that those brought to justice also stand, in some way, for far more in terms of what Nazism meant. Slogans such as "The dead endow us with an obligation" (*Die Toten verpflichten*) were evident not only on many memorials, but also in brochures and reports, with an active use of the verb implying agency beyond the grave, functioning to bind the living and the departed in a form of moral covenant, and endowing survivors with an active legacy for their mission in the present and future. A classic statement of this view of a community binding the living and the dead was provided, for example, by members of the VVN in the context of a trial of industrialists who had exploited forced laborers. They spoke "out of a sense of the duty that we owe not only to our dead in Germany but also in the whole of Europe": "In the name of the 300,000 survivors and the 500,000 dead of the German resistance movement, as well as the 11 million dead in the prisons, jails, concentration camps, and the many labor camps, … but above all in the name of the millions of forced laborers from all the countries of Europe, who were obliged to come as slave laborers to be used in the German armaments industry, we raise our voice and accuse the Nazi activists present here of crimes against humanity."[13] The statement of a sense of an imagined community of experience, speaking with a single "voice," could hardly be articulated more clearly. Here it is shaped, in large part, by a Socialist notion of the international solidarity of workers as a class, irrespective of nation.

The preconditions for the further shaping of such communities of experience varied with their social and political profiles. Some were in line with SED goals, such as those related to left-wing suffering and resistance, while others were harder to sustain on anything other than on an individual basis—as in the case of individuals persecuted on grounds of homosexuality, or, rather differently, relatives of victims of the "euthanasia" program.[14] Others had a less well-defined sense of community, particularly if they had previously been marginalized or occupied interstitial locations, such as those designated "mixed race" (*Mischlinge*). By contrast, those with an unambiguous sense of Jewish identity, whether rooted in a sense of kinship and descent, or in religious commitment as well, belonged to an already well-established community with a developed organizational and institutional network. The global post-Holocaust Jewish community increasingly saw the "Jewish catastrophe," or Shoah, as a defining collective trauma. It also, more problematically for East German Jews, had significant and politically salient bases in Israel and the United States, ensuring continual complications in the relationships between the SED leadership and Jewish East Germans.[15]

Individual survivor accounts were inflected by the changing context of discussion; even in the early postwar years, narratives already bore the marks of dominant discourses. Far from "keeping silent," survivors often had their stories actively elicited by the VVN. Many survivors had been in a relatively protected category, such as "mixed marriages" in which partners had refused to divorce them; despite being deported to forced labor camps, they managed to survive appalling conditions. Even so, many reported losing close family members in Auschwitz, Theresienstadt, Buchenwald, and elsewhere; no one was entirely unmarked by privation and bereavement. Individual stories often make for tragic reading. Many used the word "hell" to describe the places to which they had been deported, or, more generally, the ways in which their lives had been made unbearable; others reiterated the inexpressibility of their experiences and their emotions. Many had now become distrustful of fellow Germans. Some could recount ways in which people had helped protect or save them; but it is clear that they had also suffered from the way in which others had progressively excluded them from local society, ceasing to greet them, calling them names, and treating them roughly.[16] Some had been actively betrayed by former friends, neighbors, and acquaintances, who delivered them into the hands of the Gestapo or *Schutzstaffel* (SS). As one survivor put it, "That this should have an effect on the spirit probably does not need to be mentioned explicitly."[17]

There are variations in the individual details of these anguished stories. In ways similar to early testimonies in other locations—the interviews carried out in Displaced Persons camps in the Western zones by the American psychologist David Boder, for example, or the testimonies collected by the Jewish Historical Institute in Warsaw—early accounts lacked the wider framing, informed by lengthy reflection and secondary knowledge subsequently acquired, so evident in later accounts. But people were clearly already aware of some of the desired features of a Communist master narrative, even if they could not quite mold their own stories to fit this narrative. One Jewish survivor providing a report on his experiences for the VVN, for example, pointed out explicitly that, as the only Jew in his locality, he was under constant surveillance and persecuted solely on grounds of "race," making it "right from the start quite impossible to engage in any illegal [political] activity."[18] A brief report by Kurt R, written on 17 February 1948 in a predominantly political and nonemotional tone, was something of an exception. A "half-Jew," he was also a Socialist in the Social Democratic Party (SPD), and was arrested and imprisoned twice for his illegal activities. His fully Jewish father, also politically active, was gassed in Auschwitz. Kurt R himself became a member of the SED, the trade union organization (FDGB), and the VVN. His account ends on a political note about his lifelong devotion to "the eradication (*Ausmerzung*) of all former activist forces of the NSDAP who endanger our young democracy," a task to which he had committed himself entirely.[19] Such a refrain would become typical in the GDR, though the terminology and organizational frameworks changed over time.

Those who had suffered under Nazism for their left-wing political views had the easiest job of shaping personal experiences into the official narrative framework, now seizing the opportunity to "build anew." This is particularly evident in memoirs penned at a later date. Olaf B, for example, had been imprisoned on "death row" in Plötzensee and Brandenburg prisons, after being betrayed for his part in Communist resistance organizations.[20] When released at the end of the war, Olaf B, who had previously been active in Berlin's Piscator Theater, immediately started to work for a "democratic" (that is, Communist-controlled) radio station, based initially in what was to become West Berlin. The politically committed Olaf B followed the Communist radio station when it subsequently moved to the Soviet sector. This kind of "in-migration" to the Communist East is rarely noted—and was, of course, minimal compared to flight westward—but Olaf B was in some ways typical of those prepared to continue the "good fight" under Communist auspices. He rapidly became a committed GDR citizen, religiously devouring (and regurgitating to anyone who would listen) the SED official newspaper, *Neues Deutschland*, and, despite chronic ill health arising from lengthy imprisonment, threw himself into building up the new state. His memoirs and memories are framed accordingly.[21]

But the vast majority of East Germans were not survivors of Nazi persecution, let alone active anti-fascists. People who had been mobilized to support Hitler's "national community" and fight against "Bolshevism" constituted quite different, more prevalent communities of experience, whose own experiences were often at odds with the dominant narratives. Moreover, the SED portrayed itself, not without some justification, as more energetic in pursuit of former Nazis than the other two Third Reich successor states, West Germany and Austria (the latter, after 1955, being particularly dilatory in this area). Former NSDAP functionaries, SS and Gestapo officers, as well as prison and concentration camp guards, were, despite notable exceptions, on the whole more actively brought to account in the GDR than elsewhere (as indeed were many other individuals who were simply politically inconvenient or unlucky).[22]

Many former Nazi perpetrators sought to evade being brought to justice in the GDR, either by fleeing to the West in the hope of greater leniency, or by keeping their heads down and even, in many instances, changing their identity. The reactions of people accused of having been Nazi perpetrators betray many similarities. Common tropes include the claims that they "knew nothing about it," were "not responsible," had only "obeyed orders," that others had either committed the act in question or had given the orders to commit the act. Defendants often claimed in attempted mitigation that they had committed specific "good deeds": giving bread to a starving prisoner or slave laborer, for example, or "saving a Jew."[23] Such claims often had some basis, given widespread investment in a kind of "insurance policy" by those belatedly seeking to earn anticipated gratitude and potentially useful testimonials once it was clear that the war was lost. But while there has been extensive research on former Nazis in West Germany, we still know relatively little about how stories among former perpetrators developed over time in the GDR. Conversion did not always lead to redemption, if the crimes were sufficiently serious and were unearthed and brought to trial. There are some remarkable instances of apparently outstanding GDR citizens, rewarded repeatedly for their activism at work and their political commitment, whose former lives were not revealed until a quarter century or more after the end of the war. Rudolf Zimmermann, for example, was an "ideal" GDR citizen until 1967, when he came to the attention of the GDR authorities as a witness in the trial in West Germany of Walter Thormeyer, Zimmermann's former boss in the Mielec Gestapo headquarters in Poland. Thormeyer, who had held a senior position both ordering and carrying out mass murder, received a relatively lenient sentence in the Federal Republic; Helmut Hensel, Thormeyer's predecessor, who had been in charge of deportations and associated murders that took place in March 1942, was never brought to account in West Germany, despite full knowledge of his identity and whereabouts. Yet their underling Zimmermann, despite his model life as a GDR citizen, his humble social origins, and his evident later contrition, was sentenced to life imprisonment in the GDR, a term that he did, in fact, serve until his death two decades later.[24] A few former Nazis even made it to the 1980s before their identities were discovered, including, for example, former SS-Obersturmführer Henry Schmidt, who had participated in Gestapo repression in Dresden and was responsible for the ghettoization of around 985 Germans of Jewish descent, as well as the deportation of 723 to Theresienstadt and Auschwitz; he was only brought to trial in 1987.[25] Others led apparently unremarkable lives until their deaths; in one case, for example, it was only when a son who had fled to the West returned for his father's funeral that the identity of a former Ravensbrück guard, who was locally known as a benign neighbor and well-behaved citizen, was publicly revealed.[26]

The majority of Germans fit none of these categories, of course. For the most part, Germans who were not directly and actively involved in the Nazi system of persecution had accommodated themselves, in one way or another, to the changing demands of Nazism and war, prioritizing personal survival through appalling times. Many had compromised in some way with the Nazi regime; others, even if they had been opposed to or ambivalent about Nazism, had no great love for the Communist dictatorship that replaced it; many had been more enthusiastic, certainly at some times and on some issues, while still being fearful of the violent consequences of war for family members and friends. Their transitions from Nazism to communism demonstrate a different kind of complexity. The following example stands for many.

Ursula B, born in 1912, was the daughter of a landowner. In 1932, at the age of twenty, she joined the NSDAP. Her husband, also in the party, had already been a member of the SS when she first met him. During the last years of the war, and in the early postwar years, Ursula B wrote an extensive diary in the form of letters to her husband, who had gone missing in action on the Eastern front in the winter of 1943. It is clear from this diary that she was a well-integrated member of local society and unthinking upholder of the Nazi "racial community" (*Volksgemeinschaft*). On 30 April 1944, for example, she recounted a particularly shocking incident. It had come to Ursula B's notice that a French prisoner of war and forced laborer, Jacques, was becoming "ever more impertinent" (*immer frecher*). She now warned her female employees against any kind of friendship with him: "you must always bear in mind that you are German girls and he is a prisoner of war."[27] After listening to this prohibition of any intimacy, one of the castigated "German girls," Erika, went upstairs and hanged herself. She left a note for her parents to the effect that, having fallen in love with Jacques, with whom any friendship was now forbidden, "life has lost its meaning for me." Jacques, too, was now beyond himself with grief, and "flung himself on the ground, threw himself onto the girl, kissed her and cried inconsolably," expressing his love for her. Ursula B went on to recount in her diary how she reported the incident the next day to the local functionary: Jacques was immediately arrested and deported that same night. Thus, Ursula B comments, she now lacked not just one but two workers: "We drew a line under it all and spoke as little as possible about it."[28] This silencing was significant—and symptomatic. It was certainly the case that Ursula B had successfully repressed explicit discussion, if not private memories, of this incident—as of so many other aspects of her life in the Third Reich. Her reaction was probably quite typical.

Much later, on the occasion of her seventieth birthday in 1982, Ursula B wrote her memoirs for her children and grandchildren. As we shall see in the next section, these memoirs told a rather unexpected and different story of her life. In any event, Ursula B was one of those who eventually made a successful transition to life in East Germany, becoming a model GDR citizen by the 1980s—but not from an easy starting point.

Transformation and Transmission

Over time, the narratives of the past that were prevalent among communities of experience were augmented and displaced by differing interpretations among emergent communities of connection and identification. Given a dominant narrative downplaying grassroots complicity in the crimes of Nazism, a relatively guilt-free paradigm developed both among those who had been adults at the time of Nazism and among those too young to have experienced this period directly. It seems primarily to have been the generation of those caught in the middle, the "1929ers," who were, in some cases, plagued by a sense of shame and commitment to "building anew," as in the well-known case of novelist Christa Wolf.[29]

In the process of adjusting to new structures and ways of life, and despite many difficulties and tensions along the way, former Nazis could become apparently well-adjusted GDR citizens. Some were clearly opportunists, adapting their outward behavior to the demands of the times, though retaining an inner sense of resentment about the radical transformation of their lives. Others seem, as in the case of Rudolf Zimmermann, to have undergone a genuine transformation—until and unless discovered by the authorities and forced to account for a particularly brutal past. But in many cases, it was not merely behavior but also *frameworks* of perception that changed along the way: aspects of the social construction of self-representation and memory are evident in a wide variety of ego-documents across time.

Ursula B offers a striking example of this process. Her memoirs were written in the GDR for her family rather than for official purposes; the constraints to conform to a particular format, all too evident in the "Veterans' Reports" and other autobiographical materials periodically elicited by the SED and the mass organizations, were clearly not uppermost in her mind. The pressures and difficulties Ursula B and her children experienced in the early years of the GDR were not downplayed in any way. As a former Nazi and member of the privileged landowning classes, the immediate postwar years were very difficult for Ursula B, something she does not gloss over. She begins the section of her memoirs dealing with this period of her life with the phrase: "Bad times began."[30] She recounts how they had to share their house with thirteen refugee and expellee families with "very many children," and how her own children were discriminated against at school: they were refused entry to the high school classes that prepared them for the university entry examination (the *Abitur*), and had to take the training and apprenticeship route instead.[31]

Both the shape and the contents of the memoirs are nevertheless reminiscent of accounts produced in more obviously political contexts. In line with other "conversion narratives," Ursula B describes her transformation into an active member of a collective farm (LPG). Her life history in the GDR is recounted primarily in terms of her working life and her wider societal activities and political involvement; her children play a large role in the account, suggesting her success in combining motherhood and productive work. This is, in short, the voice of an active and independent woman, a classic female GDR citizen.[32] Ursula B even appears grateful for the typically Communist system of awards and honors: she recounts with pride how, by the time of writing on her seventieth birthday, she had collected a total of twelve orders of merit and innumerable citations for excellent work or contributions to the social and cultural activities and organizations in which she had been active.

How did Ursula B navigate this transition at a personal level? Following the emotional trauma and deep biographical rupture of losing her beloved husband, and after several years of battling her way through the challenges of early postwar life and looking after her young children, Ursula B finally had a personal breakdown—at which point her diary broke off. She seems to have emerged from this a changed woman; both in her behavior, demonstrated through commitment to the new Communist society, and in her autobiographical account.

But this transformation was only sustained at the price of some startling omissions from her later self-representation. In her memoirs, Ursula B succeeded in finding a degree of personal resolution of the ruptures in her life by constructing an apparent narrative continuity where, in the light of contrasting sources, there was clearly, in fact, major dissonance. She does this in two ways.

In the first place, she almost entirely ignores the Nazi era, glossing over any complicity in National Socialist practices. She suggests that, despite early—and forgivable—enthusiasm for Nazism, she had quickly become oppositional. While in 1933 they had hoped Hitler would "help agriculture," and she was happy to take on a role in the League of German Girls (BdM), the story of the violent suppression of the so-called *Röhm Putsch* in June 1934—the infamous "Night of Long Knives"—allegedly constituted a turning point, after which she had increasing doubts about the "Movement": "I was supposed to gain further qualifications in the Hitler Youth organization but refused and got into difficulties. At the same time my brother-in-law lost his civil service job, because he had belonged to the SPD."[33] She does not say what the alleged "difficulties" were, jumping conveniently over her own continuing conformity and effectively claiming innocence by association, appealing vicariously to her brother-in-law's commitment to social democracy. The fact that both she and her husband were members of the NSDAP is not mentioned, nor her husband's membership in the SS; the incident in which she unintentionally precipitated the suicide of her employee and the arrest and deportation of her forced laborer finds no place in her memoirs either. Such silencing of—and an initial failure to recognize—complicity in everyday Nazism was widespread among postwar Germans in both East and West.

Secondly, Ursula B is able to construct continuity by emphasizing the primacy of her concern for her children, doing always what she feels is what is best for them: not only during the Third Reich and the early postwar years, but also in the new, Communist society. Having experienced disadvantages and some pain in the transitional period, Ursula B makes, in the end, a strikingly successful transition to the new regime.

Not every unthinking former supporter of Hitler's regime made such a successful transition to active participation in the microstructures of the GDR. And historians do not always have the sources that make it possible to juxtapose earlier and later self-narratives in this way. Yet autobiographical accounts and oral history interviews with East Germans carried out both before and after 1990 revealed a widespread capacity for a relatively guilt-free description of their own involvement and that of their family members in the Nazi system.[34] East Germans tended to recount their own roles in the Third Reich in a matter-of-fact, un-self-critical way. Innumerable sources bear witness to the priority given in most people's lives to the survival and well-being of themselves and the close members of their families, with variations depending on how the individual life cycle coincided with major historical turning points. Few of the sources betray any sense of guilt or anguish about their own role in the Nazi past, even when they explicitly record (at the time or later) their "knowledge" of the consequences of racism for the victims of the Nazi regime.[35] The case of Ursula B offers a clear example of an ordinary Nazi becoming a good GDR citizen—by not thinking too hard about politics, or considering issues much beyond her own family's well-being. This, too, was probably typical on both sides of the Wall—in the West as much as in the East. But there was a significant difference with respect to the implications for subsequent communities of connection and identification, and hence for intergenerational transmission of the legacies of Nazism.

The difference was again rooted in the distinctive context. Whereas in the West the challenges of "1968" led members of a younger generation to confront their parents' generation (if not actually their own parents) about the Third Reich, this was not the case in the GDR, both because of the structure of the system and the character of the dominant historical narratives. By the later 1960s, the growth of the Stasi and the increased capacity of state repression meant that "1968," even with the added resonance and proximity of the Prague Spring, could not mean the same as it did in West Germany at this time. And while many were aware of the inadequacies of the anti-fascist narrative as an accurate account of the past, they were, at the same time, effectively exonerated from having to deal with the question of guilt. Increasingly, the challenges of the present seemed to reduce the significance of the past: the Wall, and not the Nazi past, became the salient defining event for younger East Germans.

The dominant narrative about Nazism was, over time, increasingly concerned with contemporary political interests. International considerations—in different ways in the GDR than in West Germany—were of overriding importance to the SED leadership, which vociferously critiqued prominent West Germans for their roles in the Third Reich, as in the notorious "Brown Books" and the campaigns against Hans Globke, Theodor Oberländer, Heinrich Lübke, and others.[36] Competition with the West was complemented by a concern about regaining status internationally, even where this was primarily symbolic. (This was not unlike Adenauer's priorities, but was expressed differently.) For example, the report on an official visit by GDR dignitaries to the Warsaw ghetto memorial in 1963 revealed that the major concern was that East Germans should be internationally accepted rather than shunned; considerable pride was expressed in the fact that the GDR delegation was given a place of honor, physically, in front of the Israeli and French delegations.[37] Drawing attention to the plight of Jews under Nazism was never entirely absent from East German historiography, but was bound up with tensions in interpretation and phraseology, even in the changed historiographical climate of the 1970s and 1980s.[38] Questions of world peace often took precedence, even when the focus was on bringing former Nazis to justice. GDR newspapers drew striking contrasts, characterizing West Germany as a state that harbored former Nazis and failed to bring them to trial in adequate numbers. As the *Berliner Zeitung* proudly proclaimed in October 1987, the GDR had squarely faced up to the past, but "[n]ot with talk about compensation" and "[n]ot with the attempt to buy oneself out" of the legacies of the mass murder of innocent millions. Not content with these unfavorable allusions, the *Berliner Zeitung* went on to underline the contrast even more explicitly: while West Germany was the self-proclaimed successor state to the Third Reich, the GDR was "the executor of the legacies of the victims of fascism… Their legacy is here, every hour of every day, a reality in all the actions" of the state.[39]

Such political instrumentalization was often obvious to older generations. Those who remembered the end of the war as defeat rather than as "liberation" continued to mutter at official commemoration ceremonies in the 1980s.[40] For the vast majority of GDR citizens, however, dealing with the challenges of the present became far more significant than chewing over an officially guilt-free past. Former "victims of fascism" and survivors of Nazi persecution could be equally distanced and cynical about official interpretations. Some even made use of the state's rhetoric for private ends, as when Ilse J, the daughter of a Jewish mother and an "Aryan" father, mobilized her "Jewishness" to attain permission to visit an uncle, a Holocaust survivor, in the West.[41] Until the later

1980s, when SED policies evolved, it was clear to many people of Jewish descent, whether or not they were also religious, that SED attitudes toward Jews could hover between ambivalent and difficult—if not, on occasion, downright hostile. Political instrumentalization could thus be counterproductive. But, for the most part, it also served to block off for members of a younger generation any direct confrontation with their parents' involvement.

Nor were the alleged legacies of the past transmitted in any direct, unidirectional way across generations within families, even those where the parental generation had truly been "anti-fascist" at the time and had not merely claimed this in retrospect. It is striking how many political activists and critics of the GDR in the 1970s and 1980s were children of people who had been, and often remained, prominent in the Communist movement. This generation, born in the decade after the war, often became increasingly frustrated as young adults by the failure of the SED regime to realize in practice the ideals and principles which they had been brought up to believe: Monika Maron, Anette Kahan, Vera Lengsfeld (Wollenberger), stand out as exemplary for this pattern.[42] It was life in the GDR and the failures of the anti-fascist state to live up to its ideals, not the legacies of Nazism, that were key to the shift from the lessons propagated by the dominant community of experience in the SED regime to different patterns of identification among the next generation. Norbert B, born in 1940, was brought up by a committed Communist, Olaf B (discussed earlier). Norbert came from a family with a variety of political views.[43] His grandfather was a "big capitalist" who had owned, among other enterprises, shops in Berlin and a margarine factory in England, and had traveled widely across Europe, apparently pursuing women almost as much as trade. One uncle supported nationalist causes, and, in due course, became a member of the NSDAP and possibly the SS. His life ended under mysterious circumstances: according to the family narrative, he was shot by partisans at the end of the war. An aunt was on friendly terms with a "Nazi bigwig" in Hamburg, to whom Olaf B probably owed his life: this Nazi was able to "pull strings" in Berlin, and apparently had Olaf B's death sentence transmuted into a lengthy term of imprisonment. As a child, Norbert B accepted his father's position on the left, but the turning point came with the erection of the Berlin Wall in 1961. At first he thought this would be a temporary measure, as in June 1953, when the borders were tightened and then relaxed again. But now, at the age of twenty-one, it was clear to Norbert that things were different, and, as he put it, "from this day on I began to hate this system," despite his father's firm beliefs.[44] Typical of his generation—the most disaffected generational cohort in the GDR—Norbert B was among the first called up to do military service in the National People's Army (NVA). This, too, proved to be a formative experience, but one that pulled him in contradictory directions and forced him to establish personal priorities. While performing patrol duties on the German-German border, Norbert had an opportunity to escape to the West, with a high chance of success and relatively little by way of personal risk. But he chose not to escape. His whole life rapidly "went through his head," with vivid thoughts of a girl whom he loved and with whom he could envisage a future if he stayed, as well as the consequences if he fled for his parents, brother, and sister, from whom he would likely never hear again. In the end, these typical family considerations—relating to both current and future families—weighed more heavily in the balance than the chance of freedom.[45] Norbert subsequently became increasingly oppositional. He was the sole member of his family to take this stance, the "black sheep" in a family of committed SED members; he steadfastly resisted all pressures to join the SED, and even thinks, upon reflection years later, that he earned some respect for taking this stance. Even so, his thinking betrayed very strong left-wing preferences, including a critique of Western materialism and individualism based on his experiences in united Germany after 1990.

East Germans reacted in a variety of ways to the various rubbing points where the intrusions and demands of the state intersected with what they saw as their private lives. There were, for example, significant variations in reactions to the building of the Wall, according to a person's age at the time, ties with friends and relatives in the West or with a "lost *Heimat*" in the former German territories of Eastern Europe, proximity to or distance from Berlin, social background, work and professional prospects, religiosity and political orientation. But for all the variations, life in "actually existing socialism" presented innumerable challenges with which East Germans found varying modes of accommodation, given the lack of realistic alternative options.[46] Meanwhile, the official rhetoric of anti-fascism allowed younger generations to grow up with a degree of ignorance or confusion about the roles of ordinary Germans in the Third Reich. They generally tended to have a sense of a guilt-free past, unlike their contemporaries in the West who had grown up in the shadow of an official culture of shame. Questions surrounding the Holocaust did become more openly problematized in the 1970s and 1980s; historians such as Kurt Pätzold placed it firmly on the GDR historiographical agenda, though wrapped in a Marxist interpretation that provided exoneration for workers and peasants. The American television miniseries *Holocaust*, screened in West Germany in 1979, was also watched in the GDR, giving rise to some muted debate as well as dismissive comments to the effect that East German films had already dealt with these issues many times over the years, and Jewish questions came increasingly to the fore in official memorial sites. The question of transmission is complex, however, and the interrelations among family narratives, increasingly transnational cultural representations, and GDR official scripts need to be more fully explored.[47]

The Legacies of the Past in Comparative Context

The distinctive structural circumstances of the GDR had a significant impact—first, on what kinds of subjectivities were or could be heard in public, and on how people were prepared to express and represent their own past, and second, on what the modes of intergenerational transmission were likely to be.

In the GDR, there was a disjuncture between the radical official break with and rejection of the past, and the relatively muted attention that questions about involvement in Nazism appear to have received within families and in informal communities of connection and identification. Former Nazis were brought to trial and prosecuted in East Germany; there was a higher turnover of elites than in the West; and anti-fascism was proclaimed as the dominant narrative of identification. Yet open debates about personal experiences and involvement in Nazism were largely kept off the public agenda. In the alleged "Country of Readers GDR" (*Leserland DDR*), works of creative literature were often seen as an alternative forum for masked debate on sensitive issues. While countless novels and films dealt, of course, with the Nazi period (including the persecution of the Jews), it was relatively rare for an individual to face up to the personal significance of the transition from Nazism to communism, and to recognize the roots of the GDR present in the Nazi past in the complex and sophisticated, even ambiguous manner that Christa Wolf did in her 1976 masterpiece, *Kindheitsmuster* (*Patterns of Childhood*). Jurek Becker's novel *Bronsteins Kinder* (*Bronstein's Children*), which problematized the treatment of the Nazi past in East German everyday life, was only published in 1982 *after* he had moved to West Berlin. The official narrative of pride in the anti-fascist legacy seems to have obviated, in a self-serving way, the need for much private soul searching or generational clashes over the question of guilt. The individual troubles of Holocaust survivors in the GDR—medical difficulties, pension requests—appeared in letters to authorities; but no widespread "culture of victimhood" emerged in the GDR comparable to that in the United States in the last two decades of the twentieth century, where there was an explosion of memoir writing and oral history projects alongside what Norman Finkelstein controversially dubbed the "Holocaust industry."[48] The communities of connection and identification that developed in the West, providing markets and audiences for survivor narratives decades after the war, did not develop in the GDR. Nor were there serious challenges to the earlier myth of national resistance, in contrast to developments in France from the early 1970s onward, following Marcel Orphül's 1969 film detailing French collaboration, *The Sorrow and the Pity* (banned from being shown on television until over a decade later), and the publication in 1972 of Robert Paxton's unusually significant historical work on Vichy France.[49] It may be argued that the myth of anti-fascist resistance was maintained until the fall of the SED regime, despite growing explicit concern with issues of Jewish suffering and popular anti-Semitism in works of East German historians such as Kurt Pätzold, because the GDR was a Communist state. Yet, for all the difficulties with respect to the postwar treatment of Jews and representations of the Holocaust in Poland, even there some key and critical questions began to be raised in the 1980s.[50] And while the 1985 creative masterpiece of the French filmmaker Claude Lanzmann, *Shoah*, unleashed ferocious debates in Poland about its critical representation of the roles of Polish bystanders, there seem to have been few echoes of any such debate in the GDR. What active discussions there were in the GDR beyond the official sphere (e.g., within and among the groups of political activists under the protective umbrella of the Protestant churches) focused on contemporary questions of world peace, the environment, the economy, human rights, as well as gay and lesbian issues—all of which had to do with the challenges of the present, not the "unmasterable past." Paradoxically, the significance of the Nazi past remained vibrant in SED official rhetoric, looming large in rituals of remembrance and reckoning, but seemed to have waned in salience in the private sphere.[51]

In West Germany, by contrast, there was a public culture of shame and responsibility, as the self-proclaimed legitimate successor state to the Third Reich. Particularly from the later 1960s onward, the West German media fostered a vehemently contested process of "coming to terms with the past." Yet, in practice, the West German record was curiously at odds with this open public debate. Following the foundation of the Ludwigsburg Central Office in 1958, considerable effort was expended in exploring Nazi crimes; but despite massive interest in the Eichmann, Auschwitz, and other trials of the 1960s, the record shows that, in West Germany, relatively few former Nazis were actually brought to court and even fewer convicted—and those who were often received remarkably light sentences.[52] Former Nazis were reintegrated nearly seamlessly in West Germany, and voices arguing for "drawing a *Schlussstrich* (line under the past)" were heard in public, alongside those challenging such demands. The vehement discussions of the 1980s onward—Bitburg in 1985, the "historians' dispute" (*Historikerstreit*) in 1986–87, the commemoration in 1988 of the November pogrom of 1938, and further controversies in the 1990s—have drawn widespread attention.[53] Without needing to rehearse the familiar ground of West German debates on "mastering" the past, it is fair to say that, by the time of what are often called the "second" and "third" generations, the dominant community of identification in the united Federal Republic was overwhelmingly one of identification with the plight of the victims—despite or perhaps precisely because of a strong sense of connection with the perpetrators. The metaphorical children and grandchildren of the "perpetrator generation" included not only those who finally sought to talk to their grandfathers on the occasion of the controversial traveling Wehrmacht exhibition in the mid 1990s, which exposed the complicity of the German army in the atrocities committed on the Eastern Front, but also those who strongly supported the unique monument of national shame, the Memorial to the Murdered Jews of Europe, inaugurated in May 2005 in the heart of united Germany's capital city, Berlin. These were predominantly "Western" concerns, at a time when East Germans found themselves primarily having to focus on "overcoming" their more recent dictatorial past. In the GDR, such a strong community of identification with the victims failed to develop because of the partially blocked lines of connection. The dominant official culture of pride in the anti-fascist legacy, rather than the Western public culture of shame and responsibility for the Nazi past, had effectively "dealt with" a past that no longer remained the most salient issue for younger generations of East Germans, who were more concerned with the present and future.

The significance of the past has frequently been explored by historians through analysis of public rituals and topographies of remembrance, cultural and political representations of the past. This needs to be combined now with a more thorough exploration of the ways in which different groups variously interacted with, sustained, and were affected by dominant narratives. Missing from many accounts of changing subjectivities is an exploration of the ways in which "private" and "public" intersect, mutually affect each other, and change over time. What is significant to remember, how it is remembered, and even the extent to which different aspects of a particular past remain significant, continually shift as people accommodate themselves to the demands of a later present. And sociopolitical circumstances and institutional structures, with differing patterns of power and dominant interests, further serve to filter and foster distinctive patterns of what is on the agenda of "memory."

Research on the complex legacies of the Nazi past in the GDR, beyond the official representations, is only just beginning. This will shed a different light than that offered by approaches focusing primarily on political instrumentalization of the past. Preliminary consideration of these questions suggests, paradoxically, that the anti-fascist state succeeded, to some considerable degree, in drawing attention away from the fact that the GDR was also a post-Nazi state, a feature decreasingly significant both in the eyes of its citizens at the time and in those of historians later on. At the same time, engagement with the challenges of the present—whether in terms of personal survival through accommodation with the structures of power or in opposition or self-distancing—turned those who were heirs of the Third Reich into East Germans for whom 1945 really did begin to look like a "zero hour" (*Stunde Null*).

Suggested Readings

Bauerkämper, Arnd. *Das umstrittene Gedächtnis. Die Erinnerung an Nationalsozialismus, Faschismus und Krieg in Europa seit 1945*. Paderborn, 2012.

Berger, Stefan, and Bill Niven, eds. *Writing the History of Memory*. London, 2013.
Frei, Norbert, ed. *Transnationale Vergangenheitspolitik. Der Umgang mit deutschen Kriegsverbrechern in Europa nach dem Zweiten Weltkrieg*. Göttingen, 2006.
Fulbrook, Mary. *Dissonant Lives: Generations and Violence through the German Dictatorships*. Oxford, 2011.
Niethammer, Lutz, Alexander von Plato, and Dorothee Wierling. *Die volkseigene Erfahrung. Eine Archäologie des Lebens in der Industrieprovinz der DDR*. Berlin, 1991.
Niven, Bill. *Facing the Nazi Past: United Germany and the Legacy of the Third Reich*. London, 2003.
Nothnagle, Alan. *Building the East German Myth: Historical Mythology and Youth Propaganda in the German Democratic Republic, 1945-1989*. Ann Arbor, M.I., 1999.
Olick, Jeffrey, Vered Vinitzky-Seroussi, and Daniel Levy, eds. *The Collective Memory Reader*. Oxford, 2011.
Rosenthal, Gabriele, ed. *The Holocaust in Three Generations*. London, 1998.
Rückerl, Adalbert. *NS-Verbrechen vor Gericht. Versuch einer Vergangenheitsbewältigung*. Heidelberg, 1982.
Stoltzfus, Nathan, and Henry Friedlander, eds. *Nazi Crimes and the Law*. Cambridge, 2008.
Weinke, Annette. *Die Verfolgung von NS-Tätern im geteilten Deutschland. Vergangenheitsbewältigungen 1949-1989*. Paderborn, 2002.

Notes

1. Discussed further in Mary Fulbrook, "Historians and Collective Memory," in *Writing the History of Memory*, eds. Stefan Berger and Bill Niven (London, 2013).
2. Pierre Nora, "The Era of Commemoration," in *Realms of Memory, Vol. III: Symbols*, trans. Arthur Goldhammer (New York, 1998), 609–37. The historical literature on remembrance is too large to cite here, but see, e.g., Jay Winter, *Remembering War: The Great War between Memory and History in the Twentieth Century* (New Haven, C.T., 2006); Jay Winter, *Sites of Memory, Sites of Mourning: The Great War in European Cultural History* (Cambridge, 1995); James Young, *The Texture of Memory: Holocaust Memorials and Meaning* (New Haven, C.T., 1993).
3. See, e.g., Harald Welzer, Sabine Moller, and Karoline Tschuggnall, *"Opa war kein Nazi." Nationalsozialismus und Holocaust im Familiengedächtnis* (Frankfurt am Main, 2002); Lawrence Langer, *Holocaust Testimonies: The Ruins of Memory* (New Haven, C.T., 1993); Geoffrey Hartman, ed., *Holocaust Remembrance: The Shapes of Memory* (Oxford, 1994).
4. This research is part of an Arts & Humanities Research Council (AHRC)-funded collaborative project under the direction of the author at University College London (UCL): "Reverberations of War: Communities of Experience and Identification in Germany and Europe after 1945." I am grateful to the AHRC for its support of this project.
5. The latter two categories, connection and identification, are distinct from but bear some relation to the notions of "post-memory" and "prosthetic memory." See Marianne Hirsch, *Family Frames. Photography, Narrative and Postmemory* (Cambridge, M.A., 1997); Marianne Hirsch, "The Generation of Postmemory," *Poetics Today* 29/1

(2008):103–28; Alison Landsberg, *Prosthetic Memory: The Transformation of American Remembrance in the Age of Mass Culture* (New York, 2004).
6. See, e.g., Mark Mazower, *Hitler's Empire: Nazi Rule in Occupied Europe* (London, 2009); Timothy Snyder, *Bloodlands: Europe between Hitler and Stalin* (London, 2011); Robert Gildea, Olivier Wieviorka, and Anette Warring, eds., *Surviving Hitler and Mussolini* (Oxford, 2006).
7. See Norbert Frei, *Vergangenheitspolitik* (Munich, 1996); Robert Moeller, *War Stories: The Search for a Usable Past in the Federal Republic of Germany* (Berkeley, 2001).
8. See Thomas Fox, *Stated Memory: East Germany and the Holocaust* (Rochester, N.Y., 1999); Jeffrey Herf, *Divided Memory: The Nazi Past in the Two Germanys* (Cambridge, M.A., 1997); Mary Fulbrook, *German National Identity after the Holocaust* (Oxford, 1999). Also see Andreas Agocs's contribution to this volume.
9. See Alan Nothnagle, *Building the East German Myth: Historical Mythology and Youth Propaganda in the German Democratic Republic, 1945-1989* (Ann Arbor, M.I., 1999).
10. David Cesarani and Eric Sundquist, eds., *Challenging the Myth of Silence* (London, 2012).
11. See Zoe Waxman, *Writing the Holocaust: Identity, Testimony, Representation* (Oxford, 2006); Annette Wieviorka, *The Era of the Witness*, trans. Jared Stark (Ithaca, N.Y., 2006).
12. See, e.g., BArch, DY 55/V 278/4/142, Eine bescheidene Anfrage an das Kreis- bezw. Landes-Sekretariat der VVDN [sic] betreffs des Mordsturms Laudin, 10 March 1953.
13. BArch, DO 1/32729, VVN Nebenkläger, Dresden, 12 January 1949.
14. See, e.g., BArch, DO 1/32563, letters from relatives of people killed in Neuruppin, passim.
15. See David Tompkins's chapter in this volume.
16. BArch, DY55/V278/96, Berichte ehem. Rassisch Verfolgter, passim.
17. BArch, DY55/V278/96, Bericht für die Forschungskommission, Heinz C., 14 February 1948.
18. BArch, DY55/V278/96, Ludwig S, Meine Erlebnisse während des Naziregimes, n.d.
19. BArch, DY55/V278/96, Kurt R, Tatsachenbericht über meine illegale Tätigkeit von 1930 bis 1945, 17 February 1948.
20. Olaf B, *TU Station. Bericht aus faschistischen Kerkern* (Berlin, 1981).
21. Olaf B's son Norbert (pseudonym), in discussion with the author, 2005.
22. See, e.g., Arnd Bauerkämper, *Das umstrittene Gedächtnis. Die Erinnerung an Nationalsozialismus, Faschismus und Krieg in Europa seit 1945* (Paderborn, 2012); Jürgen Danyels, ed., *Die geteilte Vergangenheit. Zum Umgang mit Nationalsozialismus und Widerstand in beiden deutschen Staaten* (Berlin, 1995); Norbert Frei, ed., *Transnationale Vergangenheitspolitik. Der Umgang mit deutschen Kriegsverbrechern in Europa nach dem Zweiten Weltkrieg* (Göttingen, 2006); Adalbert Rückerl, *NS-Verbrechen vor Gericht. Versuch einer Vergangenheitsbewältigung* (Heidelberg, 1982); Nathan Stoltzfus and Henry Friedlander, eds., *Nazi Crimes and the Law* (Cambridge, 2008); Annette Weinke, *Die Verfolgung von NS-Tätern im geteilten Deutschland. Vergangenheitsbewältigungen 1949-1989* (Paderborn, 2002).
23. See, e.g., BArch, DO 1/32729, VVN Nebenkläger, 12 January 1949, 7; on the memory strategies of a former Nazi functionary in West Germany, see Mary Fulbrook, *A Small Town near Auschwitz: Ordinary Nazis and the Holocaust* (Oxford, 2012).

24. BArch DP3/1588, Protokoll, 25 April 1968, fol. 228–29; Anklageschrift, 3 May 1968, fol. 232ff.; BArch DP3/1587, Hensel's statement of 6 October 1967.
25. BArch, DP3/1614, Oberstes Gericht der DDR, 1. Strafsenat, Urteil, 21–22 December 1987; Bezirksgericht Dresden, 1. Strafsenat, Urteil, September 1987; DP3/2273, passim.
26. Norbert B (pseudonym), in discussion with the author, summer 2006.
27. Kempowski Bio (KB), 2910/2, Ursula B diary entry of 30 April 1944.
28. Ibid.
29. See further Mary Fulbrook, *Dissonant Lives: Generations and Violence through the German Dictatorships* (Oxford, 2011).
30. KB, 2910/1, Ursula B memoirs, 11.
31. KB, 2910/1, Ursula B memoirs, 12.
32. See also Lutz Niethammer, Alexander von Plato, and Dorothee Wierling, *Die volkseigene Erfahrung. Eine Archäologie des Lebens in der Industrieprovinz der DDR* (Berlin, 1991).
33. KB, 2910/1, Ursula B memoirs, 7.
34. For pre-1990 accounts, see Niethammer, *Volkseigene Erfahrung*, which concentrates on a distinctive generational group. See also Fulbrook, *Dissonant Lives*.
35. Gertraud T (pseudonym), in discussion with the author, summer 2006.
36. See further Fulbrook, *German National Identity*.
37. BArch, DY 30/IV A2/2.028/110, Kurzbericht über die Teilnahme an Ghetto-Feiern in Warschau, n.d., and Bericht über die Durchführung der Beschluüsse zum 20. Jahrestag des Warschauer Ghetto-Aufstandes, n.d., attached to letter of 9 May 1963.
38. See, e.g., Helmut Eschwege, *Fremd unter meinesgleichen. Erinnerung eines Dresdner Juden* (Berlin, 1991), 184–211, on the difficulties he encountered researching, writing, and publishing *Kennzeichen J. Bilder, Dokumente, Berichte zur Geschichte der Verbrechen des Hitlerfaschismus an den deutschen Juden 1933-1945* (Berlin, 1966).
39. BArch, DO 1/32778, *Berliner Zeitung*, 3–4 October 1987.
40. See further Fulbrook, *Dissonant Lives*.
41. Ilse J (pseudonym), in discussion with the author, summer 2007.
42. Anetta Kahane, *Ich sehe was, was du nicht siehst. Meine deutschen Geschichten* (Berlin, 2004); Vera Lengsfeld, *Von nun an ging's bergauf... Mein Weg zur Freiheit* (Munich, 2007); Monika Maron, *Pawels Briefe* (Frankfurt am Main, 1999).
43. Norbert B, in discussion with the author, summer 2006.
44. Ibid.
45. Ibid.
46. For further discussion and references, see Andrew Port's Introduction and chapter in this volume; Mary Fulbrook, *The People's State: East German Society from Hitler to Honecker* (London, 2005).
47. For a fascinating example, see chapter 18 of Bettina Völter and Gabriele Rosenthal, "We Are the Victims of History: The Seewald Family," in *The Holocaust in Three Generations*, ed. Gabriele Rosenthal (London, 1998).
48. Norman Finkelstein, *The Holocaust Industry: Reflections on the Exploitation of Jewish Suffering* (London, 2000); see also Peter Novick, *The Holocaust and Collective Memory: The American Experience* (London, 1999).
49. Robert Paxton, *Vichy France, Old Guard and New Order, 1940-1944* (New York, 1972). On developments in France, see, e.g., the epilogue of Julian Jackson, *France: The Dark*

Years 1940-1944 (Oxford, 2001); Henri Rousso, *The Vichy Syndrome: History and Memory in France since 1944*, trans. Arthur Goldhammer (Cambridge, M.A., 1994).
50. On developments in Poland, see, e.g., Robert Cherry and Annamaria Orla-Bukowska, eds., *Rethinking Poles and Jews: Troubled Past, Brighter Future* (Lanham, M.D., 2007); Czesław Madajczyk, *Die Okkupationspolitik Nazideutschlands in Polen 1939-1945* (Berlin, 1987; shortened version of orig. Polish, 1970); Antony Polonsky, ed., *My Brother's Keeper: Recent Polish Debates on the Holocaust* (London, 1990).
51. See further Fulbrook, *Dissonant Lives*.
52. Rückerl, *NS-Verbrechen vor Gericht*; Devin O. Pendas. *The Frankfurt Auschwitz Trial, 1963-1965: Genocide, History, and the Limits of the Law* (Cambridge, 2006); Rebecca Wittmann, *Beyond Justice: The Auschwitz Trial* (Cambridge, M.A., 2005).
53. See, e.g., Fulbrook, *German National Identity*; Ilya Levkov, ed., *Bitburg and Beyond: Encounters in American, German and Jewish History* (New York, 1987); Astrid Linn, 'Noch heute ein Faszinosum…' *Philipp Jenninger zum 9. November 1938 und die Folgen* (Münster, 1990); Charles Maier, *The Unmasterable Past: History, Holocaust, and German National Identity* (Cambridge, M.A., 2003); Bill Niven, *Facing the Nazi Past: United Germany and the Legacy of the Third Reich* (London, 2003).

CHAPTER 2

Divisive Unity
The Politics of Cultural Nationalism during the First German Writers' Congress of October 1947

ANDREAS AGOCS

During his closing speech at the First German Writers' Congress in October 1947, one of the event's organizers, the editor Günther Birkenfeld, made an emphatic statement: "We Germans don't have much more left than our language and our culture. At this congress I've gained the tragic and painful impression that we already no longer speak a common language and that the German language is on its way to split into two dialects, an eastern and a western one."[1] This emotional declaration summed up the tragic failure of a congress that had been meant to be a demonstration of unity by German writers and intellectuals trying to counter the looming division of Germany. Instead—at least according to the official GDR historiography—it became a cultural cornerstone of the East German state established two years later.[2]

Conceived by anti-fascist intellectuals in the Soviet-licensed "Kulturbund zur demokratischen Erneuerung Deutschlands" (Cultural League for the Democratic Renewal of Germany), the First German Writers' Congress, which was held in occupied Berlin, has become a symbol for the emerging cultural Cold War. More than twenty years after the end of this conflict, it invites us to rethink many assumptions about the origins of the German division—especially as it concerns the relationship between culture and politics, on the one hand, and between international and domestic German tensions, on the other. Did the gradually intensifying political division in Germany in the years from 1946 to 1948 correspond to an incipient split of German "national culture" that would later culminate in efforts to construct a distinct GDR culture? Was this cultural division brought about by increasing antagonism among the occupation powers, or was it inherent in positions and unresolved tensions among German intellectuals that played out independently of the Cold War?

Scholarship in the East and West has tended to describe the First German Writers' Congress as the last attempt at intellectual unity among German writers at the beginning of the Cold War.³ In West Germany, for example, the literary historian Waltraud Wende-Hohenberger cites the official GDR literature, maintaining that "there was unity and unanimity among the numerous participants ... the 'congress centered fully on a clear and unambiguous avowal of the democratic unity of Germany.'"⁴ In a similar vein, the literary scholar Manfred Jäger, who left the GDR in 1955 to publish in West Germany, calls the congress a "symbol" that demonstrated how "the Germans' willingness to meet and engage in dialogue (*Begegnungsbereitschaft*) was gradually subverted by the confrontation between the Western powers and the Soviet Union."⁵ These interpretations paint a picture of well-meaning German intellectuals and writers engaged in a possibly naïve, but certainly futile, attempt to stem the political current by espousing their own model of cultural unity—an attempt that ultimately broke down in the face of more powerful and divisive political forces. Moreover, this assumption seems to confirm the hackneyed idea of a century-old bifurcation of culture and politics in Germany, and thus runs the risk of reiterating the myth of the nonpolitical German intellectual who places aesthetic over political concerns.⁶

Standard historical interpretations also imply that the Cold War was carried to the intellectuals in occupied Germany by forces from "without," embodied by the opposing non-German participants at the congress: the American journalist Melvin J. Lasky and the Soviet writers Vsevolod Vishnevski and Valentin Kataïev. While the East German historiography condemned a perceived American attempt to use the event as a staging ground for anti-Soviet propaganda, the U.S. historian David Pike notes the "belligerence" of the Soviet representatives who "descended upon the congress." Pike emphasizes that "the tenor of remarks made there both by the Russians [*sic*] and the German Communists certainly suited the hardline policies developing in connection with the SED conference in late September," a step toward the further Stalinization of the Soviet Zone of Occupation (SBZ).⁷

While there is no doubt that the congress took place in a climate of escalating Cold War tensions, the dominant interpretations tend to separate the intellectual concerns of the congress's participants from the political objectives of the Cold War rivals. By placing the congress of 1947 in a wider thematic and chronological context, this essay argues that older cultural debates among German intellectuals preceded and paved the way for the split that occurred during the congress. Even before the outbreak of open tensions between East and West on the third day of the event, the congress exposed rifts and unresolved conflicts within Germany's cultural scene that reached back to at least 1933. Accordingly, the congress and its failure need not only to be interpreted as an episode in the Cold War, but also be placed in a discussion of the continuities and ruptures of intellectual and cultural traditions in the GDR after 1945. In particular, the following will argue that the congress organizers' concept of "anti-fascist humanism" was not merely a Stalinist tool, but rather the continuation of a distinctive German idea of national culture. This unacknowledged cultural nationalism ran counter to the political trends of the Cold War, but it could also be transformed into the divisive rhetoric of the East-West confrontation.

The First German Writers' Congress and the Traditions of Anti-fascist Humanism

Originally planned for July, the First German Writers' Congress took place 4–8 October 1947 in the eastern sector of occupied Berlin and drew more than 280 participants from Germany and abroad. The event came on the heels of the Truman Doctrine, the consolidation of the Bizone (which united the British and American zones of occupation), the introduction of the Marshall Plan, and the formation of the Communist Information Bureau (Cominform) in September 1947.[8] Because the SED was not officially a Communist party, it did not take part in the formation of the Cominform. The congress was nevertheless staged at a time when, in an attempt to consolidate their leadership, Communist parties all over Eastern Europe were trying to woo Western intellectuals. As party member Wolfgang Leonhard observed at the second SED Party Conference of September 1947, "The thesis of a separate road to Socialism was not officially set aside, but ... [i]n contrast with the period of 1945–46, our links with the Soviet Union were now openly proclaimed."[9] The prospect of a united Germany seemed more and more tenuous.

Despite—or because of—these hardening divisions, the congress was meant to be a signal of unity among German intellectuals in East and West. Officially sponsored by the SED and the Soviet Military Administration in Germany (SMAD), the congress was the brainchild of Communist functionary and intellectual Alexander Abusch and the anti-fascist poet and playwright Günther Weisenborn. Both intellectuals were leading members and activists in the Kulturbund, a Soviet-licensed organization founded in 1945 as an officially nonpartisan coalition of anti-fascist intellectuals.[10] The Kulturbund's coalition between liberals and Communists was anchored in the common emphasis on Germany's "humanist tradition"—understood as the heritage of Johann Wolfgang von Goethe, Heinrich Heine, and other classical eighteenth- and nineteenth-century writers, but also subsuming Martin Luther and Karl Marx. This broadly defined cultural concept served as the glue that patched over political differences and thus provided a blueprint for postwar Germany's cultural renewal, ostensibly the official mission of the Kulturbund. The conception of the First Writers' Congress—as well as the discussions that took place there—need to be understood in this context. For its planners within the Kulturbund, the congress was designed as a continuation of the pre-1945 German anti-fascist coalitions, even though, by 1947, this ideal was already in the process of being replaced with official Soviet attacks on Western modernism, combined with the Zhdanov-inspired defense of "bourgeois humanist culture" against Western "formalism" all over Soviet-occupied Eastern Europe.[11]

The event's main organizers were Weisenborn and Birkenfeld, as representatives of the Association for the Protection of German Writers (Schutzverband Deutscher Autoren [SDA]), an organization that defended the professional interests of writers. Birkenfeld was also the editor of the literary journal *Horizonte* and one of the more outspoken liberal Kulturbund board members. While the SDA had planned on a meeting of authors to discuss mainly technical and professional questions, it was the Kulturbund that envisioned a congress of writers whose statements of unity would provide an alternative to the increasingly divisive political discussions at the time. The result would be a "renewal" of German culture within Europe after the Nazi catastrophe.

Weisenborn had conceived the basic themes of the congress. The first day was to honor the victims of fascism and discuss the contributions of exile writers, the second day was dedicated to the debate of ideological issues, and the third day was to conclude the event with a public declaration and an "appeal to the world."[12] It was Abusch who gave this basic scheme a more concrete shape. He understood the congress as a continuation and revival of the politicized meetings of exile writers during the Nazi period, especially the Schutzverband Deutscher Schriftsteller (SDS) congress in Paris in 1938, where anti-fascist German exile writers had collectively and publicly condemned Nazism and fascism. Like the Paris conference, the Berlin congress was to represent the anti-fascist, humanist "other Germany" to the wider world by declaring responsibility for the Nazi past, and to demonstrate the attempt by anti-fascist humanist intellectuals to renew German culture.

The letters of invitation that the SDA sent out to writers in the East and West expressed the hope "that this gathering will demonstrate to Germany and the world that we are actively working for the renewal of German literature in a spirit of cosmopolitanism."[13] The response to the congress's invitations was mixed. Prominent German writers and intellectuals declined to attend, among them Thomas Mann, Alfred Döblin, and Karl Jaspers. Attempts at recruiting prominent international figures such as John Steinbeck and Louis Aragon failed. A number of writers from the Soviet Union, Czechoslovakia, and Yugoslavia, as well as from Great Britain, attended. To ensure the participation of all four occupation powers, the SDA, which was seen as more interested in technical matters and which was well represented in the Western zones, was declared the congress's main organizer. This was important because the Western Allies already had well-founded reservations about the Communist influence on the Kulturbund.[14]

The Cold War at the Congress

The list of speakers and discussion leaders was carefully balanced to represent all four occupation zones and all political persuasions. Still, Weisenborn and Birkenfeld could not prevent the blowup of Cold War tensions on the third day of the congress. The confrontation was triggered by a speech by the American representative, Melvin J. Lasky, who was, at the time, the Berlin correspondent for *Partisan Review* and the substitute at the congress for the much better known John Steinbeck. According to GDR literary scholar Ursula Reinhold, the journalist Lasky was "sneaked" into the program by Birkenfeld as a counterweight to the Soviet speakers.[15] The fact that Lasky, who spoke fluent German, was the Berlin correspondent for small U.S. journals that "normally could have never afforded a foreign correspondent" gave rise to the unconfirmed suspicion among German Communists that Lasky's speech was orchestrated and paid for by the U.S. government. In fact, and unlike the Soviet authorities, the U.S. Office of the Military Government in Germany (OMGUS) considered the congress a "German-only" event that did not warrant any heightened initiative.[16]

Lasky's speech on cultural freedom initially found undivided applause and approval—for example when he described the damage that the Nazi period had inflicted on German culture: "I am convinced that [German] writers and artists—even if not the people as a whole—have nothing but fear and disgust for a totalitarian society." Lasky then went on to praise American society for being founded on the principle of cultural freedom and the "contest of ideas." He also mentioned violations of this principle in America in the past, e.g., the censorship of works by James Joyce before, and of Leon Trotsky during, the war.[17] Lasky's speech ended in tumultuous disturbances, however, when he not only condemned Nazi practices, but also declared his solidarity with artists in the Soviet Union who suffered from censorship at home. His remarks were accompanied by applause, but also by exclamations of disapproval and outrage. When Lasky mentioned the concrete cases of Sergey Eisenstein and GF Alexandrov, the atmosphere became so turbulent that Birkenfeld interrupted the speech to appeal for quiet and tolerance. It took a while until the uproar finally subsided and Lasky could resume his speech, all the while interrupted by exclamations of "Bravo," "fewer lies," and "violation of guest privilege."[18]

The American journalist was able to finish his address with the following words: "In all countries on earth the great writer has always been to some extent a revolutionary fighter… He carried the seed of rebellion and revolt into people's minds and hearts. Respectable citizens, official powers, the authorities, and tradition, if they had been farsighted enough, would have immediately recognized him as their enemy."[19] This ending of Lasky's speech was greeted by enthusiastic applause—even by Ricarda Huch, the congress's honorary president. In contrast, the Soviet delegation, led by Lieutenant Colonel Alexander Dymshits, the SMAD cultural officer—who had invested a great deal of personal effort in the congress's success—had already protested by conspicuously leaving the room during the speech.

Ironically, Lasky and Dymshits could have found much common ground under different circumstances. Both men were intellectuals of Jewish descent with an affinity for German culture and proficiency in the German language. As a former Trotskyist and member of the New York Left, Lasky also deeply believed in the political function of the arts.[20] While Lasky had critically commented on censorship in the United States, Dymshits had used his influence to restrain the censorship of German writers in the SBZ.[21] All of this counted for little in Berlin in the fall of 1947, however. During the afternoon sessions of the same day, Soviet writer Valentin Kataïev commented on the Lasky speech, "I'm glad that I have finally seen the face of a living warmonger [*Kriegsbrandstifter*]. Back home in the Soviet Union we don't have any of those types." To the audience's applause Kataïev compared Lasky's "lies" to the methods of Joseph Goebbels.[22]

Lasky's speech was also fiercely debated among the German participants: defended by most representatives of the Western zones, attacked by many of the Kulturbund intellectuals. The outbreak of Cold War tensions at the congress also dominated press coverage of the event, in the Western as well as in the Eastern occupation zones. While Soviet-licensed newspapers, such as the *Tägliche Rundschau*, sharply attacked Lasky's contribution as a deliberate provocation, the U.S.-licensed *Tagesspiegel* printed the speech almost in its entirety as an affirmation of Western cultural values.[23] The French-licensed *Kurier* made the strongest effort to cover the intellectual debates at the conference, but even this paper compared the congress with "Babylon."[24] The First German Writers' Congress's main objective—the restoration and demonstration of intellectual unity across East and West—had failed. As its only achievement the event could point to the passing of two unanimous resolutions: one against anti-Semitism and the other for the repatriation of exile intellectuals. But these voices of unity and reconciliation were drowned out by the noises of the Cold War.

The anti-Semitism resolution was introduced by the writer and KPD functionary Hermann Duncker, who reflected in his speech on his experiences in U.S. exile: "My years in America have made a strong impression on me. When we got news about what was happening in Germany ... the most horrible things must surely have been the atrocities of anti-Semitism. And it was even worse when ... American friends showed us accounts of anti-Semitism flourishing again in Bavaria and other places."²⁵ Duncker's appeal for a resolution against anti-Semitism met with unanimous support and the discussion it triggered seemed to be free of the East-West differences that characterized interpretations of the Holocaust in the Federal Republic and the GDR in later years.²⁶ Two days after Duncker's speech, the German-Jewish literary scholar Hans Meyer, whose family had been killed in Germany, complained that the resolution had faded into the background after the Lasky incident: "It has been disturbing for me to read parts of the press coverage about our congress. I would have assumed that Duncker's request for us to take up the fight against anti-Semitism should have been the headline of all newspapers.... But this was not the case."²⁷ Meyer's reproach was greeted with applause. Yet, this reminder about the main victims of Nazism struck a contrasting note at an event that otherwise emphasized German anti-fascist martyrdom.

"The Home of the Poet": Anti-fascist Exile or Inner Emigration?

The Lasky incident ended up as the congress's most publicized event in the press of all four occupation zones. Yet, the ground for the confrontation had already been prepared by debates among German intellectuals that reached back long before 1947 and that centered on the meaning and political implications of a specific German anti-fascist humanism. Specifically, three interrelated subjects of debate had already divided German postwar intellectuals before the outbreak of East-West tensions: the contrast between German anti-fascists in exile and "inner émigrés"; the wider meaning of the German catastrophe; and the role of a renewed German culture in postwar Europe. Taken together, these conflicts weakened the vision of an all-German cultural nationalism espoused by anti-fascist writers and enabled it to be blended into Cold War politics and GDR "foundation myths."

The concept of the Kulturbund had originally been designed by KPD intellectuals in exile in Moscow, especially by its first president, the poet Johannes R. Becher.²⁸ Yet, in accordance with official Soviet occupation policy, the Kulturbund made great symbolic and practical efforts after its creation in June 1945 to bridge the gap between German returnees from exile, on the one hand, and the large number of artists who had withdrawn into the proverbial "inner emigration" in Nazi Germany, on the other. In a highly publicized event, for example, Becher made 83-year-old Gerhart Hauptmann the Kulturbund's honorary president. Because the Nazis had allowed the renowned dramatist to stay in Germany, Becher's gesture was symbolic for the Kulturbund's rehabilitation of controversial "inner émigrés," such as the novelist Hans Fallada.²⁹ Even without the Cold War, the congress revealed that the rift within the German intellectual community—between the "other Germany" of exiles and resisters, and the conformists and inner émigrés—was still wide open. In fact, those unresolved tensions surfaced memorably at the congress during a passionate debate surrounding speeches by the novelist Elisabeth Langgässer, a representative of the "inner emigration," and Alfred Kantorowicz, a former exile who had also pursued illegal underground activities during the Third Reich.

Langgässer and Kantorowicz's speeches revealed that by 1947, after the experiences of dictatorship and exile, two distinct aesthetic positions had developed among German intellectuals: Langgässer's continued espousal of a Catholic-Christian concept of art was in marked contrast to Kantorowicz's "politically concrete definition of art and literature."[30] Although she was baptized as a Catholic, Langgässer's paternal descent had made her a "half-Jew," according to National Socialist racial logic. She was allowed to stay in Germany legally, but, because of her background, suffered publication bans and other discriminatory actions. In her speech at the congress, Langgässer declared that "the home of the poet is language." Since Nazi propaganda had appropriated the German language to an unprecedented extent, writers who had stayed in Germany had been as much in exile as their colleagues who had left for foreign countries. For now, Langgässer demanded that language be granted "a period of peace and silence."[31] In contrast to this emphasis on reflection and language—which Langgässer maintained was not be confused with a retreat into an "inner life"—Kantorowicz, a veteran of the Spanish Civil War, reminded his audience of the times when writers had exchanged "the typewriter for the machine gun"—without ceasing to be writers.[32] While novelists such as Langgässer distinguished between their political and artistic identities, Kantorowicz—as well as Weisenbusch, Abusch, and other representatives of anti-fascist resistance and exile—believed that the identities of "writer" and "resistance activist" could not be separated.

The two speeches triggered an intense discussion among the congress participants about the moral equivalence of inner and outer emigration and about the merit of literature published between 1933 and 1945 in Germany. The writer Karl Schnog, who had spent five years in Dachau and Buchenwald, was the first to express his resentment of the inner émigrés: "I find it inappropriate that we put the clever and tolerably decent ones, who kept working under the Hitler regime with little or no blemish, almost on the same level with the ones who were real fighters."[33] Greta Kuckhoff, the widow of the executed poet and resister Adam Kuckhoff, chimed in by attacking Langgässer's "dangerous idea" about giving language a "grace period" in response to National Socialism: "Our authors and poets must not be silent at this time, they need to say the right thing."[34] On the third day of the congress, the poet Eva Richter-Schoch came to the defense of the inner émigrés: "During the first two days of this congress, I have gotten the terrible feeling that a new *Übermensch* writer is being envisioned here. He is supposed to be politically immaculate, he's supposed to be a fighter. You know, when I closed my eyes, I sometimes thought I was back in Hitler's days, because that's what Hitler demanded from his writers."[35]

Not for the first—or last—time, it was the young philosopher and writer Wolfgang Harich who made the most provocative points, laying bare not only the gap between inner émigrés and exiles, but also the generational differences at a congress that was meant to be a display of unity. Harich, who had already fiercely attacked conservative writers such as Ernst Jünger in the Kulturbund journal *Aufbau*,[36] entered the discussion not as an inner or outer émigré, but "from the perspective of someone who had come of age in Germany in those twelve years [of Nazi dictatorship]. Today, I sometimes ask myself, why did I not become a Nazi?" Harich ascribed his anti-fascist and pacifist convictions to the reading of books that had been published before 1933, and to exile publications that had been illegally distributed in Nazi Germany. The writings of inner émigrés did not have the same effect: "If I had had to depend on this literature, I might as well have turned into a staunch SS trooper." Harich's remarks elicited laughter and led to an uproar.[37]

The 1947 congress revealed two conflicting interpretations of the humanist intellectual: either as someone who resisted attempts at politicization, or as someone who actively effected political change—with the machine gun as much as with the typewriter. Initially these different positions reflected the different experiences of inner émigrés, on the one hand, and of exiles and resisters (many of them of a younger generation), on the other. The escalating conflict between the Western Allies and the Soviets did not *create* these divisions, but instead transformed them into ideological statements defining the two Cold War camps: the liberal understanding of artistic freedom in the West left room for the independence of artistic identities from political identities and activities. In contrast, the emerging state in the East—which was based on an ostensible alliance among intellectuals, workers, and farmers—rejected the idea of purely aesthetic concerns as remnants of bourgeois thinking. By 1947, both of these developing positions had become incompatible with the notion of German national unity based on humanist culture.

From Existentialism to Anti-formalism

There were other indicators that the pre-1945 consensus, based on a broad definition of anti-fascist humanism, was breaking apart even without the direct influence of the superpowers. In the spring of 1947 the Kulturbund organized a debate entitled, "Is There a Special German Intellectual Crisis?" Kulturbund member Ferdinand Friedensburg, the head of the Christian Democratic Union (CDU) in the SBZ, introduced the discussion by asserting that "the serious spiritual disease that our people went through ... is not merely a German matter, but ... is part of a general intellectual and cultural crisis that afflicts humankind at large."[38] The KPD functionary Abusch—who had joined the board as "ideological coordinator"—disagreed, contending that "we cannot simply declare the intellectual crisis in Germany as identical with the ... symptoms of crisis in the rest of the world." German intellectuals had the responsibility "to comprehend the causes for the German catastrophe and to understand the specific German guilt for it as a precondition for democratic renewal."[39]

The difference between Abusch's position and the view of Nazism as symptomatic of a wider crisis of the West formed an important intellectual backdrop for the political conflicts that erupted at the First Writers Congress. Abusch had defined the Kulturbund's concept of a Socialist humanism in his book *Irrweg einer Nation* (A Nation's Wrong Track), written in Mexican exile during the war. His concept of Socialist humanism was essentially a fusion of classical German culture with Marxist insights about the historical-materialist context of its production. Without materialist-dialectical analysis, he argued, humanism would turn into Nietzschean cultural criticism, lose its connection to the working class, and eventually become the anti-humanism that had bolstered the rule of German Junkers, "monopoly capitalists," and, ultimately, fascists.[40]

The publication in 1946 of Abusch's book by Aufbau, an East German publishing company, was, to some extent, a response to the liberal historian Friedrich Meinecke's take on German history in *The German Catastrophe*, published earlier that year in the Western zones. Meinecke had spent the Nazi years in inner emigration after critical statements about the Nazis had forced him to resign as chair of the *Historische Reichskommission* and as editor of the *Historische Zeitschrift*.[41] *The German Catastrophe* was meant to provide intellectual guidance and leadership for a traumatized nation. Meinecke interpreted National Socialism as the catastrophic culmination of the modern era's two converging "waves": the national and the Socialist mass movements. This "universal process of transformation in the West" made the German catastrophe a question that went beyond Germany and affected the fate of the occident as a whole: "The *Hitlermenschentum* (Hitler-humanity) ... was made possible by a shifting of the inner forces in man, which had been occurring since the age of Goethe, and which can also be understood as a disruption of the inner balance between rational and irrational forces."[42]

Meinecke argued that the Nazi dictatorship was not foreordained but "could have been successfully prevented"—something that, for Meinecke, implicated the German people for having brought Hitler to power in the first place: "A unique personality and a unique constellation succeeded in rising to power and in forcing the German people, for a limited time, on an errant path... For the German people this provides the reassuring opportunity and responsibility to purify themselves from the horrors they experienced." For the purification of the German mind, Meinecke envisioned the foundation of *Goethegemeinden* (Goethe communities) in all major cities and towns, which, through public readings, would carry the "living testimonies of the great German mind ... into the audience's hearts."[43]

In an *Aufbau* article that appeared in January 1947, Abusch launched a sharp refutation of Meinecke's liberal arguments. He condemned the discussion of a "collective guilt of the West" and of "a general European spiritual crisis" for evading questions about specific German guilt for Nazism and for neglecting an investigation of Nazism's causes, especially its materialist-economic aspects.[44] Abusch's critique of Meinecke was part of a wider attack against perceived attempts at subsuming the recent German past under a wider "spiritual crisis of the West." An *Aufbau* issue from June 1946 contained an attack on Martin Heidegger, which not only condemned his moral conduct under the Nazis, but also linked it to his leading role in the development of modern existentialism.[45] Subsequent *Aufbau* articles also assailed the existentialism of French resistance icons Jean-Paul Sartre and Albert Camus.[46] These critiques were variations of Abusch's view of existentialism as a "philosophical fad" (*Modephilosophie*) and as a "philosophy of exaggerated subjectivism."[47] It is important to note that Abusch's critique of existentialism was based on its alleged lack of attention to Germany's specific responsibility for the recent past. Even though grounded in specific German problems, this critique would, in the late 1940s, be subsumed under the Stalinist "formalism debate," which condemned existentialism together with all other forms of "bourgeois" thought and artistic expression.[48] Existentialism and humanism, the ideological pillars of what James Wilkinson called the "intellectual resistance" in Europe, had apparently ceased to provide anti-fascist unity.

At the congress, it was once more Wolfgang Harich who took up Abusch's criticism of the leading philosophical trends. Harich's target was the philosopher Karl Jaspers and his use of terms such as "mass existence, mass order, mass organization, and bureaucratic rule." According to Harich, Jasper's assessment of mass society in his 1930 work *Die geistige Situation der Zeit* (The Spiritual Situation of the Times) had prepared the way for the retreat into the "inner life" (*Innerlichkeit*) that had been so conducive to Nazi rule. In allusion to Jasper's influential postwar tract on the concept of collective guilt, Harich lashed out: "And the same Herr Jaspers has now written a brochure on the question of guilt, in which he tries to deflect the real moral question of general responsibility for fascism by talking about a general guilt of human existence."[49] In short, then, the debate over the existentialist diagnosis of the "spiritual crisis of Europe," which had already been the subject of discussions in the Kulturbund and in *Aufbau*, had reached the congress and merged with the older conflict between inner emigration and activist resistance or exile.

German Culture after the War

At the same time that the anti-fascist consensus was falling apart under political pressures, young intellectuals such as Harich were dismantling the ideological and philosophical foundations of humanist cultural renewal. Other discussions at the congress suggested that this project was based on an understanding of an "other" German culture that had not only survived twelve years of Nazi rule and war untainted, but also still enjoyed the same international respect as before. If the reconciliation of German exiles and inner émigrés was one of the congress's objectives, another one was Germany's "readmission" into the international cultural scene after more than a decade of either forced or self-imposed exclusion. Weisenborn's opening speech put this in dramatic terms: "We turn to the great powers of this earth and solemnly appeal to them for the end of [our] intellectual isolation… We reach out to the world and appeal to the men of thought and intellect. We will fight and keep the voice of conscience alive so that future generations will be able to say: a call went out from Germany, and we heard it and heeded it."[50]

Weisenborn's sentiment reflected an inherent contradiction in the Kulturbund's concept of German cultural renewal—a project that many speakers at the congress explicitly compared to the Protestant Reformation. While the speakers explicitly condemned the nationalism of the Nazis and appealed to universal and cosmopolitan values, many also expressed their pride in German culture and a sense of its special mission in healing the wounds of war in Europe. Weisenborn's statement can thus be described as an expression of unacknowledged "cultural nationalism," heightened by the pressures of the budding Cold War. Rather than taking sides in the Cold War, many writers of Weisenborn's generation believed in a "third way" involving a regenerated German culture based on the cultural traditions of the pre-Nazi past. This vision was supported by some of the foreign speakers, such as the Yugoslav writer Jovan Popović. The former partisan earned widespread applause at the congress when he declared that "Goethe, Heine, and other great German poets were not to be found in the knapsacks of Hitler's soldiers—we found ham and silk stockings in them. But Goethe was carried in the knapsacks of the Yugoslav freedom fighters, and he was read just as much, or almost as much, as Tolstoy's *War and Peace*… Therefore nobody should hold German culture in contempt, because German culture was not on the side of the fascists: it was on the side of those who fought against fascism."[51]

In trying to heal the deep rift that Nazism's legacy had opened up between Germany and the rest of the world, Weisenborn and his cohorts underestimated the differences in perspective between German anti-fascists and writers from other countries. Weisenborn's mixture of anti-fascist ideology, internationalism, and the sense of a German universal mission—a blend that also characterized much of the early Kulturbund rhetoric—seemed to conflate the sense of German victimization at the hands of the Nazi regime with the barbarism that Germany had inflicted on other countries during the war. In 1947, the rest of the world showed little inclination to heed calls that went out from Germany, whether by anti-fascists or other intellectuals. As Hermon Ould, the British general secretary of the International PEN Club, commented on Weisenborn's speech, "I'm not sure if the Germans are aware of how strong the sentiments against them still are, especially in those countries that have suffered from German occupation, e. g., France and Czechoslovakia."[52] Clearly the project of German cultural renewal made little impression on non-German intellectuals, who, unlike the Kulturbund activists, did not list German culture among Nazism's primary victims.

Why were anti-fascist intellectuals such as Weisenborn seemingly blind to the fact that the postwar constellation left little room for their brand of cultural nationalism—which, as we have seen, had already been wrought with conflict and division even before Lasky entered the stage? One answer arguably lies in the first part of Weisenborn's speech, which was entitled "On the Death and the Hope of Poets." Weisenborn compared the experiences of his generation, i.e., the experience of total war and mass slaughter, with the generation of Andreas Gryphius and Hans Jakob Christoph von Grimmelshausen, the poets of the Thirty Years' War. Asserting that "being a poet in Germany is a dangerous profession," Weisenborn, not unlike Kantorowicz, explicitly compared the activity of writing to the act of political resistance.[53] The writers' congress—and the desire for German unity—was the expression of an aesthetic self-understanding that linked artistic production and anti-fascist resistance identity.

The generation of Weisenborn, Abusch, and Kantorowicz, all born around 1900, had come of age in a period of intense politicization of culture—German culture in particular.[54] For writers like Kantorowicz, the editor of the journal *Ost und West*, the belief in German cultural unity was inextricably bound up with their identities as anti-fascist resisters.[55] Even without the Cold War, this specific sense of German and artistic identity would have been hard to maintain. The year 1947, which marked the failure of the German Writers' Congress, also saw the birth of the *Gruppe 47* (Group 47) in the Western occupation zones. The writers in this informal group were not interested in restoring pre-1933 traditions of cultural unity, calling instead for a radical break with German tradition, often through the adoption of Anglo-American literary models.[56] Younger than those in Weisenborn's generation, these writers' formative experiences had occurred not in exile or resistance, but as young Wehrmacht draftees and Allied POWs. In the future Federal Republic, it would be writers such as Alfred Andersch and Heinrich Böll, with their American-style prose and far-reaching critiques of all authority, who would wield more cultural influence than Weisenborn or Kantorowicz, who held on to their failed dreams of anti-fascist solidarity and German national unity.

Almost as if to signal the official end of this project, a "tormented" Günther Birkenfeld informed the congress participants on the event's final evening of a decision by the American and British occupation authorities to prohibit the Kulturbund's activities in their zones.[57] The congress co-organizer declared that he identified with the American understanding of democracy, not with that of "the great Eastern democracy." At the same time, however, Birkenfeld condemned the end of the Kulturbund in the West because "we Germans don't have much more left than our language and our culture"—a language that was supposedly in the process of being broken up into Eastern and Western dialects. With applause from the audience, Birkenfeld proclaimed that he would stay in the Kulturbund "until he would no longer be able to speak his mind as freely" as in his journal *Horizonte*.[58]

Developments that took place after the failure of the congress demonstrated that its objective of humanist cultural renewal in East and West was incompatible with Stalinist Cold War strategies—not a component of it. Appeals to SMAD officials by Heinz Willmann, the Kulturbund's general secretary and a leading SED member, to apply for a Western license were finally denied by the Soviets in 1949: they had, by this point, lost all interest in the Kulturbund's existence as an all-German organization.[59] Similarly, in 1948, the SED turned down Kantorowicz's request for financial subsidies for his struggling *Ost und West* journal, which ceased in December 1949. By then, the formation of two German states had made his project—to serve as the voice of an all-German anti-fascist tradition—as obsolete as an all-German Kulturbund or an all-German Writers' Congress.[60]

Anti-fascist Humanism and Cultural Nationalism in the GDR

East Germany's "transition from antifascism to Stalinism" in the years from 1947 to 1953 went hand in hand with the diminishing significance of the Kulturbund.[61] Cultural activities in the last phases of the SBZ (such as the planning of the centenary events commemorating the 1848 revolution) had already shifted from the Kulturbund to the SED's own "cultural departments" and "central cultural committees."[62] At the first Cultural Congress of the SED in May 1948, Anton Ackermann redefined humanism for the future GDR: "Marxism is the new, real Humanism."[63] The Kulturbund, established by Communists and non-Communists to restore German cultural unity on the basis of the country's humanist tradition, became an SED mass organization that, along with a host of other institutions that carried out "cultural mass work" (*kulturelle Massenarbeit*), served to "channel cultural life where possible to ensure that people do not engage in activities that could challenge or undermine the [party's] leadership."[64]

Harich—who in 1957 would himself become the victim of a purge following the end of the political thaw initiated by Soviet leader Nikita Khrushchev's 1956 "secret speech"—may have anticipated this new understanding of the relationship between culture and politics in his critical response to Lasky's speech at the First German Writers' Congress.[65] During a seemingly unrelated discussion on the day after Lasky's speech, Harich alluded to the American's closing statement about the writer as "revolutionary fighter" (a phrase that seemed, incidentally, to echo Kantorowicz's demand for the writer occasionally to trade his typewriter for the machine gun): "It was said this morning that the writer needs to take an oppositional stance, unconditionally, at all costs... I disagree. In a place where positive, constructive, and progressive developments are unfolding, the writer needs to be supportive, and, under the condition that the state is a state of the people, he must also be state-affirming (*staatserhaltend*), if I may use this term."[66] Six years later in June 1953, when confronted with the protests of workers in East Berlin, the Kulturbund's board (led by Becher and Abusch) seemed to take Harich at his word by affirming the organization's loyalty to the GDR and to the leadership of the SED.[67] The tradition of anti-fascist humanism had evolved from a project of cultural renewal to a conservative institution that defended a centralized party dictatorship against a popular uprising.

The SED had also begun to organize meetings and conferences of party members who were writers—and who had, since 1950, increasingly been represented within the Kulturbund by the newly established German Writers' Association (*Deutscher Schriftsteller-Verband*, or DSV)—and no longer the SDA, another symbol of pre-1945 anti-fascist unity that had since become irrelevant. Even more than the Kulturbund, the DSV, under Abusch's leadership, was little more than an extension of the SED's cultural department, especially after the purges of reform-minded functionaries in 1956. The DSV was established in July 1950 at the Second Writers' Congress, an event staged in direct response to Lasky's anti-Communist "Congress for Cultural Freedom" held in West Berlin earlier that year.[68] The Second Writers' Congress had little in common with its predecessor's attempt to bridge the political divide with appeals to cultural unity, but was squarely grounded in the political dynamics of the Cold War. By the time of the Fourth German Writers' Congress in 1955, the official agenda did not include any reference to an all-German national literature. Rather, the congress was designed to "raise the ideological and artistic quality of our [the GDR's] literature, in order to make our literature an even more efficient means for the formation of our workers' consciousness (Socialist education)."[69] For this purpose, the organizers did not appeal to Germany's pre-1933 traditions of classical humanism, but instead called for an "intensified effort" by GDR writers to "acquire and master the techniques of Socialist realism."[70] The critiques of existentialism and modernism that had been one of the undertones of the First German Writers' Congress had, by then, already deteriorated into the Stalinist campaign against "formalism" and "cosmopolitanism."[71]

The vision underlying the First Writers' Congress—the vision of a regenerated humanist German culture that would provide national unity and counter political division—remained a chimera. While the liberal and Communist intellectuals on the board of the early Kulturbund had viewed the congress as a vehicle to restore a cultural German unity shattered during the 1920s and 1930s, the SED cadres who later shaped cultural policies in the GDR would transform anti-fascism and classical German culture from pillars of a renewed and reunified Germany into cultural-ideological justifications for Germany's political division. By the early 1950s, both anti-fascism and the staging of writers' congresses had become tools in the construction of a specific East German national identity.[72] An exception to this development was the Wartburg Congress of July 1954, a meeting initiated by Protestant pastor Otto Riedel with the authorization of Becher, the GDR's first minister of culture by this time. A former member of the Confessing Church during the Third Reich, Riedel envisioned a meeting of writers from East and West and a manifestation of cultural unity at the site where the Bible was first translated into German. Riedel seemed concerned about the SED's involvement in his planned exchange of ideas, which, Riedel wrote the DSV general secretary, was not supposed to be about "party-political speeches."[73]

The conference was seen as a success—despite the absence of the most prominent West German writers—and there was no Lasky scandal at the Wartburg. The conference's guiding principle—a *Bekenntnis der Teilnehmer* (Confession of Participants)—was prominently signed by Anna Seghers, Alfred Kurella, and other icons of anti-fascist resistance and exile:

> In the hour of German need, we, German poets and writers, have met at the Wartburg to listen and talk to each other.
> This is the place where Wolfram von Eschenbach and Walther von der Vogelweide sang, ... where Luther created the German language, where a new people [*Geschlecht*] strove for a new fatherland.
> We stand by the enduring forces of humanism and call on everybody of good will not to let up in their effort for a unified Germany...
> Regardless of our political and ideological differences, we jointly affirm the unity of our fatherland, which we will serve in peace.[74]

The language of the confession displayed all the hallmarks of the speeches at the First Writers' Congress. Its rhetoric of German martyrdom, the belief in the regenerative power of German culture, and its evocation of the Protestant Reformation as a symbol for German national unity and postwar renewal echoed Weisenborn's opening speech "On the Death and Hope of Poets" (*Von Tod und Hoffnung der Dichter*) at the 1947 congress.[75]

The SED must have sensed that the Wartburg meeting's interpretation of German culture, and especially its acknowledgement of "political and ideological differences," constituted a potential threat. As a result, the DSV assigned the organization of the next meeting to the East German CDU, whose general secretary, Gerald Götting, made sure that "the next Wartburg circle [would] not be conducted under Riedel's leadership." Under Götting's and the East-CDU's direction, future Wartburg meetings would flout the GDR's purported tolerance of Christian artists—while forestalling even the possibility that critical statements would be voiced.

Conclusion

The First German Writers' Congress in 1947 was a focal point of many controversies and debates that preceded the Cold War and the East-West split in Germany. Rather than disrupting or destroying the unity of German intellectuals—which, in their own understanding, was based on common prewar traditions of anti-fascism and German culture—the politics of the Cold War exploited preexisting fault lines, such as the rift between exiles and inner émigrés, as well as the different interpretations of modernist thought and the question of German guilt. The congress also exposed a peculiar concept of cultural nationalism among German intellectuals, one fed by the prewar experiences of the anti-fascist generation and a rather vague definition of German humanism that would supposedly bridge political differences and restore Germany's standing in Europe after the Third Reich.

There is barely a trace of the all-German cultural nationalism on display at the First Writers' Congress at the SED-staged congresses that followed after 1950—or, for that matter, in the GDR's official memory culture, which celebrated an exalted version of anti-fascism and Communist resistance.[76] As for Germany's humanist tradition, SED cultural policy eventually chose classical Weimar to represent the cultural heritage of the GDR's "Socialist national culture," e.g., at the celebrations in 1955 that marked the 150th anniversary of Friedrich Schiller's death.[77] During the last two decades of the GDR, the activities of the National Research and Memorial Sites of Classical German Literature (*Nationale Forschungs- und Gedenkstätten der klassischen deutschen Literatur*, or NFG) in Weimar represented Weimar humanism less as a symbol for all-German traditions, but rather as the GDR's alternative to an ostensibly Americanized and materialist consumer culture in the West.[78]

Yet, the debates at the First Writers' Congress, as well as their continuations, transformations, and distortions in the GDR, also illuminate the concept of anti-fascism and its complex history. In his study of the founding of the GDR, Gareth Pritchard has demonstrated "how effective Stalinism proved at manipulating, exploiting and eventually neutralizing the idealism of the German Left."[79] The Communist participants at the congress, such as Abusch, Weisenborn, and Harich, were not naïve idealists, of course. Nor did they merely cynically exploit the notion of humanist renewal as a vehicle for Stalinist one-party rule. Rather, Abusch's Socialist-humanist critique of Meinecke and Harich's understanding of the engaged, post–Third Reich German intellectual seem to address Mary Fulbrook's question of the extent to which the East German dictatorship was "supported by belief in higher ideals, and a determination to tolerate imperfections and distortions in the difficult circumstances of the post-Nazi present, in the hope of building a truly better future."[80]

Interpretations that describe the rhetoric of anti-fascism and Socialist humanism merely as tools that aided the SED regime's consolidation of power and long-term stability neglect the complex intellectual, social, and generational frontlines that fed into these concepts and that burst to the surface at the 1947 congress. The developments that took place after the division of Germany also suggest that the ideas of anti-fascist cultural unity at the First Writers' Congress were more than just a cynical instrument in the Stalinization of East Germany. While the vision of the congress's organizers proved illusionary, the workers' and farmers' state that claimed the congress as one of its cultural cornerstones never seemed very comfortable with the congress's brand of cultural nationalism—and took pains not to let it reemerge outside the tight control of the SED.

Lastly, the analysis of the anti-fascist cultural nationalism at the congress and later in the GDR contradicts interpretations of apolitical German intellectuals whose obsession with purely cultural or aesthetic problems left them exposed to the dark machinations of politics.[81] Culture did not surrender to politics at the congress: the two were inextricably intertwined in a series of divisive and unresolved debates that did not begin or end with Lasky's speech at the congress.

Suggested Readings

Clark, Mark W. *Beyond Catastrophe: German Intellectuals and Cultural Renewal after World War II, 1945–1955*. Lanham, M.D., 2006.

Davies, Peter. *Divided Loyalties: East German Writers and the Politics of German Division, 1945–1953*. London, 2000.

Dietrich, Gert. *Politik und Kultur in der Sowjetischen Besatzungszone Deutschlands (SBZ) 1945–1949. Mit einem Dokumentenanhang*. Berlin, 1993.

Fulbrook, Mary. *Anatomy of a Dictatorship: Inside the GDR, 1949–1989*. New York, 1995.

Gansel, Carsten. *Parlament des Geistes: Literatur zwischen Hoffnung und Repression, 1945–1961*. Berlin, 1996.

Herf, Jeffrey. *Divided Memory: The Nazi Past in the Two Germanys.* Cambridge, M.A., 1997.
Jäger, Manfred. *Kultur und Politik in der DDR, 1945–1990.* Cologne, 1995.
Naimark, Norman M. *The Russians in Germany: A History of the Soviet Zone of Occupation, 1945–1949.* Cambridge, M.A., 1995.
Pike, David. *The Politics of Culture in Soviet-Occupied Germany, 1945–1949.* Stanford, C.A., 1992.
Port, Andrew I. *Conflict and Stability in the German Democratic Republic.* New York, 2007.
Pritchard, Gareth. *The Making of the GDR, 1945–53: From Antifascism to Stalinism.* Manchester, 2000.
Schivelbusch, Wolfgang. *In a Cold Crater: Cultural and Intellectual Life in Berlin, 1945–1948.* Trans. Kelly Berry. Berkeley, C.A., 1998.
Scott-Smith, Giles. "'A Radical Democratic Political Offensive': Melvin J. Lasky, Der Monat, and the Congress for Cultural Freedom." *Journal of Contemporary History* 35/2 (2000): 263-80.
von Richthofen, Esther. *Bringing Culture to the Masses: Control, Compromise and Participation in the GDR.* New York, 2009.
Wilkinson, James D. *The Intellectual Resistance in Europe.* Cambridge, M.A., 1981.

Notes

1. Ursula Reinhold, Dieter Schlenstedt, and Horst Tanneberger, eds., *Erster Deutscher Schriftstellerkongreß. 4.– 8. Oktober 1947* (Berlin, 1997), 418.
2. Seminal accounts published in the GDR include Karl-Heinz Schulmeister, *Auf dem Wege zu einer neuen Kultur. Der Kulturbund in den Jahren 1945–1949* (Berlin, 1977); Gerhard Schmidt, *Der Kulturbund zu Frieden und Demokratie in den Jahren 1948/49. Ein Beitrag zur Vorgeschichte der Gründung der Deutschen Demokratischen Republik. Teil 1 and Teil 2* (Berlin, 1984).
3. See, e.g., Waltraud Wende-Hohenberger, ed., *Der erste gesamtdeutsche Schriftstellerkongreß nach dem Zweiten Weltkrieg: im Ostsektor Berlins vom 4. bis 8. Oktober 1947* (Frankfurt am Main, 1988); Gert Dietrich, *Politik und Kultur in der Sowjetischen Besatzungszone Deutschlands (SBZ) 1945–1949. Mit einem Dokumentenanhang* (Berlin, 1993), 96–101; cf. Carsten Gansel, *Parlament des Geistes. Literatur zwischen Hoffnung und Repression, 1945–1961* (Berlin, 1996), 41–92. The complete speeches and discussion protocols of the congress were published in Reinhold et al., *Schriftstellerkongreß*.
4. Wende-Hohenberger, *Schriftstellerkongreß*, v, quoting from Schulmeister, *Auf dem Wege*.
5. Manfred Jäger, *Kultur und Politik in der DDR, 1945–1990* (Cologne, 1995), 18–19.
6. See, e.g., Wolf Lepenies, *The Seduction of Culture in German History* (Princeton, 2006).
7. David Pike, *The Politics of Culture in Soviet-Occupied Germany, 1945–1949* (Stanford, 1992), 376.
8. See Christoph Kleßmann, *Die doppelte Staatsgründung. Deutsche Geschichte, 1945–1955* (Göttingen, 1982), 182–84.
9. Wolfgang Leonhard, *Child of the Revolution*, trans. CM Woodhouse (London, 1979), 363.
10. For accounts of the Kulturbund's establishment and the role of the Soviet Union, see Pike, *Politics of Culture*; Norman M. Naimark, *The Russians in Germany: A History of*

the *Soviet Zone of Occupation, 1945–1949* (Cambridge, M.A., 1995), 400–408. See also Magdalena Heider, *Politik—Kultur—Kulturbund. Zur Gründungs- und Frühgeschichte des Kulturbundes zur demokratischen Erneuerung Deutschlands, 1945–1954 in der SBZ/DDR* (Cologne, 1993); Dietrich, *Politik und Kultur*; Wolfgang Schivelbusch, *In a Cold Crater: Cultural and Intellectual Life in Berlin, 1945–1948*, trans. Kelly Berry (Berkeley, 1998), 72–106.

11. See Günter Erbe, *Die Verfemte Moderne. Die Auseinandersetzung mit dem "Modernismus" in der Kulturpolitik, Literaturwissenschaft und Literatur der DDR* (Opladen, 1993), 59; see also Pike, *Politics of Culture*, 376.
12. See Reinhold et al., *Schriftstellerkongreß*, 20.
13. Letter of Invitation for Heinrich Berl, 14 July 1947, in Reinhold et al., *Schriftstellerkongreß*, 487.
14. Reinhold et al., *Schriftstellerkongreß*, 24–25.
15. Ibid., 49.
16. Giles Scott-Smith, "'A Radical Democratic Political Offensive': Melvin J. Lasky, *Der Monat*, and the Congress for Cultural Freedom," *Journal of Contemporary History* 35/2 (April 2000): 265. Lasky's later activities as editor of the journal *Der Monat* and as initiator of the anti-Communist "Congress for Cultural Freedom" were indeed financed by the CIA.
17. Reinhold et al., *Schriftstellerkongreß*, 296–98.
18. Ibid., 300–301.
19. Ibid., 301.
20. See Scott-Smith, "'Political Offensive,'" 267–68.
21. See Naimark, *Russians in Germany*, 460; Giles McDonogh, *After the Reich: The Brutal History of the Allied Occupation* (New York, 2007), 224.
22. Reinhold et al., *Schriftstellerkongreß*, 336.
23. See "Kulturelle Freiheit," *Tagesspiegel*, 8 October 1947.
24. *Der Kurier*, 9 October 1947. See also Wende-Hohenberger, *Schriftstellerkongreß*, 95.
25. Reinhold et al., *Schriftstellerkongreß*, 219.
26. Besides David Tompkins's essay in this volume, see Jeffrey Herf, *Divided Memory: The Nazi Past in the Two Germanys* (Cambridge, M.A., 1997); Jürgen Danyel, ed., *Die geteilte Vergangenheit. Zum Umgang mit Nationalsozialismus und Widerstand in beiden deutschen Staaten* (Berlin, 1985); see also Bill Niven, "The Sideways Gaze: The Cold War and Memory of the Nazi Past, 1949–1970," in *Divided, but Not Disconnected: German Experiences of the Cold War*, ed. Tobias Hochscherf, Christoph Laucht, and Andrew Plowman (New York, 2010), 49–62.
27. Reinhold et al., *Schriftstellerkongreß*, 415.
28. For a biography of Becher and his artistic and political visions, see Alexander Behrens, *Johannes R. Becher. Eine politische Biographie* (Cologne, 2003); cf. Jens-Fietje Dwars, *Abgrund des Widerspruchs. Das Leben des Johannes R. Becher* (Berlin, 1998).
29. See Schivelbusch, *Cold Crater*, 84–88.
30. Wende-Hohenberger, *Schriftstellerkongreß*, xvii. For a brief sketch of Kantorowicz's biography, see Beate Ihme-Tuchel, "Alfred Kantorowicz," in *Opposition und Widerstand in der DDR. Politische Lebensbilder*, ed. Karl Wilhelm Fricke, Peter Steinbach, and Johannes Tuchel (Munich, 2002), 258–64.
31. Reinhold et al., *Schriftstellerkongreß*, 137, 141.
32. Ibid., 144, 145.
33. Ibid., 153.

34. Ibid., 156.
35. Ibid., 324. On Greta Kuckhoff, see the essay by Sayner in this volume.
36. See Wolfgang Harich, "Ernst Jünger und der Frieden," *Aufbau* 2/6 (1946): 556–70.
37. Reinhold et al., *Schriftstellerkongreß*, 158–59. For reactions to Harich's speech, see also "Erster deutscher Schriftsteller Kongreß," *Tagesspiegel*, 8 October 1947.
38. "Gibt es eine besondere Deutsche Geistige Krise?" *Aufbau* 3/4 (1947): 305.
39. Ibid., 309, 307.
40. See Alexander Abusch, *Der Irrweg einer Nation* (Berlin, 1946), esp. 139, 161.
41. See Mark W. Clark, *Beyond Catastrophe: German Intellectuals and Cultural Renewal after World War II, 1945–1955* (Lanham, M.D., 2006), 15; see 15–43 for Meinecke's career and ideas both before and after 1945.
42. Friedrich Meinecke, *Autobiographische Schriften, Werke, Band VIII*, ed. Eberhard Kessel (Stuttgart, 1969), 325–31, 376.
43. Ibid., 388, 420, 443.
44. Abusch also criticized Meinecke's version of humanist cultural renewal: the establishment of Goethe communities. See Alexander Abusch, "Die deutsche Katastrophe," *Aufbau* 3/1 (Jan. 1947): 2, 8.
45. See Henri Mougin, "Wie Gott in Frankreich: Heidegger unter uns," *Aufbau* 2/6 (1946): 579–84.
46. See J. Alvarez de Vayo, "Die Existenzialphilosophie und ihre politischen Folgen. Bemerkungen über Jean-Paul Sartre," *Aufbau* 2/11 (1946): 1158–61.
47. Alexander Abusch, "Gibt es eine besondere deutsche Krise?" (1947) in *Kulturelle Probleme des sozialistischen Humanismus. Beiträge zur deutschen Kulturpolitik, 1946–1961 (Schriften, Band III)* (Berlin, 1962), 41.
48. For the Europe-wide significance of humanism and existentialism for postwar concepts of intellectual renewal, see James D. Wilkinson, *The Intellectual Resistance in Europe* (Cambridge, M.A., 1981).
49. Reinhold et al., *Schriftstellerkongreß*, 160–61.
50. "'Von Tod und Hoffnung der Dichter.' Rede Auszüge von Günther Weisenborn," *Berlin am Mittag*, 6 October 1947.
51. Reinhold et al., *Schriftstellerkongreß*, 134.
52. "Gespräch mit Hermon Ould," *Berlin am Mittag*, 6 October 1947. The reference to Czechoslovakia seems to be a strategic choice, given the still open-ended political situation there.
53. See "'Von Tod und Hoffnung der Dichter.'"
54. See Detlev J. K. Peukert, *Die Weimarer Republik. Krisenjahre der klassischen Moderne* (Frankfurt, 1987).
55. On Kantorowicz's journal see Ewald Birr, *Ost und West, Berlin 1947–1949. Bibliographie einer Zeitschrift* (Munich, 1993); see also Alfred Kantorowicz, *Deutschland-Ost und Deutschland-West. Kulturpolitische Einigungsversuche und geistige Spaltung in Deutschland seit 1945* (Münsterdorf, n.d.). On the influence of the prewar experiences on this generation's understanding of democracy in East and West, see also Sean Foner, "Für eine demokratische Erneuerung Deutschlands. Kommunikationsprozesse engagierter Demokraten nach 1945," *Geschichte und Gesellschaft* 33 (2007): 228–57.
56. On surveys of the cultural developments in early postwar West Germany, see, e.g., Jost Hermand, *Kultur im Wiederaufbau. Die Bundesrepublik Deutschland, 1945–1965* (Munich, 1986); Hermann Glaser, *Kulturgeschichte der Bundesrepublik Deutschland. Bd. 1: Zwischen Kapitulation und Währungsreform, 1945–1948* (Munich, 1985).

57. See Schivelbusch, *Cold Crater*, 98.
58. *Der Kurier*, 9 October 1947. See also Reinhold et al., *Schriftstellerkongreß*, 417–18.
59. See SAPMO—BArch DY 27/1395, letter of Heinz Willmann to the deputy Soviet commander of Berlin, Colonel Jelisarow, 29 September 1949.
60. See Birr, *Ost und West*, 10–11.
61. See Gareth Pritchard, *The Making of the GDR, 1945–53: From Antifascism to Stalinism* (Manchester, 2000).
62. See Dietrich, *Politik und Kultur*, 65–72, 112–13.
63. "Marxistische Kulturpolitik. Rede Anton Ackermanns auf dem Ersten Kulturtag der SED in Berlin, 7. Mai 1948," in *Um die Erneuerung der deutschen Kultur: Dokumente zur Kulturpolitik, 1945–1949*, ed. Gerd Dietrich (Berlin, 1983), 266.
64. Esther von Richthofen, *Bringing Culture to the Masses: Control, Compromise and Participation in the GDR* (New York, 2009), 2, 3. For a broader analysis of the role of the Kulturbund and other mass organizations in the GDR's "contours of power," see Mary Fulbrook, *Anatomy of a Dictatorship: Inside the GDR, 1949–1989* (New York, 1995), 58–61.
65. For a brief account of Harich's role as a GDR dissident, see Beate Ihme-Tuchel, "Wolfgang Harich," in Fricke et al., *Opposition und Widerstand*, 216–23.
66. *Erster Deutscher Schriftstellerkongreß*, 350.
67. See BArch-SAPMO, DY 27/916, "Erklärung des Kulturbundes zur loyalen Haltung der Intelligenz," 3 July 1953.
68. See Gansel, *Parlament des Geistes*, 158, 161.
69. ZK der SED, Abt. Kunst. Sekretariatsvorlage zum IV. Schriftstellerkongreß (11 June 1955), published in Gansel, *Parlament des Geistes*, 342–45.
70. Ibid., 343.
71. See Mathias Judt, ed., *DDR Geschichte in Dokumenten. Beschlüsse, Berichte, interne Materialien und Alltagszeugnisse* (Berlin, 1998), 295ff.
72. The East German Akademie der Künste (Academy of the Arts) was another cultural institution that initially promoted German unity before being transformed into an SED tool whose role was to help establish a GDR cultural identity; see Peter Davies, *Divided Loyalties: East German Writers and the Politics of German Division, 1945–1953* (London, 2000).
73. Pfarrer Riedel to DSV Secretary Gustav Just, 3 March 1954, quoted in Gansel, *Parlament des Geistes*, 227.
74. "Wartburg-Treffen. Bekenntnis der Teilnehmer (Juli 1954)," published in Gansel, *Parlament des Geistes*, 406.
75. It was also strikingly reminiscent of Becher's more famous speech at the inauguration of the Kulturbund in June 1945. See Deutscher Kulturbund, *Manifest und Ansprachen von Bernhard Kellermann [et al.] gehalten bei der Gründungskundgebung des Kulturbundes zur demokratischen Erneuerung Deutschlands am 4. Juli 1945 im Haus des Berliner Rundfunks* (Berlin, n.d.).
76. See Mary Nolan, "Antifascism under Fascism: German Vision and Voices," *New German Critique* 67 (Winter 1996): 33–55.
77. See Gunther Mai, "Sozialistische Nation und Nationalkultur," in *Weimarer Klassik in der Ära Honecker*, ed. Lothar Ehrlich and Gunther Mai (Cologne, 2001), 29–76.
78. See Lothar Ehrlich, Gunther Mai, and Ingeborg Cleve, "Weimarer Klassik in der Ära Honecker," in Ehrlich and Mai, *Weimarer Klassik*, 18.
79. Gareth Pritchard, *The Making of the GDR, 1945–1953* (Manchester, 2000), 229.

80. Fulbrook, *Anatomy of a Dictatorship*, 11. Even though the ideal of anti-fascism appealed to many East German intellectuals until the last years of the GDR, Andrew I. Port contends that workers and farmers in East Germany "who openly compared the methods of the SED to those of the Nazis ... obviously remained immune to official claims that the GDR represented a dramatic break with and positive alternative to National Socialism." See Andrew I. Port, *Conflict and Stability in the German Democratic Republic* (New York, 2007), 273. Cf. John C. Torpey, *Intellectuals, Socialism, and Dissent: The East German Opposition and Its Legacy* (Minneapolis, 1995).
81. Wolf Lepenies speaks of the "overrating of culture at the expense of politics." See Lepenies, *Seduction of Culture*, 8.

CHAPTER 3

Communicating History
The Archived Letters of Greta Kuckhoff and Memories of the "Red Orchestra"

JOANNE SAYNER

Anti-fascism was the cornerstone of ideology in the German Democratic Republic (GDR). In the fiercely dichotomized debates about East German history that have erupted since 1989, it has been dismissed as merely a state-imposed doctrine, as an ideology with no links to the population, and as a hypostatized cult of the dead.[1] As such, anti-fascism has become part of the "totalitarian" narrative, seen not as the opposite of an oppressive dictatorial regime, but instead as its symptomatic (and emblematic) result.[2] Even in work by those historians who have advocated a more carefully differentiated approach to the East German past, there often persists a monolithic understanding of anti-fascism.[3] Based on previously unpublished archival sources and taking a Foucauldian approach, the following essay examines constructions of anti-fascist subjectivity in the life-writings of Greta Kuckhoff in order to present a more complicated picture of the term *anti-fascism*.[4]

Born in Frankfurt an der Oder in 1902 into a Catholic lower-middle-class family, Greta Kuckhoff studied philosophy and economics at the University of Berlin. She then spent two years at the University of Madison in Wisconsin, where she pursued a doctorate in sociology. On her return to Europe she worked in various capacities as a freelance translator before taking up a post at the University of Frankfurt am Main, where she worked for Karl Mannheim at the Institute for Social Research. Her research career was cut short in March 1933, when the Nazis closed the Institute in Frankfurt; she was away at the time on a study trip at the London School of Economics, but then returned to Germany and worked as a freelance translator and interpreter in Berlin for, among others, the Nazi Racial Policy Office (*Rassenpolitisches Amt*). She was involved in the first published English translation of Adolf Hitler's *Mein*

Kampf. But at the same time, she was also a member of the anti-fascist resistance group named the "Red Orchestra" (*Rote Kapelle*) by the Nazis.

The "Red Orchestra" was actually composed of different groups across Europe, often with little or no contact with each other.[5] The Nazi nomenclature suggested a supposed Communist connection. In fact, those working with Kuckhoff in Berlin came from many different sociopolitical backgrounds. Half of the members of the group were women, which was unusual. Beginning in 1933, they concentrated on practical, pedagogical resistance, disseminating anti-fascist leaflets and information about the horrific reality of the Nazi regime, and helping those targeted by the state. More contentiously, some members of the group were later involved in transmitting information to the Soviet authorities. Attempts to establish radio contact with Moscow were, however, an "unmitigated disaster, since the equipment supplied by the Soviets was defective," and the information that they did succeed in passing along to the Soviet embassy about German war plans was not believed.[6] The members of the Berlin circle were arrested in autumn 1942 and Kuckhoff's husband and friends were subsequently executed as traitors.[7] Initially condemned to death, Kuckhoff herself survived the end of the war after her sentence was commuted to ten years imprisonment. From 1945 she worked in various high-level administrative positions in the Soviet Zone of Occupation (SBZ) and later the GDR, becoming the first head of the state bank in 1950 and later vice president of the Council of Peace (*Friedensrat der DDR*). Throughout her life, she endeavored to get the activities of the members of the Berlin "Red Orchestra" commemorated in a way that she thought properly reflected their actions and priorities.

As part of her commemorative work, Kuckhoff wrote letters. Her archived papers (*Nachlass*) contain thousands of letters sent to more than 1,200 individuals and institutions. Preserved as transcripts of letters sent, originals received, and copies gathered from other sources, many of these are addressed to key figures involved in writing histories of anti-fascist resistance and, more specifically, the role of the "Red Orchestra."[8] In this chapter, these letters are read as one of many new sources available since unification that offer new ways of interpreting the group. As a form of life-writing, letters are a memory genre in which not only the identities of the writer, but also those of her addressees are represented. Although often associated with notions of spontaneity, immediacy, and revelation, letters are no less constructed than any other genre—as is shown by the numerous drafts in Kuckhoff's papers. Her letters epitomize a dialogical process of remembering that is found throughout Kuckhoff's work: she challenged and contradicted understandings of anti-fascism that she encountered in popular histories in East and West Germany, as well as beyond. It is for this reason that the letters are so significant. Through them it is possible to trace diachronically and synchronically not only dominant and competing understandings of anti-fascism, but also to highlight competing forms of subjectivity upon which such understandings were based. The letters represent different approaches to anti-fascist pasts and, as such, suggest different ways of being anti-fascist in the writers' past, present, and future. After examining the usefulness of discourse analysis for an investigation of such subjectivities, the essay looks at how selected letters communicate (resistant) anti-fascist histories, tracing competing claims to memory, experience, and authority in these texts—and suggesting how such claims problematize models of and approaches to the GDR that downplay individual agency.

Discursive Frames

Although controversial, contested, and often contradictory, Michel Foucault's writings provide a useful framework for understanding anti-fascism in the past and present. Above all, his combined focus on issues of history, power, and subjectivity are extremely productive for examining aspects of the East German state and its contemporary reception. Foucauldian discourse analysis combined with feminist cultural studies approaches, which focus on political reflection and possibilities for change, inform the following analysis of Kuckhoff's unpublished archival material.[9]

Foucault's work draws fundamental attention to the use of language in a specific historical context. It emphasizes the "local intelligibility of actions which are meaningful within specific alignments of power,"[10] thus pointing toward contextualized understandings of GDR anti-fascism and the eclecticism of practice.[11] No one text or individual will provide the "key" to understanding anti-fascism, of course, but such an analysis can highlight the cumulative effect of different knowledges, individuals, and institutions involved in the production of anti-fascist discourse. It allows for consideration of the competing economic, political, sociological, and cultural understandings of anti-fascism.

Conceptualizations of discourse are fundamental to Foucault's approach. Discourse can be understood as "ways of constituting knowledge, together with the social practices, forms of subjectivity and power relations which inhere [within them]."[12] It insists on the relevance of material practice. It places an emphasis on institutions *and* individuals as social actors, as well as on the interactions among them. History writing, and specifically anti-fascist histories, are examples of "historically situated fields of knowledge," i.e., discursive formations, with power relations inherent in them.[13] History writing is not just about the texts themselves, but the institutional conditions of their production, dissemination, and reception. Such discursive formations offer subject positions with which an individual may identify and adopt through repeated practice: anti-fascist histories provide anti-fascist personalities, which subjects can assume consciously and unconsciously.

A Foucauldian analysis sensitizes us to the numerous sites of power within culture, both symbolic and material.[14] In this model, power is not simply imposed from the "top down," but instead is transmitted by and through all historical agents. Power is a "strategy that maintains a relation between the sayable and the visible."[15] However, because power is "co-constituted by those who support or resist it,"[16] such agents are able to challenge, or reverse, the discourse if "there is a space between the position offered by a discourse and individual interest."[17] While repeated anti-fascist discourse disciplines individuals, producing subjected and—to speak using Foucault's language—"practiced" bodies, resistance is nevertheless an integral part of the discourse.

With respect to the GDR, this is in no way to downplay the centralized system of power, the very real bodily harm that symbolic or material resistance might have provoked, or the attempted imposition of a "Socialist consciousness" (*sozialistisches Bewusstsein*) by the political elite. But discourse explicitly goes beyond "a general system of domination exerted by one group over another."[18] Instead, it insists upon a relationship of interdependence of these propagandistic state powers and those intersecting with it. Rather than seeing the Socialist state as a "discursive prison" (*Diskursgefängnis*),[19] such an approach allows us to get beyond simplifying dichotomies that insist upon either state manipulation of its citizens, or on the outright rejection of any influence of such "strategic communication."[20]

The following essay looks at the ways in which competing versions of anti-fascism were "made sayable" in Kuckhoff's letters. Rather than seeing dominant GDR state discourse as merely prescriptive and repressive, it examines the ways in which Kuckhoff's letters engaged with the meanings attached to anti-fascist resistance at specific points in time. Looking at just a few of her confrontations with writers of popular history in East and West Germany allows us to consider "the subject positions made possible within [her] texts,"[21] i.e., the positions offered by the "plurality of resistances" in her understanding of anti-fascism.[22] This is not simply to understand discourse analysis as a focus on textuality. It is, however, to use literary historical analysis in order to challenge blind spots in current conceptualizations of anti-fascism. As such, this essay offers another "small piece in the mosaic of the still-to-be-written cultural history of antifascism."[23]

Writing Popular Histories

Kuckhoff's papers contain many transcripts of letters she sent. Because she also preserved letters she received, this means that it is possible to reconstruct many of the exchanges she had about writing the histories of the "Red Orchestra"—an undertaking notable for the lack of involvement by academic historians.[24] Indeed, until the 1980s, the narratives in widespread circulation in East and West Germany were based, for the most part, on newspaper and journal articles, popular history books, television, and film. It is the longevity of the emphases in these texts—emphases subsequently challenged by historians after German unification in 1990—that makes Kuckhoff's correspondence and her attempted intervention so significant.

In 1947 Kuckhoff began a correspondence with Wilhelm Flicke, who was writing two books linked to her resistance group: a history of the Nazi surveillance service (*Abhördienst*), and a novel about the "Red Orchestra." Kuckhoff had met with Flicke in Nuremberg, where she was about to record her testimony against Manfred Roeder, the Nazi judge who had sentenced many of her group to death. Flicke told her that he himself had been a member of the Social Democratic Party (SPD), but that, during the Nazi regime, he had worked as a surveillance technician and had been given the task of writing a history of the "Red Orchestra" using Gestapo files.[25] The reason the Nazis had requested this, he said, was so that after Germany's ultimate triumph in the war, Hitler could explain to the German people why victory had been so hard won and had involved so many losses.[26] For his part, Flicke said that he wrote the manuscript because he believed that after German defeat, and once the population had freed themselves from "Nazi intoxication," they would "hunger for the truth."[27] Writing to Flicke shortly after their meeting, Kuckhoff told him that his work had made an impression on her, but that his manuscript had also left her feeling uneasy because of his reliance on Nazi sources and because of his ability to represent only one side (i.e., the Nazi side) of the story. She expressed concern that he should also convey "the genuine political and human motivations [of the group] with the same thoroughness."[28] She said that she had spoken to a publisher in the Soviet zone who was more interested in the novel than in the historical text. Making reference to her own political capital and the fact that her name was well known, she proposed getting the book published in the Soviet zone and offered to act as an intermediary.[29]

In his reply, Flicke suggested that he first complete the novel and then send it to her for comment before they think any further about publication. He added that he would particularly value her input with regard to the court case, about which he had found little material but which Kuckhoff had witnessed herself. In terms of the general direction of his narrative, he referred to already opposing characterizations of the group and suggested a way to combine these: "We can't portray the work of the group as that of an espionage organization. On the other hand, we also can't make a one-sided epic song of inner resistance out of it without mentioning the other side ... because then we certainly would run the risk that one day someone will appear and claim: No, children, things were quite different! What counts here is finding a dramatic synthesis. That must at least be attempted with a good will effort."

Concerning the historical text, he wrote that the American authorities had already expressed an interest in the manuscript and that he was negotiating a contract. He sent her the preface and introduction of this book to read but, in a remarkably forthright admission about the influence that current political conditions had on his text, maintained: "Because the current manuscript is geared towards the American psyche, it remains to be considered, of course, whether one makes certain changes, deletions, or additions depending on the country in which it is published. For the moment I want to wait and see what the immediate future brings in terms of developments in international relations (*zwischenstaatliche Entwicklung*). If the hoped-for détente occurs, then another revision can easily be done." Three months later, Kuckhoff wrote Flicke in response to the preface and introduction he had sent her. Her letter contained some fairly stringent criticism of his work, but this was partly mitigated by flattery, as well as by her directing her comments at other recently published texts. The letter begins: "I find your writing and your train of thought about the issues interesting, particularly the fact that you also recognize the difficulties resulting from the tense international situation, which stands in the way of a just and accurate evaluation of everything."[30] Kuckhoff lamented that a book about the underground had recently been published by Allen Welsh Dulles, which was, in her opinion, "completely wrong" about the "Red Orchestra."[31] Kuckhoff considered Dulles's book to be particularly important because it was the first one about German resistance published in North America.[32] It portrayed resistance group leaders Harro Schulze-Boysen and Arvid Harnack as spies who had only begun their resistance work *after* the German invasion of the Soviet Union.[33] In her comments to Flicke she complained, "It obviously makes us bitter because we know that evidence is available that clearly proves the falsity of such claims." Couching her criticism of Flicke's work in terms of prevailing political conditions, she wrote, "The forewords that you enclosed might have been correct when you wrote them, but today they seem to be particularly dangerous. Germany's political maturity has not increased but decreased." She criticized in particular any tendency—notwithstanding his comments in an earlier letter to her—to portray the group only as spies and insisted that the members had worked since 1933—and not just since the beginning of the war—to liberate Germany from the Nazis and preserve "Germany's sovereignty." She concluded that any text that did not make this its focal point was simply wrong. It seems that their correspondence came to an end at this point.

Flicke's partly fictionalized text was published in West Germany in 1949. It first appeared in serial form in a West German newspaper and then as a novel called *The Red Orchestra Spy Ring: Freely Retold According to the Facts* (*Spionagegruppe Rote Kapelle: In freier Bearbeitung den Tatsachen nacherzählt*).[34] At the time of its publication, Kuckhoff wrote to Franz Dahlem, the head of the SED's "West Commission," that the other survivors of the resistance group objected in particular to Flicke's portrayal of the group as part of "a large, ideologically sound network of agents … in Berlin," and that they advocated an official protest. She wrote that she was herself less sure that a protest would be a good idea because, she said, it could degenerate very quickly into a clash before any proper historiographic work had been done on the group. But she also asked him whether she, as someone with a certain institutional standing, should get involved in this matter herself.[35] The response from GDR authorities was that a public confrontation would be "inexpedient."[36] This is not to say that there had been no previous work done in the Soviet zone on the group. A text written by Klaus Lehmann with the support of survivors had been published by the Union of those Persecuted by the Nazi Regime (VVN) in 1948.[37] But in the ensuing battle to shape public memory of the group, it was Flicke's text, which was based on Gestapo files, that was used by others, particularly those in the West writing about the group.[38]

In the early 1950s several Western publications characterized the members of the "Red Orchestra" as traitors and promoted the idea that a "spy ring" still existed and was a danger to the Federal Republic.[39] A series of articles was published in *Der Fortschritt* called "The Secret of the Red Orchestra." The articles were framed by two pictures: one of a person hanging from a noose in 1942—and one that was still to be filled (presumably in the 1950s). The implication was obviously that survivors like Kuckhoff who had escaped the death penalty should still be "brought to justice." This was followed by a 1951 series in *Stern* magazine entitled "Red Agents among us," which included a photograph of Kuckhoff as head of the GDR state bank and a caption saying that this position had been a "reward for loyal service" during the war.[40] A book by former Nazi judge Manfred Roeder was published in 1952, followed by books by Gerhard Ritter in 1954 and David Dallin in 1956.[41] All three denied the group the status of resistance, and such claims of betrayal pervaded the early histories of West Germany. Publications that portrayed the resistance in a more differentiated, positive light, including Günther Weisenborn's *Der lautlose Aufstand* from 1953, were less common.[42] Weisenborn, himself a former member of the "Red Orchestra," had been a regular correspondent of Kuckhoff's since the end of the war. While she disagreed with several aspects of his portrayal, including his naming of the group as the "Schulze-Boysen/Harnack-Organization"—which, she argued, focused unduly on only two (male) members, they remained friends for decades and worked together to commemorate the group.[43]

Since 1948 Kuckhoff had immersed herself in work for the emerging GDR state. Her correspondence shows that she was clearly aware of the texts being published in West Germany and of the personal attacks against her, but she decided not to intervene.[44] It is clear from one particular letter in her papers that what finally prompted her to respond was not a polemical Western publication but rather one that appeared in the East and tested her loyalty to the

GDR.[45] In 1955 she wrote to SED General Secretary Walter Ulbricht in response to his recently published book on contemporary history, *Zur Geschichte der neuesten Zeit*:[46]

> Dear Comrade Ulbricht,
> For reasons of political discipline, I have done nothing over the past ten years—following a first failed attempt—to explain the peculiarity of our resistance work (Dr Harnack, Schulze-Boysen) based on my knowledge, and to point out the problems connected to it. I was convinced that one day, after studying the documents that are undoubtedly available and by talking at length to me, the party would carry out an evaluation and, at the appropriate moment, release ... the principal findings about the nine-year struggle. Now that your book about the German working class during fascism has been published, I have compared its portrayal with my own experiences and found that I have to comment on it.[47]

She went on to take issue with many elements of Ulbricht's narrative, including his emphasis on the role played by the leadership of the German Communist Party (KPD) in the resistance. This, she agrees, may well have been the case if one considers the "resistance as a whole," but it was not the case for her own group. She criticized the absence of any detailed consideration of the "Red Orchestra," insisting that "not mentioning it does not simply make it go away," but that that merely allowed West German historians to write their own polemical histories. She added that the group's emphasis on certain activities had not been correctly represented by him. She then listed what were, according to her, the characteristics of the anti-fascist fight, including the fact that it had started in 1933 when the group decided to stay in Germany rather than go into exile; she also added that it involved cooperation among a diverse group of people, not all of whom were Marxists. Her emphasis on the diversity of political viewpoints was strengthened in the subsequent drafting process. The letter thus pursued a dual strategy of reinforcing the narrative of the political status quo (the necessity of political discipline, an awareness of a current struggle, and a belief in the party) but, at the same time, challenged Ulbricht himself, e.g., pointing to the fact that Ulbricht had left Germany to go into exile, denying the leadership of the KPD in the inner-German resistance, and complicating the narrative about Communist motivations for resistance. The letter's closing request—that they should meet to discuss the way in which the group was being remembered in the GDR—was not, based on the available archival sources, acknowledged.

Two years later Kuckhoff noted with dismay that Flicke's text had been republished in the West by his niece shortly after his death.[48] This substantially altered version, which emphasized even more forcefully the group's supposed role as spies for the Soviet Union, was also translated into French.[49] In the GDR itself, several texts published around this time profiled members of the "Red Orchestra" group and emphasized the diversity of their motivations for resisting, including their political and religious ones.⁵⁰ Others reverted to the homogenizing narratives of Ulbricht's text, often through direct quotation.⁵¹ Throughout the 1960s Kuckhoff wrote repeatedly to East German state figures and members of the SED Politburo requesting that she, as one of the few surviving members, be actively involved in conducting research on the group.⁵² In an interview and in subsequent correspondence with Russian historian Lew Besymenski, Kuckhoff refuted several times the increasing portrayal in the GDR of "Red Orchestra" activities as simply spying (*Kundschaftertätigkeit*).⁵³ But her work was made all the more difficult at this point by the intervention of one of the most powerful institutions in the GDR: the infamous Ministry for State Security (MfS, or Stasi).

Shared Narratives of the Cold War

As Johannes Tuchel has pointed out, the year 1965 marked a sea change in East Germany in terms of public discussion of wartime resistance.⁵⁴ The MfS—after learning of Besymenski's intention to write a book on the "Red Orchestra" and of the Soviet Union's plan to produce a film with DEFA, the East German film studio—became heavily involved in directing the commemoration of a group that seemed ideally suited for propaganda purposes. The Department of Propaganda (*Agitation*) had, since the start of the year, begun collecting documents about the group with the aim of producing a book with Dietz, a major East German publishing house. It seems that Kuckhoff's previous interventions must have had some impact because, as Tuchel suggests, the head of the department, Günther Halle, had intended that Kuckhoff write a foreword for the book. There is evidence that Mielke spoke to Kuckhoff about this on 22 November 1965, according to Tuchel, who remarks that this was the beginning of several exchanges between the Stasi and Kuckhoff "that would not always run smoothly."⁵⁵ Two letters written by Kuckhoff to Erich Honecker before and after Mielke's visit suggested what some of the points of contention were—points that go to the very heart of her understanding of anti-fascism. On 15 October 1965 she wrote to Honecker after friends in Moscow and West Germany had sent her an extract from Valentin Bereschkov's memoirs, which had appeared in the Soviet journal *Novyj Mir* and in which he described how German anti-fascists had been able to warn the Soviet Union of the impending invasion during World War II—a warning not taken seriously by Soviet authorities.⁵⁶ In this letter to Honecker, Kuckhoff was able to maintain a critical stance toward the Soviet authorities while, at the same time, emphasizing her own work with Russian historians. This was not the only time she referred to mistakes by Soviet authorities in a letter to Honecker. In December of that year she wrote him the following:

> I have a request: that you let me know whether or not I have understood you correctly. I understood that the comrades researching the resistance should let me examine the available files and that you would try to get hold of the files in our partner country [the Soviet Union] for evaluation. I repeat my request once again: it matters a great deal to me to get an evaluation from the party about this group in particular, because my husband—along with many old comrades—and our friends fought for years (from at least '33) to help with educational work (*Überzeugungsarbeit*) and to make a substantial contribution to the anti-Hitler Coalition. I am the only survivor (as far as I know) who knew both the Harnacks and Schulze-Boysen and [Wilhelm] Guddorf, along with [John] Sieg. Since 1945 it has been a ... matter of concern to me to gain clarity about certain events that considerably unsettled the comrades and friends in charge, so that one can present a more balanced portrayal (not so that one reveals everything)—which could also certainly help today, in many respects, to win new companions in the struggle (*Kampfgefährte*) and allow for a fair evaluation [of the group's wartime activities].
>
> Com[rade] Mielke told me that I would be "astounded" by the amount of material and he sent very friendly comrades to me who asked me questions but, nevertheless, did not bring me any material. The young comrade who has been directly entrusted with the research knows all about the available literature—but so do I.[57]

Referring to the recycling of incorrect historical accounts in the West German, English, French, Polish, and Soviet historiography, the letter then asked for Honecker's support in obtaining evidence that would help clarify certain facts to be employed as part of a useable history: "I hoped that a historically intelligent representation would first lay the foundations for a more personal one." Pointing once again to Flicke's republished text, Kuckhoff claimed, "If nothing at all had been published, I could ultimately understand that nothing should be published by our side either—but I have not thought that for at least the last decade now." She drew again on her own firsthand experience to make the case that she should be allowed to speak her mind about the documents currently kept in "a certain ministry." The letter then returned to the "certain events" that had caused the members of the group disquiet—referring in particular to the "assignment" (*Auftrag*) set for her by Arvid Harnack. It was Harnack who had, before his execution, given Kuckhoff the task of finding out why the Soviet authorities had been so careless with the resisters' names—a carelessness that ultimately led to their arrest. At the same time, and using the same tone of reassurance earlier used in the letter to Ulbricht, she concluded by referring to the "high degree of discipline and restraint" that she had shown about this issue for the last twenty years. There is, once again, no evidence of a reply in her papers.

A year later, in 1966, the Institute for Marxism-Leninism (IML) published the fifth volume of the *History of the German Working-Class Movement* (*Ge-*

schichte der deutschen Arbeiterbewegung). This narrative transformed the small, informal resistance circle around Schulze-Boysen and Harnack into one of the largest European anti-fascist resistance organizations.[58] Whereas Kuckhoff had been stressing diversity and educational work, dominant GDR discourses increasingly emphasized coordinated leadership by the KPD and links to the Soviet Union. Despite an obviously fraught relationship between Kuckhoff and representatives of key GDR institutions, the state's reticent attitude toward her involvement suddenly changed in 1966 when Winfried Martini (a former member of the Nazi Foreign Office) published a series of articles in the conservative West German newspaper *Die Welt*.[59] The Berlin group of the "Red Orchestra" was the focus of the first three articles and was referred to throughout as a Communist spy ring. Martini focused his attention on the women of the group, beginning with Ilse Stöbe, who had been his secretary. In discussing her appearance, her taste in men, and her weakness for luxuries, he attributed no political or humanist motives to her resistance activities, but instead maintained that they were born merely out of her love for a fellow resister.[60] While he did mention the diverse backgrounds of the Berlin circle in a subsequent article, the implication was that the Communist members had led a naïve group of non-Communists to their deaths. He labeled a former Nazi colleague of Arvid Harnack a fanatic and dismissed the large number of women in the group as merely characteristic of Soviet spy rings in general.[61] He described resister Erika von Brockdorff as someone who "went laughing to the guillotine," and Kuckhoff herself as someone who "began to 'sing' after her arrest."[62] Following the publication of the series, Kuckhoff received a letter from the SED asking for her immediate help in persuading GDR historian and fellow resister Heinrich Scheel to draft a response that could be published in the West in the "anti-fascist" newspaper *Die Tat*. In a negative reply she wrote, "I myself do not think that one should offer a polemical opinion now; rather, it is much better to write a serious article that clearly conveys our position." She pointed out that she had been attempting to do just that for the past twenty years.[63]

It was not only in the East that Kuckhoff refused to cooperate in such rushed public refutations. Correspondence with surviving group members in the West, such as Günther Weisenborn, was vitally important to her, but she rejected certain Western collaborations that, she felt, still drew inappropriately on Gestapo sources, and, in particular, on the testimony of Nazi judge Manfred Roeder. A notably acerbic exchange occurred between her and *Spiegel* editor Heinz Höhne following a series of articles that appeared in the magazine in 1968. These articles were a combination of translated extracts from a book published in French one year earlier by Gilles Perrault (*L'orchestre rouge*), and articles written by Höhne himself.[64] The pieces were first serialized in the magazine and then published as a single volume in 1970.[65] Höhne wrote that he needed to supplement Perrault's work with his "own research" because the former was limited in its portrayal of the Berlin group. In an intriguing "memo" (*Hausmitteilung*) that appeared in the first edition of the *Spiegel* texts, the author portrayed history writing as a contemporary drama in which the surviving "Red Orchestra" members were conspiring to prevent the truth from being told. He claimed that Kuckhoff and Weisenborn, among others, had refused to provide him with information. In the article that followed, Höhne described himself as someone working with an array of historical sources that confused more than enlightened. He did not position himself on the side of the former Nazis, anti-Communists (like Roeder and Flicke and the historian Ritter), and more right-wing authors (such as those whose work appeared in *Der Fortschritt* and *Stern*), or on the side of surviving members who, he said, remained uncooperative because they wanted the group's actions to be understood simply (*nur noch*) as political resistance. Taking Kuckhoff and Weisenborn as exemplary "apologists" who refused to give detailed information about their contact with the Soviet Union, he accused their testimony of being disingenuous. He clearly situated the Berlin group within a Soviet spy ring that had been formed between 1937 and 1939, and that had had links to Belgium and France—something vigorously disputed by survivors. Höhne's narrative echoed, in many ways, Flicke's earlier letters to Kuckhoff: while claiming to be objective, he, in fact, combined many of Flicke's assertions with pieces written by Nazi judge Roeder.

Hans Coppi argues that Höhne made numerous factual errors, including the incorrect attribution of certain radio transmissions to the group.[66] Höhne's texts nevertheless became decisive for perpetuating the resisters' representation in the West as Communists, spies, and traitors. What is notable, however, is that Höhne was able to make his case sound more convincing because of the distorted emphasis that East German publications similarly placed themselves on the group's contact with the Soviet Union. In fact, he drew on major GDR newspapers and journals such as *Neues Deutschland, Junge Welt,* and *Für Dich* to support his argument. For Kuckhoff it was, therefore, a cruel irony that the emphasis on espionage that she found so offensive in West German (and Nazi) sources was also present in many of the publications that appeared in the East. In several of her letters—and notwithstanding Höhne's claims to the contrary—Kuckhoff denied that anyone from *Der Spiegel* had been in contact with her to ask for information, but reaffirmed that even if they had been, she was not prepared to appear alongside Roeder "as a source."[67] In response to a letter from Kuckhoff, Höhne expressed sarcastic regret that she was not willing to cooperate with him in his work on the group, but attributed this to the fact that she believed that "only a Marxist could write about this group."[68]

Martini and Höhne's texts were probably the clearest examples of what Hans Coppi calls the "grey zone of moralising clichés about spying and betrayal" that characterized West German writing about the group during the 1960s.[69] But there were exceptions, such as the prominent West German author Ingeborg Drewitz's 1968 work on Adam Kuckhoff.[70] A lengthy correspondence had already taken place between Kuckhoff and Drewitz before this short piece appeared,[71] and it emphasized many of the points that Kuckhoff had been advocating herself, such as the diverse political backgrounds of the group and the start of their resistance as early as 1933. It also mirrored the critical position taken by Kuckhoff about remembrance in both East and West Germany. Drewitz referred to the "odium of betrayal" and anti-Communist tenor maligning the group in the Federal Republic, something she interpreted as a sign of a society "evading its past." In the GDR, she claimed, the prescriptive nature of some forms of commemoration—such as the "inviolability of memorial days" (*Gedenktagsunantastbarkeit*)—had led to a lack of "serious academic attempts at interpretation."[72] But with a circulation of only 400 copies, Drewitz's publication simply did not enjoy the same prominence as Höhne's *Spiegel* articles.

By the end of the 1960s, the Soviet Union had posthumously awarded honors to many of those executed, as well as to some surviving members of the group. In collaboration with the Stasi, Moscow constructed a narrative asserting that the "Red Orchestra" had been spies for Soviet intelligence authorities. This allowed for the creation of a *joint* anti-fascist past. As Tuchel points out, the fact that the majority of those commemorated had never had any such connection to the Soviet authorities was of no interest to the Stasi.[73] These alleged links were further emphasized in—and represented visually in the publicity posters, as well as encapsulated in the title of—the 1970 DEFA film *klk an ptx: Die Rote Kapelle*. Kuckhoff was not invited to contribute to the film—despite living in close proximity to the film's producers, Claus and Wera Küchenmeister, and despite the fact that she was played in the film by an actress.[74]

Kuckhoff was, nevertheless, involved with a text that was published jointly later that year by the IML and MfS under the names of Karl Heinz Biernat and Luise Kraushaar. It included biographies, letters, and photographs of members of the group, and Kuckhoff was indeed consulted.[75] In Tuchel's detailed examination of the publishing history of this book—which he summarizes as "a very successful piece of Mielke's politics of history" (*Mielke'scher Geschichtspolitik*)— he refers to criticism that Kuckhoff made of the first edition, and that was noted by the MfS: "Comrade Kuckhoff said that the historical facts are correctly portrayed, for the most part, but the people involved in the resistance fight must be portrayed 'more warmly' and their motives for participating in the resistance must be brought out more clearly. She refers particularly to the women who were illegally active in the organization."[76] It was clear from these comments that Kuckhoff had continued her strategy of positively noting that work was being done—while, at the same time, criticizing *how* it was being done.

Contested Commemoration

While Kuckhoff did her best to benefit from the increased publicity and interest in the group in the 1960s, she continued to work on what might be seen as a parallel but intersecting path of commemoration: writing, speaking, and sometimes successfully publishing work that contradicted the dominant narratives and instead emphasized the educational resistance work of the group. She also focused on why that was significant in terms of "anti-fascist" politics for contemporary Germany. She wrote articles for the East German journal *Die Weltbühne* on individual members of the group and on the importance of the Holocaust as a motivation for resistance.[77] In 1972, she published her autobiography, which went through several reprintings and translations,[78] and replied to dozens of letters by young people in the GDR and the Soviet Union in response to the group's increased public profile following the film and the appearance of her autobiography.[79] These diverse types of life-writing were forms of commemoration that she had already begun in the immediate postwar period (along with numerous speeches and radio broadcasts), and that she would continue to pursue until her death in 1981.[80] In all of these activities she challenged a reductive understanding of the resistance that incorrectly emphasized Communist leadership and insisted on the necessity of talking to people with diverse political beliefs. Despite enjoying some public success, Kuckhoff's letters suggested that she remained disillusioned by the official state response. In 1975 she wrote to Honecker, "Haven't we exaggerated the spying element? ... It already took long enough before we were able to shine a little light on the work of our comrades... But, in the meantime, many prejudices about 'spying' have taken root because of the many hostile texts that had been published in the interim."[81] She pleaded for a "proper" recognition of the group's work during the year marking the thirtieth anniversary since liberation.

These letters showed that Kuckhoff was continually challenging depictions of the resistance group on both sides of the so-called Iron Curtain. They provide further proof of the connections between the politics of remembering the Nazi past and anti-fascist resistance in both postwar German states, of the "osmotic and, at the same time, diffuse way in which the histories of the states were linked."[82] From a historiographic point of view, what is interesting is that the focus of the representations in the East and West on espionage marginalized the main work the group was involved in, namely, the writing and dissemination of anti-fascist leaflets and posters. Hans Coppi writes that this "form of educational activity (*Aufklärungstätigkeit*) was unthinkable for the intelligence service groups set up by Moscow in Western Europe because it was too dangerous."[83] Kuckhoff and her fellow resisters believed that such dangerous educational work would make it possible to awaken people to the horror of fascism, combat national and racial stereotypes, and form collaborative political projects for the future. It was a belief that many of the resisters paid for with their lives.

Kuckhoff's letters suggest that she remained convinced about the continued possibilities of such writing: that, by drawing on the supposed intimacy of the letter, she could persuade others using reasoned argument and thus shape the emerging historiography on resistance. Her efforts ultimately failed because her narrative did not fit within the polarized discourses of the Cold War, which, in their own ways, reiterated the original Nazi narrative. Since unification, work has been done to dismantle such monolithic interpretations and thus complicate this history.[84] But Kuckhoff's papers shows that there is still a wealth of information to be uncovered about the writing of anti-fascist resistance histories and that more consideration should be given to the individual and collective anti-fascist understandings that were subsequently built upon them. Life-writings, such as Kuckhoff's letters, are invaluable in this process because they focus attention on the ways in which certain memories became part of wider historical narratives. The rhetorical strategies they employ show how certain anti-fascisms were—or were not—"made sayable" within prevailing power relations in both postwar German states.

Kuckhoff's letters reiterated the fact that she supported the East German state, yet, at the same time, consistently challenged the way in which it represented anti-fascism. She was certainly in a privileged position that emboldened her to attempt to engage and persuade high-profile state and party figures in correspondence. Her political capital derived from her role in the anti-Nazi resistance and from her subsequent roles in the East German state apparatus. As such, her writings allow for a discussion of diverse forms of antifascism that continued through 1945 and beyond, and that are often not considered in contemporary discussions. Notwithstanding attempts since the mid 1990s to provide more differentiated narratives about the GDR, there is still a persistent reduction of anti-fascism to dominant SED discourse.[85] On the one hand, there are repeated claims about a complete lack of coalescence between official anti-fascist discourse and personal memory[86]—on the other, about the wholesale "unthinking" identification of GDR citizens with state anti-fascism as a way of avoiding guilt and any critical examination of the Nazi past.[87] Dismissing anti-fascism merely as a symptom of totalitarianism marginalizes the "points of resistance" that were, as the foregoing examination of Kuckhoff suggests, undoubtedly present.[88] As Helmut Peitsch points out, the historical commission headed by Martin Sabrow called for more research on "areas of individual self-determination" and "forms of identification" in the GDR.[89] On the basis of actual examples such as Kuckhoff's life-writings, it is possible "to ground" the debate about anti-fascism and thus provide an analysis that does not rely on an *ostalgic* backlash, or simply on an insistence on individual stories of success (*geglückte Privatbiographie*).[90] Kuckhoff did not succeed, in

Foucauldian terms, in reversing dominant anti-fascist discourse. But her writings provide traces of an anti-fascist "way of being" that challenged monolithic and reductive narratives about the past. This, in turn, helps to complicate and question the narratives of the present.

Suggested Readings

Barck, Simone. *Antifa-Geschichte(n). Eine literarische Spurensuche in der DDR der 1950er und 1960er Jahre.* Cologne, 2003.
Beattie, Andrew. *Playing Politics with History: The Bundestag Inquiries into East Germany.* New York, 2008.
Clarke, David and Ute Wölfel, eds. *20 Years On: Remembering the German Democratic Republic.* Basingstoke, 2011.
Claussen, Christoph. *Faschismus und Antifaschismus. Die nationalsozialistische Vergangenheit im ostdeutschen Hörfunk (1945-1953).* Cologne, 2004.
Coppi, Hans, Jürgen Danyel, and Johannes Tuchel, eds. *Die Rote Kapelle im Widerstand gegen den Nationalsozialismus.* Berlin, 1994.
Danyel, Jürgen. *Die geteilte Vergangenheit. Zum Umgang mit Nationalsozialismus und Widerstand in beiden deutschen Staaten.* Berlin, 1995.
Großbölting, Thomas, ed. *Friedensstaat, Leseland, Sportnation? DDR-Legenden auf dem Prüfstand.* Bonn, 2010.
Hook, Derek. "Discourse, Knowledge, Materiality, History: Foucault and Discourse Analysis." *Theory Psychology* 11 (2001): 521–47.
Foucault, Michel. *The Will to Knowledge: The History of Sexuality: Vol. One.* Trans. Robert Hurley. London, 1998.
Fraser, Nancy and Linda Gordon. "A Genealogy of Dependency: Tracing a Keyword of the U.S. Welfare State." *Signs* 19/2 (1994): 309–36.
Kendall, Gavin and Gary Wickham. *Using Foucault's Methods.* London, 2000.
Tuchel, Johannes, ed. *Der vergessene Widerstand. Zu Realgeschichte und Wahrnehmung des Kampfes gegen die NS-Diktatur.* Göttingen, 2005.
Weedon, Chris. *Feminist Practice & Poststructuralist Theory,* 2nd ed. Oxford, 2001.
Weisenborn, Günther. *Der lautlose Aufstand.* Hamburg, 1953.

Notes

1. Olaf Groehler, "Zelebrierter Antifaschismus," *Journal Geschichte* 5 (1990): 46–55; Dan Diner, "On the Ideology of Antifascism," trans. C. Bundermann, *New German Critique* 67 (1996): 123–32; Herfried Münkler, "Überholen ohne einzuholen. Deutsche Gründungserzählungen im Leistungsvergleich," *Blätter für deutsche und internationale Politik* 40 (1995): 1179–90; Raina Zimmering, *Mythen in der Politik der DDR* (Opladen, 2000); Birgit Müller, "Erinnerung in der DDR," *Dossier Geschichte und Erinnerung* (2008), Bundeszentrale für politische Bildung (http://www.bpb.de/themen/IBOVZC.html) (accessed 11 March 2010); Annette Leo, "Keine gemeinsame Erinnerung: Geschichtsbewusstsein in Ost und West," *Dossier Geschichte und Erinnerung* (2010), Bundeszentrale für politische Bildung (http://www.bpb.de/themen/JH31QR.html) (accessed 11 March 2010).

2. For a persuasive critique of this process, see Andrew Beattie, *Playing Politics with History: The Bundestag Inquiries into East Germany* (New York and Oxford, 2008).
3. For example, Corey Ross, *The East German Dictatorship: Problems and Perspectives in the Interpretation of the GDR* (London, 2002), 178–81.
4. This chapter is part of a larger project on Greta Kuckhoff, entitled *Reframing Antifascism: Genre, Memory and the Life Writings of Greta Kuckhoff* (forthcoming).
5. Hans Coppi, "Die 'Rote Kapelle' im Spannungsfeld von Widerstand und nachrichtendienstlicher Tätigkeit. Der Trepper-Report vom Juni 1943," *Vierteljahreshefte für Zeitgeschichte* 44/3 (1996): 436.
6. Michael Burleigh, *The Third Reich: A New History* (London, 2000), 671.
7. Hans Coppi, Jürgen Danyel, and John Tuchel, eds., *Die Rote Kapelle im Widerstand gegen den Nationalsozialismus* (Berlin, 1994).
8. Kuckhoff's "Nachlass," which is held at the Federal Archives (*Bundesarchiv*) in Berlin-Lichterfelde, is referred to in the following as BArch N2506. It was confiscated by the Stasi at the time of her death in 1981; the Federal Archives were recently able to bring together Kuckhoff's extensive papers and begin cataloguing them. This process was completed in April 2010. My thanks to archivist Ulf Rathje for his continued support during the course of my research.
9. Though the extent to which Foucault's work allows for a "criticalist" stance that emphasizes political utility is contested, I understand his writings in this way. See Derek Hook, "Discourse, Knowledge, Materiality, History: Foucault and Discourse Analysis," *Theory Psychology* 11 (2001): 522. See also Nancy Fraser and Linda Gordon, "A Genealogy of Dependency: Tracing a Keyword of the U.S. Welfare State," *Signs* 19/2 (1994): 310–11.
10. Joseph Rouse, "Power/Knowledge," in *The Cambridge Companion to Foucault*, ed. Gary Cutting (Cambridge, 2005), 111.
11. Gavin Kendall and Gary Wickham, *Using Foucault's Methods* (London, 2000), 123.
12. Chris Weedon, *Feminist Practice & Poststructuralist Theory*, 2nd ed. (Oxford, 2001), 105.
13. Rouse, "Power/Knowledge," 96.
14. Christoph Claussen, *Faschismus und Antifaschismus. Die nationalsozialistische Vergangenheit im ostdeutschen Hörfunk (1945-1953)* (Cologne, Weimar, and Vienna, 2004), 53.
15. Kendall and Wickham, *Using Foucault's Methods*, 49.
16. Rouse, "Power/Knowledge," 112.
17. Ibid.
18. Michel Foucault, *The Will to Knowledge: The History of Sexuality: Volume One*, trans. Robert Hurley (London, 1998), 92.
19. Martin Sabrow, "Geschichtskultur und Herrschaftslegitimation. Der Fall der DDR," in *Verwaltete Vergangenheit. Geschichtskultur und Herrschaftslegitimation in der DDR*, ed. Martin Sabrow (Leipzig, 1997), 11.
20. Claussen, *Faschismus und Antifaschismus*, 54.
21. Hook, "Discourse, Knowledge, Materiality, History," 527.
22. Foucault, *The Will to Knowledge*, 96.
23. Simone Barck, *Antifa-Geschichte(n): Eine literarische Spurensuche in der DDR der 1950er und 1960er Jahre* (Cologne, Weimar, and Vienna, 2003), 19.
24. Johannes Tuchel makes this point about the GDR, but the same can also be said for the Federal Republic. See Johannes Tuchel, "Das Ministerium für Staatssicherheit und

die Widerstandsgruppe 'Rote Kapelle' in den 1960er Jahren," in *Der vergessene Widerstand. Zu Realgeschichte und Wahrnehmung des Kampfes gegen die NS-Diktatur*, ed. Johannes Tuchel (Göttingen, 2005), 256.
25. BArch N2506/63, Report by Kuckhoff, n.d.
26. BArch 2506/31, Wilhelm Flicke to Greta Kuckhoff, 27 April 1947; BArch N2506/30, Greta Kuckhoff to Franz Dahlem, 15 June 1949.
27. BArch 2506/31, Wilhelm Flicke to Greta Kuckhoff, 27 April 1947.
28. BArch N2506/31, Greta Kuckhoff to Wilhelm Flicke, 28 March 1947.
29. Ibid.
30. BArch N2506/31, Greta Kuckhoff to Wilhelm Flicke, 30 June 1947.
31. Allen Welsh Dulles, *Germany's Underground* (New York, 1947).
32. BArch N2506/35, Greta Kuckhoff to Gerhard Köster, 22 September 1949.
33. Dulles *Germany's Underground*, 100–101.
34. Wilhelm Flicke, *Spionagegruppe Rote Kapelle. In freier Bearbeitung den Tatsachen nacherzählt* (Kreuzlingen, 1949).
35. BArch N2506/30, Greta Kuckhoff to Franz Dahlem, 15 June 1949.
36. BArch N2506/30, Franz Dahlem to Greta Kuckhoff, 23 June 1949 and subsequent undated letter.
37. Klaus Lehmann, *Widerstandsgruppe Schulze-Boysen/Harnack* (Berlin, 1948). There is a copy of this in Kuckhoff's papers, but no indication of what she thought about the text. It profiles only the men in the group. See also Rudolf Pechel, *Deutscher Widerstand* (Zurich, 1947).
38. Coppi, "Die Rote Kapelle im Spannungsfeld," 434.
39. Hans Coppi and Geertje Andresen, eds., *Dieser Tod paßt zu mir. Harro Schulze-Boysen—Grenzgänger im Widerstand. Briefe 1915-1942* (Berlin, 2002), 11.
40. "Das Geheimnis der Roten Kapelle," *Der Fortschritt* (1950); "Rote Agenten unter uns," *Der Stern* (6 May 1951–1 July 1951). No authors are named in the bylines of these articles. Friends of Kuckhoff sent her the articles, copies of which are preserved in BArch N2506/55.
41. Manfred Roeder, *Die Rote Kapelle. Aufzeichnungen des Generalrichters Dr. M. Roeder* (Hamburg, 1952); Gerhard Ritter, *Carl Goerdeler und die deutsche Widerstandsbewegung* (Stuttgart, 1954). There is a damning report in Kuckhoff's papers about this book; it was presumably written by Kuckhoff. See BArch N2506/299, "Betrifft: Goerdeler-Buch von Prof. Ritter," n.d.; David Dallin, *Die Sowjetspionage. Prinzipien und Praktiken* (Cologne, 1956).
42. Günther Weisenborn, *Der lautlose Aufstand* (Hamburg, 1953).
43. There is an extensive correspondence between the two in BArch N2506/59.
44. BArch N2506/34, Armin Gerd-Kuckhoff to Greta Kuckhoff, 17 July 1951, and Kuckhoff to Gerd-Kuckhoff, 25 July 1951; BArch N2506/262, Greta Kuckhoff to Mathilde Hell, 16 August 1951.
45. For an extended discussion of this letter see Joanne Sayner, "Verehrter Gen. Ulbricht: Negotiations of Self and Socialist Identity in Greta Kuckhoff's Letters," in *The Self in Transition: East German Autobiographical Narratives*, ed. David Clarke and Axel Goodbody (Amsterdam, 2012).
46. Walter Ulbricht, *Zur Geschichte der neuesten Zeit* (Berlin, 1955), 18–33.
47. BArch N2506/58, Greta Kuckhoff to Walter Ulbricht, 1955.
48. Wilhelm Flicke, *Agenten funken nach Moskau* (Wels, 1957).
49. BArch N2506/56, Victor Alexandrov to Julius Mader, 9 November 1965.

50. Walter A. Schmidt, *"Damit Deutschland lebe". Ein Quellenwerk über den deutschen antifaschistischen Widerstandkampfes 1933-1945* (Berlin, 1958). This text reproduces extracts from Lehmann's book, along with additional biographical information.
51. These are collated in BArch Sg Y4/V1/15, Ruth Seydewitz, *Wo das Leben ist* (Berlin, 1956); *Zur Geschichte der deutschen antifaschistischen Widerstandsbewegung 1933-1945. Eine Auswahl von Materialien, Berichten und Dokumenten* (Berlin, 1958); Heinrich Scheel, "Die Rolle der Befreiungskriege in der illegalen Widerstandsliteratur—Dargestellt am Beispiel der Widerstandsgruppe Schulze-Boysen/Harnack und 'Innere Front,'" in *"Das Jahr 1813". Studien zur Geschichte und Wirkung der Befreiungskriege* (Berlin, 1963); Carlheinz von Brück, *Im Namen der Menschlichkeit. Bürger gegen Hitler* (Berlin, 1964).
52. BArch N2505/199, Greta Kuckhoff to Hermann Mattern [sic], 10 September 1964; BArch N2506/199, Greta Kuckhoff to Albert Norden, 25 December 1964.
53. BArch N2506/28, Greta Kuckhoff to Lew Besymenski, 12 December 1965.
54. Tuchel, "Das Ministerium für Staatssicherheit," 235.
55. Ibid., 236. For further details on Kuckhoff's contact with the MfS, see Sayner, *Reframing Antifascism*.
56. BArch N2506/33, Greta Kuckhoff to Erich Honecker, 15 October 1965.
57. BArch N2506/33, Greta Kuckhoff to Erich Honecker, 6 December 1965.
58. Coppi and Andresen, *Dieser Tod*, 14; see also Tuchel, "Das Ministerium für Staatssicherheit," 234.
59. Wilfried Martini, "Deutsche Spionage für Moskau 1939 bis 1945," Parts I–XI, *Die Welt*, October 1966.
60. Wilfried Martini, "Meine Sekretärin, die Geheimagentin. Ein Funkspruch entlarvte Ilse Stöbes Verbindung zur 'Roten Kapelle,'" *Die Welt*, 15 October 1966.
61. Wilfried Martini, "Wer dirigierte die 'Red Orchestra'? Trotz unzulänglicher Voraussetzungen arbeitete der Agentenring lange Zeit unbehelligt," *Die Welt*, 17 October 1966.
62. Wilfried Martini, "Aufrecht ging die Agentin zur Guillotine. Das Ende der 'Roten Kapelle'—Die Vierte Abteilung in Westeuropa," *Die Welt*, 18 October 1966.
63. BArch N2506/273, Marc Spangenberg to Kuckhoff, 17 November 1966, and Kuckhoff to Spangenberg, 19 November 1966.
64. Giles Perrault, *L'Orchestre rouge* (Paris, 1967).
65. Heinz Höhne, "'ptx ruft moskau—'. Die Geschichte der Roten Kapelle," *Der Spiegel* 23–30 (1968); *Kennwort Direktor. Die Geschichte der Roten Kapelle* (Frankfurt am Main, 1970).
66. Coppi and Andresen, *Dieser Tod*, 18.
67. BArch N2506/53, Greta Kuckhoff to "Redaktion" at *Der Spiegel*, 12 June 1968.
68. BArch N2506/52, Heinz Höhne to Greta Kuckhoff, 4 July 1968.
69. Coppi, "Die "Rote Kapelle" im Spannungsfeld," 431–58.
70. Ingeborg Drewitz, *Leben und Werk von Adam Kuckhoff. Deutscher Schriftsteller und Widerstandskämpfer hingerichtet durch den Strang in Berlin-Plötzensee am 5. August 1943* (Berlin, 1968).
71. The correspondence between Kuckhoff and Drewitz can be found in BArch N2506/30.
72. Drewitz, *Leben und Werk*, 4.
73. Tuchel, "Das Ministerium für Staatssicherheit," 255.
74. See Sayner, *Reframing Antifascism*.

75. Karlheinz Biernat and Luise Kraushaar, *Die Schulze-Boysen/Harnack-Organisation im antifaschistischen Kampf*, ed. Institut für Marxismus-Leninismus beim ZK der SED (Berlin, 1970).
76. Tuchel, "Das Ministerium für Staatssicherheit," 260.
77. Joanne Sayner, "Living Antifascism: Greta Kuckhoff's Writings in *Die Weltbühne*," in *Writing Under Socialism*, ed. Meesha Nehru and Sara Jones (Nottingham, 2011), 50–70.
78. Joanne Sayner, *Women without a Past? German Autobiographical Writings and Fascism* (Amsterdam and New York, 2007).
79. BArch N2506/98.
80. Joanne Sayner, "The Organic Intellectual: The Public and Political Impact of Greta Kuckhoff 1945-1949," in *Cultural Impact: Studies in Transmission, Reception and Influence*, ed. R. Braun and L. Marvyn (Rochester, N.Y., 2010), 227–43.
81. BArch N2506/33, Greta Kuckhoff to Erich Honecker, 16 March 1975.
82. Barck, 11; Jürgen Danyel, ed., *Die geteilte Vergangenheit. Zum Umgang mit Nationalsozialismus und Widerstand in beiden deutschen Staaten* (Berlin, 1995); Jeffrey Herf, *Divided Memory: The Nazi Past in the Two Germanys* (Cambridge, M.A., 1997); *Deutsche Vergangenheiten—eine gemeinsame Herausforderung. Der schwierige Umgang mit der doppelten Nachkriegsgeschichte*, ed. Christoph Kleßmann et al. (Berlin, 1999).
83. Coppi, "Die 'Rote Kapelle' im Spannungsfeld," 437.
84. Coppi, Danyel, and Tuchel, eds., *Die Rote Kapelle im Widerstand*.
85. As discussed in Beattie, *Playing Politics with History*.
86. Münkler, "Überholen ohne einzuholen"; Herfried Münkler, "Das kollektive Gedächtnis der DDR," in *Parteiauftrag. Ein neues Deutschland. Bilder, Rituale und Symbole der frühen DDR*, ed. Dieter Vorsteher (Berlin and Munich, 1996), 458–68; Monika Flacke, ed. *Mythen der Nationen. 1945—Arena der Erinnerungen*, vol. 1.2 (Berlin, 2004), cited in Helmut Peitsch, "How Memory is Remembered: The Potsdam Memory Archive 1995-96," in *20 Years On: Remembering the German Democratic Republic*, ed. David Clarke and Ute Wölfel (Basingstoke, 2011), 357–84.
87. Leo, "Keine gemeinsame Erinnerung."
88. Foucault, *The Will to Knowledge*, 96.
89. Peitsch, "How Memory is Remembered," 357–59.
90. Thomas Großbölting, "DDR-Legenden in der Erinnerungskultur und in der Wissenschaft. Eine Einleitung," in *Friedensstaat, Leseland, Sportnation? DDR-Legenden auf dem Prüfstand*, ed. Thomas Großbölting (Bonn, 2010), 19, 22.

CHAPTER 4

Remembered Change and Changes of Remembrance
East German Narratives of Anti-fascist Conversion

CHRISTIANE WIENAND

In the aftermath of World War II, the new political rulers in the Soviet Zone of Occupation (SBZ) and in the early German Democratic Republic (GDR) not only contended with social and economic disarray, but also faced the question of how to deal with the Nazi past and those Germans living under their rule. Anti-fascism became a central ideological framework—a "founding myth" of the East German state—and a "central component of East German political culture" that was meant to contribute to the legitimization of the new political regime and to the integration of ordinary East Germans into the new political order.[1] Anti-fascist discourse was closely connected with Communist resistance against the Nazi regime, and anti-fascist Communist resistance fighters such as Ernst Thälmann were propagated as new heroes, as "saints of socialism."[2] Besides these widely told Communist anti-fascist stories, there was also a parallel, though less prominent, anti-fascist discourse that centered upon so-called anti-fascist returned Prisoners of War (POW) who claimed to have undergone an anti-fascist conversion during their captivity in the Soviet Union.[3]

The experience of war captivity shaped the memories and narrations of the past of those who returned to Germany.[4] The various narratives about captivity and subsequent return were not only produced by returned soldiers themselves, but also found expression in public representations of anti-fascist returnees in East and West Germany. One of those narratives concerned anti-fascist conversion during war captivity in the Soviet Union. In the Federal Republic, this narrative was declared to be a myth, and its protagonists were often publicly denounced early on as *Vaterlandsverräter* (traitors to the Fatherland). In contrast, the narrative of anti-fascist conversion played a significant role in official memory culture in the GDR, and was used by former Wehrmacht soldiers who sought to integrate themselves into the East German Socialist state after their return. The collapse of the GDR regime in 1989 also affected the ways in which former POWs used the anti-fascist conversion narrative in their memories, as well as the way in which the narrative was publicly dealt with in the memory culture (*Erinnerungskultur*) of unified Germany.

This essay examines the narrative of anti-fascist conversion in memories of East German POW returnees by exploring one specific case in depth. The analysis places this narrative into its historical and cultural contexts while considering the German-German perspective and taking into account the long-term impact of World War II. Based on this empirical analysis, the essay looks at how historical agents tried to deal with and make sense of the two main political and societal transformations in contemporary German history: the end of the Nazi regime in 1945 and the breakdown of the GDR state in 1989. It shows how East German returnees adopted the officially sanctioned anti-fascist narrative in order to convey their own subjective experiences of the past; this, in turn, produced individual narrations that adapted and manipulated the "established" collective narrative for personal ends.

Anti-fascist Stories in East Germany

The GDR regime and the state-controlled mass media developed a specific interest in those returning *Wehrmacht* soldiers who claimed to have experienced an anti-fascist conversion during Soviet captivity. Anti-fascist returnees could be presented by the regime as *Neue Menschen* (new men) who had returned from the USSR as friends of the Soviets, and who could help build up the new Socialist state. Anti-fascist returnees and the narrative of anti-fascist conversion fit perfectly into the wider ideological framework of the anti-fascist founding myth of the GDR and the narrative of German-Soviet friendship.[5] Within this discourse war captivity was perceived as an *Universität des Lebens* (university of life) that had fostered "the reeducation of former POWs, tainted by fascist ideology, into new men, into builders of a truly democratic and peace loving Germany."[6] The regime's interest in anti-fascist returnees was part of a wider political strategy to integrate ordinary Germans, including former members of the NSDAP, into the East German state.[7] As Frank Biess has shown in his study of returnees in the first postwar decade, the narrative of anti-fascist conversion during Soviet captivity appeared from 1948 onward in the official speeches and writings of SED functionaries.[8] This narrative also offered individual returnees the possibility of integrating themselves smoothly into the new ideological and political climate.[9] At the same time, Biess explores the discrepancies between the promotion of anti-fascist returnees as ideal citizens and existing social reality when he discusses the resentment felt by ordinary East

Germans against this anti-fascist interpretation of their experiences in Soviet war captivity.[10]

Who were these anti-fascist returnees, and upon what experiences did they ground their claim to have experienced an anti-fascist transformation during Soviet captivity? During World War II, the Soviets established "antifa schools" in which they sought to reeducate German POWs.[11] After the battle of Stalingrad in the winter of 1942–43, several high-ranking officers of the Wehrmacht and ordinary soldiers joined German Communists living in Soviet exile to found the *Nationalkomitee Freies Deutschland* (National Committee for a Free Germany).[12] The *Nationalkomitee* regarded itself as a resistance group against Adolf Hitler's regime, and in 1943 it published a manifesto in which it appealed to the German people to end the war and instead build a free and democratic Germany. The members of the *Nationalkomitee* were also involved in various propaganda activities aimed at German combatants. The *Nationalkomitee* was dissolved in the fall of 1945, yet the Soviets continued their reeducation efforts by establishing anti-fascist committees and a system of antifa schools in the POW camps.[13]

Among the anti-fascist returnees were those who had been members of the *Nationalkomitee* and those who had attended antifa schools during the war, as well as returnees who first affiliated themselves with the antifa committees in the camps or attended antifa schools only after German capitulation.[14] What connects all of these returnees is their later claim to have experienced an anti-fascist transformation during captivity. Some of the anti-fascist returnees became publicly known in the GDR as they made careers as party functionaries or in the East German army, the *Nationale Volksarmee* (National People's Army, or NVA).[15]

The narrative of anti-fascist conversion was propagated throughout the GDR after the war and reappeared in various forms in public accounts. It appeared, for instance, in popular East German TV films such as *Gewissen in Aufruhr* (Conscience in Turmoil) and the 1970s trilogy *Heimkehr in ein fremdes Land* (Return to a Foreign Country). *Gewissen in Aufruhr* was a successful 1961 film adaptation of the widely read memoirs of Rudolf Petershagen, a decorated Wehrmacht officer. The renowned East German actor Erwin Geschonneck played the lead role of Joachim Ebershagen, who reevaluated his National Socialist beliefs during Soviet captivity.[16] While Petershagen/Ebershagen represents an elderly bourgeois former Wehrmacht officer who successfully integrated himself into the postwar Socialist state, the main character of *Heimkehr in ein fremdes Land* represents a generation of East Germans who were still young when they returned from captivity.[17] These young anti-fascist returnees, embodied in the film by the character Martin Stein, were portrayed as those who actively helped to build a new Socialist society.[18] *Gewissen in Aufruhr* was the film adaption of a published autobiography, while *Heimkehr in ein fremdes Land* was based on an autobiographical novel published by Günter Görlich in 1974. Anti-fascist conversion also became a literary topos in a specific type of autobiographical GDR fiction. Well-known authors such as Hermann Kant and Franz Fühmann exemplified this branch of GDR literature.[19]

Besides East German film and fictional literature, autobiographical *Erinnerungsliteratur* (memoir literature) also featured the topos of the anti-fascist conversion. Several of these autobiographies were published by the East German publisher *Verlag der Nation*, the publishing house of the National Democratic Party (NDPD), a "block" party created as a way in which to integrate former Nazis and members of the Wehrmacht into the East German party system. The *Verlag der Nation* soon established itself as a forum for so-called *spezifische Wandlungsliteratur*, i.e., literature that thematized the anti-fascist conversion process of the middle classes, of the bourgeois intelligentsia, and of former members of the NSDAP and the Wehrmacht.[20] In the years 1966, 1968, and 1976, the *Verlag der Nation* held advisory meetings with authors, historians, and journalists to discuss the specific requirements for writing and publishing *Wandlungsliteratur*.[21] The publisher's agenda was best exemplified by its *autobiographisch-biographische Reihe* (autobiographical-biographical series), which began with the autobiography of Rudolf Petershagen in 1957. During the 1960s, the *Verlag der Nation* and other East German publishers released autobiographies written by other anti-fascist returnees, who were mainly former members of the *Nationalkomitee Freies Deutschland* and its officers' association, the *Bund deutscher Offiziere* (League of German Officers). The best-known autobiographies were the ones written by Wilhelm Adam, Egbert von Frankenberg, Otto Rühle, and Luitpold Steidle.[22]

Under SED leader Walter Ulbricht, the *Nationalkomitee Freies Deutschland* gained the status of a resistance organization, one whose founding anniversary was publicly celebrated each year. Former members were treated as anti-Nazi resistance fighters, and received tributes and honorary pensions. During the Ulbricht years, the *Nationalkomitee* and its manifesto were regarded as a major ideological precursor of the GDR and the East German constitution.[23] According to Julia Warth, the ways in which the *Nationalkomitee* was honored during the early decades of the GDR constituted a "politicized historical (*geschichtspolitischer*) myth of the Ulbricht era."[24] After Erich Honecker succeeded Ulbricht, anti-fascist returnees ceased to be a focus of national narratives. Under Honecker, in fact, the *Nationalkomitee* lost its importance as a resistance organization; the new focus was placed on Communist resistance in Germany itself, to which Honecker had belonged.[25] That shift became manifest in 1971 with the dissolution of the *Arbeitsgemeinschaft ehemaliger Offiziere* (Working Group of Former Officers); this had been an established forum for exchange among anti-fascist returnees.[26]

Despite this shift, the *Verlag der Nation* continued to publish autobiographical accounts of anti-fascist returnees. One of these was Bernt von Kügelgen's *Die Nacht der Entscheidung. Erinnerungen an Familie und Jugend* (The Night of Decision: Memories of Family and Youth), which was published in 1983; a second edition appeared in 1985, and the autobiography reached circulation figures of more than 20,000 copies.[27] In 1984, it appeared in West Germany with Pahl Rugenstein in Cologne.[28] Kügelgen's book is characteristic of the ways in which Soviet war captivity and its impact was publicly remembered in the GDR with reference to the anti-fascist conversion narrative.[29] In various letters and private documents written after unification in 1990, Kügelgen reevaluated his autobiography and his self-understanding as an anti-fascist returnee. The case of Bernt von Kügelgen demonstrates in detail the ways in which an anti-fascist returnee referred to the publicly sanctioned collective narrative of war captivity—the anti-fascist conversion narrative—and, at the same time, how he could make individual use of this narrative and his memories to serve his own personal ends. As we shall see in the next section, Kügelgen's autobiographical account, together with his private papers, provides important autobiographical source material allowing for a detailed analysis of this essay's central questions.[30]

Remembered Changes: Bernt von Kügelgen and His Anti-fascist Conversion

Bernt von Kügelgen was born in St. Petersburg in 1914 into an aristocratic German-Baltic family. He was captured near Demjansk in July 1942 while serving as a *Feldwebel* (sergeant) in the Wehrmacht. In the winter of 1942, he publicly declared himself an anti-fascist on the notice board in his POW camp. Kügelgen later joined the *Nationalkomitee Freies Deutschland*, worked as a so-called *Frontbeauftragter* (person who tried to convince German soldiers fighting on the front to surrender), and then returned to Berlin in August 1945. In the GDR Kügelgen joined the Communist Party (KPD), and later became a member of the SED; he pursued a career as a journalist and cultural functionary, for which he received high official honors.[31] Unlike other Wehrmacht officers and soldiers who also claimed to have undergone an anti-fascist conversion during war captivity, Kügelgen did not join the East German army or the NDPD. He stayed in contact with fellow former POWs through his active engagement in the *Komitee der antifaschistischen Widerstandskämpfer* (Committee of Anti-fascist Resistance Fighters) and as vice-president of the *Arbeitsgemeinschaft ehemaliger Offiziere*.

From 1957 to 1976 he served as editor-in-chief of the weekly newspaper *Sonntag*, and, beginning in 1968, worked for the Ministry for State Security as an *Inoffizieller Mitarbeiter* (informant) with the code name *Wilhelm*.[32] Kügelgen was a respected person in the GDR and, at times, much in demand as a wartime witness and former member of the *Nationalkomitee*. When the regime planned to celebrate the twenty-fifth anniversary of the *Nationalkomitee*'s creation, Kügelgen helped conceive the commemorative exhibition.[33] In the late 1980s, he was even interviewed in the West German documentary *Man nannte sie Verräter* (They were called Traitors) and invited to speak at a conference about the *Nationalkomitee* organized by the Protestant Academy of West Berlin.

Bernt von Kügelgen wrote his autobiography after retiring as editor of *Sonntag*, and at a time when he was increasingly dissatisfied about the way in which the *Nationalkomitee* was treated in official GDR memory culture under Honecker.[34] Not only was there less interest in the *Nationalkomitee*, but also a shift in official GDR memory culture in the late 1970s and early 1980s toward commemorating formerly neglected topics, groups, and dates, such as the November 1938 pogrom (*Kristallnacht*, or Night of Broken Glass) and the conspiracy of 20 July 1944.[35] Kügelgen apparently experienced the diminishing public attention given to the *Nationalkomitee* as a vilification of his past and of his self-understanding as an anti-fascist returnee and former resistance fighter. The fact that Kügelgen was dissatisfied with the way the *Nationalkomitee* and its members were officially commemorated was also a reason to demand—in vain—the publication of a third edition of his autobiography.[36]

In his autobiography Kügelgen describes his transformation and conversion from a nonpolitical *Mitläufer* (follower) of the Nazi regime into an anti-fascist and a Communist. His description contains many of the same basic features that appear in other anti-fascist conversion stories and that constitute a wider narrative of anti-fascist conversion.

Kügelgen's captivity constitutes the narrative framework and the starting point for the book. From time to time he interrupts his narration with flashbacks to his family history. Both storylines, the war captivity and his family history, culminate in a *Nacht der Entscheidung* (Night of Decision) in the officers' camp of Oranki, where he declared himself an anti-fascist.[37] In his autobiography he describes the decision to become an anti-fascist, and later a Communist, as a result of several complex stages of reflection and realization. According to his account, the first step of his conversion was a commitment to anti-fascism and a sense of enmity toward Hitler. In a second step taken while still in captivity, he began to sympathize with Socialist ideas and became a friend of the Soviets and the Soviet Union. The third step was Kügelgen's transformation into a Communist, a step that became manifest when he joined the KPD after returning to Berlin. According to Kügelgen, the decisive point in declaring himself an anti-fascist was the realization that the Wehrmacht had waged a criminal war of aggression. He came to this realization during interrogations with Soviet officers and by reading anti-fascist avowals by other German POWs.[38] He also mentions reading books by Vladimir Lenin and Joseph Stalin that served as an intellectual catalyst for this transformation process.[39] Kügelen refers as well to the insights he gained at the antifa school in Krasnogorsk and to the personal encounters he had with Soviet civilians and Soviet colleagues working as a *Frontbeauftragter*.[40] Finally, he mentions the esteem he felt for the patriotism exhibited by exiled German Communists he met during his imprisonment. Kügelgen not only connects the process of conversion to his experiences in captivity, but also emphasizes the way in which he could link these new ideas to his family's democratic beliefs prior to 1933.

The autobiography also recounts several obstacles that Kügelgen had to overcome on his way to becoming an anti-fascist. The most important one was the oath of allegiance that he and all German soldiers had personally sworn to Hitler.[41] The Soviets knew about the moral problems the oath created for German POWs, which led them to publish and distribute a pamphlet entitled *Manneswort eines deutschen Hauptmanns* (The Word of Honor of a German Captain). Written by Wehrmacht officer Ernst Hadermann, it argues that the oath was no longer binding for German soldiers, for it had been sworn not to Hitler personally, but to him as leader of the German people, a position he had—according to Hadermann—forfeited. For Kügelgen as well as other anti-fascist returnees such as Otto Rühle, Hadermann's text represented a way in which to overcome the moral bond forged by the oath.[42] Kügelgen's decision to join the *Nationalkomitee Freies Deutschland* was not part of the conversion process, but rather the expression of a conversion that had already taken place.

All in all, Kügelgen describes his conversion not as a radical change, but as a *process* in which he was able to sort out "the mosaic of reality."[43] This description of anti-fascist conversion as a process consisting of several elements and obstacles was an important narrative tool used to explain and legitimize his conversion to his readers. It was also in accordance with the requirements of the publishing house, which explicitly told its authors not to pass over conflicts they experienced along the path to anti-fascism.[44] Even though Kügelgen's autobiographical text belonged to the tradition of anti-fascist memory literature in the GDR, he explicitly distinguished himself from other anti-fascist returnees and his own work from other published autobiographies by representing himself as a member of a younger generation—a generation that was open to the new ideologies learned during war captivity, a generation that could thereby serve as a new elite for the Socialist GDR.[45]

Kügelgen's autobiography contains another narrative strand besides that of his anti-fascist transformation, namely, his family history. By choosing *Erinnerungen an Familie und Jugend* (Memories of Family and Youth) as the subtitle for his book, he explicitly referred to the memoirs of his ancestor Wilhelm von Kügelgen: *Jugenderinnerungen eines Alten Mannes* (Memories of Youth by an

Old Man), a classic work of humanist writing published in 1870. Through his choices for the subtitle and cover of his autobiography (a photo of his birthplace, St. Petersburg), as well as through the narrative flashbacks to his family history, Kügelgen explicitly emphasized his bourgeois family origins. By doing so, he stylized himself as a representative of the humanistic tradition—a tradition the GDR regime proudly embraced at the time the book appeared.[46] By making these various references to his family background, in his autobiography Kügelgen managed to combine his aristocratic-bourgeois family tradition with his anti-fascist Communist thinking—thus constituting and emphasizing his postwar identity as an anti-fascist returnee of aristocratic-bourgeois origin who represented a successful alliance between anti-fascism and the bourgeoisie. This offered readers from a similar bourgeois background an opportunity to identify themselves with the ideas propagated in his own autobiography.[47]

Kügelgen's memoirs fit officially sanctioned narratives of the past, including the anti-fascist conversion narrative and the idea of German-Soviet friendship—not only in terms of content, but also in terms of the style and language he chose. Written like a novel with direct speech and a first-person narrator, his account belonged to the existing tradition of autobiographies already published by other anti-fascist returnees.[48] But despite the similarity of narrative patterns and language, Kügelgen's description of his conversion demonstrates the way in which he also used his autobiography to serve his own ends and personal interests, i.e., to propagate his own self-understanding of his identity as an anti-fascist returnee—an anti-fascist returnee with a bourgeois background whose autobiography represents a continuation of his family tradition.[49]

GDR newspapers and journals praised Kügelgen's account of his anti-fascist conversion. Most East German reviewers, who referred to his anti-fascist conversion not so much as a political change, but rather as an intellectual change, used various terms to describe Kügelgen's narration: *Umdenken* (rethinking), *Frontenwechsel* (change of fronts), *weltanschaulicher Prozess des Anderswerdens* (ideological process of becoming different), *Entscheidung für den Fortschritt* (decision for progress), and even *Wieder- und Neugeburt des Menschlichen* (being born again or born anew).[50] The religious term *Bekehrung* (conversion) was used as well to describe his anti-fascist transformation.[51] In this way, the reviewers followed Kügelgen's own interpretation of his autobiography and his self-presentation as a representative of the humanist tradition. The tenor of the reviews suggested furthermore that anti-fascist conversion stories such as Kügelgen's were no longer regarded primarily in political terms, but rather as part of a specifically East German way of culturally dealing with the past—a way that did not need to be further legitimized or explained. Kügelgen himself saw his memoir as a political book and as a contribution to the "propagandistic fight of the cross-border media."[52] East German reviewers considered this an anachronistic attitude, for, in their opinion, there was no longer a need to continue an ideological discussion with the West by referring to anti-fascist conversion.

Contesting Change: Narratives about Returnees in the Federal Republic

In contrast to the reception in the GDR, West German reviewers and members of the Kügelgen family in the Federal Republic struggled in particular with his transformation story and its political-ideological undertones.[53] Letters from West German readers expressed differing opinions about Kügelgen's autobiography, running the gamut from severe criticism to strong approval of his story.[54] Some of the West German reception employed the type of Cold War rhetoric typical of West German discourse in the 1950s and 1960s about war captivity in the East, one in which anti-fascist returnees like Kügelgen were seen as opportunists and *Russenknechte* (servants of the Russians). In a review for the newspaper *Die Welt*, for instance, Enno von Löwenstern accused Kügelgen of opportunism, of collaboration with the Soviets, and of obscuring the Communist nature of the *Nationalkomitee*.[55]

The Cold War climate influenced the ways in which East and West Germans regarded and evaluated each other, particularly with respect to the diverging ways in which they dealt with the National Socialist past and its aftermath. The conversion of former Nazis and *Mitläufer* into democrats was a publically accepted narrative in West German society.[56] In fact, various types of democratic conversion stories involving former POWs flourished in the Federal Republic.[57] Many West Germans were at least skeptical, however, about narrations that described conversions to anti-fascism or even socialism and communism. And while anti-fascism was established as *the* crucial narrative in East Germany, an anti-Communist attitude was widespread in the West German public sphere—an attitude that influenced the narratives about the experiences of German soldiers who had returned from Soviet captivity. In addition to the West German media, West German veterans' associations, such as the *Verband der Heimkehrer, Kriegsgefangenen und Vermisstenangehörigen e.V.* (Association of Returnees, POWs and Family Members of MIAs), helped forge an image of Soviet captivity based on anti-Communist sentiment.[58] In contrast to East Germany, where the positive experience of an anti-fascist transformation became the central narrative of Soviet captivity, the bulk of West German narratives focused on the negative aspects of their experiences in the Soviet Union, such as starvation, hard labor, and disease.[59]

In a series of trials against POWs accused of having maltreated fellow prisoners (the so-called *Kameradenschinderprozesse*), which took place in the

Federal Republic between 1949 and 1964, some returnees were accused of criminal acts directly connected to their activities in anti-fascist groups during war captivity, or to their membership in the *Nationalkomitee*.[60] Members of the latter who returned to West Germany—such as the former Wehrmacht general Walther von Seydlitz-Kurzbach, who had served as vice-president of the committee—were publicly denounced in the 1950s and 1960s as traitors to the country and their comrades.[61] Some former members of the *Nationalkomitee* living in West Germany, such as the future ambassador to Israel Jesco von Puttkamer, even used their autobiographies to criticize the committee, as well as the reeducation efforts that had taken place in the Soviet camps.[62]

Only gradually did West German historians and the West German media assume a more nuanced attitude toward those who had opposed the Nazi regime during war captivity, especially those who had been members of the *Nationalkomitee*. By the 1980s, when Bernt von Kügelgen's autobiography was published, the language in which the *Nationalkomitee* was described in West Germany had become less ideologically aggressive when compared to the harsh Cold War rhetoric of the 1950s and 1960s.[63] In early 1989, West Germans vehemently debated whether the *Nationalkomitee* should be a part of the permanent exhibition of the *Gedenkstätte Deutscher Widerstand* (German Resistance Memorial) in Berlin. In the course of this debate, various arguments and criticisms developed over the previous decades were once again raised against the members of the *Nationalkomitee*: they had broken their solemn oath of allegiance and had endangered their families and friends back home. They had joined the *Nationalkomitee* out of sheer opportunism. What they had done did not really count as resistance because they had been on safe ground as German POWs in the Soviet Union. And, finally, to acknowledge the *Nationalkomitee* as a resistance group would be tantamount to honoring an autocrat like Walter Ulbricht as a resistance fighter.[64] The debate was also shaped by an academic conference organized in 1989 by the Protestant church in Berlin, as well as by two documentaries from 1989: *Roter Stern und Stacheldraht* (Red Star and Barbed Wire) and *Man nannte sie Verräter* (They Were Called Traitors), which attempted to examine the *Nationalkomitee* and its former members from a more neutral perspective.

Changes of Remembrance: Memories of Anti-fascist Returnees after 1989–90

The version of Bernt von Kügelgen's autobiography published in the GDR in 1983 and one year later in the Federal Republic was the product of various interests and agents. Kügelgen anticipated the reactions of his readers by including an explanatory part dealing with his oath of loyalty to Hitler. He followed the guidelines of the publishing house and of the two reviewers.[65] He took up familiar narrative patterns, including the anti-fascist conversion narrative, the narrative of German-Soviet friendship, as well as the narrative of a successful alliance between anti-fascism and the bourgeoisie. Finally, he combined his anti-fascist conversion story with a history of his family. Kügelgen adopted the anti-fascist conversion narrative, but adapted it to his personal needs and interests in order to create and sustain a specific postwar identity as an anti-fascist returnee living in the GDR. His anti-fascist conversion in Soviet captivity therefore constituted a foundation allowing for his self-understanding as a GDR citizen. It was only after reunification that Kügelgen began to question and even revise parts of this narrative.

Kügelgen soon realized that the fundamental political changes that took place following the collapse of the GDR limited his opportunities to reach the German public. He nevertheless continued his efforts to publish a revised version of his autobiography. The intended audience was the West German public, which, he believed, would have different attitudes about his conversion than those of his former East German readership: "It may be," Kügelgen conceded in a 1993 letter, "that those passages were too heavily focused on a GDR readership and that a reader who comes from a completely different social and political environment cannot thoroughly comprehend everything."[66] In a letter to American historian Arthur L. Smith, Kügelgen stated that his autobiography should be regarded as a product from a time in which he still believed in the "viability of Socialism."[67] Both statements indicate Kügelgen's awareness that the context in which he had written his autobiography had influenced how he interpreted and narrated the past.

Kügelgen developed several ideas for revising his autobiography, but did not do so in the end. He had intended to be more critical of the antifa school he had attended during his captivity and which, as he wrote in several letters between 1993 and 1999, had provided him with a highly idealized image of the Soviet Union.[68] He had also intended to add a "detailed footnote" about the crimes committed by Stalin, whom he had praised in his 1983 autobiography.[69] In a letter to a West German schoolteacher in 1999, Kügelgen justified his earlier beliefs and actions, claiming that when he was writing his autobiography in the early 1980s, he had drawn on his knowledge at the time of his conversion and had therefore seen no need to reflect critically upon Stalin.[70] In other letters he mentioned that his growing awareness of the truth about Stalin and the Soviet Union had been a long and painful process for him, and that the full truth about Stalin's crimes against German Communists living in Soviet exile had only become public in the final years of the GDR.[71] Faced with the new political climate in reunified Germany, Kügelgen felt the need to comment on his understanding of socialism. He remained convinced that the ideals and goals of genuine socialism were still positive and desirable. Despite all envisaged revisions, then, Kügelgen maintained his anti-fascist self-understanding and did not question the essence of his anti-fascist conversion.

Like Bernt von Kügelgen, other anti-fascist returnees—such as the authors Hermann Kant and Gerhard Zwerenz—held on to and, at the same time, questioned their anti-fascist conversion narratives under the new political circumstances of unified Germany. The two met in 1997 at a panel discussion that touched on their war captivity. Both claimed to have returned from the USSR as anti-fascists who actively wanted to participate in the erection of a new Germany. But when Kant—who had made reference to his anti-fascist conversion in his literary work—mentioned his experiences in captivity at the panel discussion, he expressed an ambivalent attitude: "Even though I learned a lot in those four years, those years were nevertheless stolen years ... and there was never anybody who would say: Please forgive us for sending you there."[72] The two novelists were antagonists who had not spoken with each other for years: Zwerenz had been expelled from the SED in 1957 and subsequently fled to West Germany, where he used his writings to criticize the East German regime. Kant stayed in the GDR and became engaged as a cultural and political functionary. Despite their political differences, Zwerenz nevertheless agreed with Kant's views about war captivity, claiming that even though they had been too young to have destroyed anything during the war, both had to "suffer in the East" and that this experience had not left them "undamaged."[73]

Given the changed political and ideological circumstances following German unification, it is no surprise that many East German returnees subsequently modified the way in which they referred to their anti-fascist past and conversion. They did not simply cast off their identity as anti-fascist returnees, but instead made use of the opportunity to break with old narratives, express new ideas, and critically reflect on previously held attitudes and beliefs.

Not all former East German returnees continued to refer to the anti-fascist conversion narrative following the collapse of the SED regime. In contrast to men such as Kügelgen, they instead emphasized the hardship and the suffering they had experienced in Soviet captivity.[74] They were backed by the West German *Verband der Heimkehrer*, which recruited East Germans after unification.[75] In oral history interviews conducted between 2005 and 2009, East German returnees claimed that their experiences in Soviet captivity—that captivity in general—had been a taboo topic in the GDR.[76] They did not mention that the anti-fascist conversion narrative was not only an accepted, but also a legitimizing narrative in East Germany—perhaps because that narrative did not reflect their own experiences of captivity—or, for that matter, what they wanted to remember. These interviews reflected not only a perspective on war captivity no longer shaped by the anti-fascist conversion narrative, but also a resurgent public narrative in post-unification Germany that sees the "Germans as victims."[77] The anti-fascist conversion narrative may have been the dominant public narrative of war captivity in the GDR, yet it represented the experiences of only a minority of East Germans who, like Bernt von Kügelgen, claimed to have returned to Germany after the war as anti-fascists.

The public representation of anti-fascist returnees has changed since unification. They appeared in various public forums in the GDR, figuring prominently, for example, in feature films. While returnees from Soviet captivity frequently appear as characters in films produced in unified Germany—such as the highly popular *Das Wunder von Bern* (The Miracle of Berne, 2003)—anti-fascist returnees as such did not make an appearance until the 2009 film *Uranberg*.[78] And when they appear, old (West) German resentment against them tends to surface—as in the 2003 documentary series *Die Gefangenen* ("The Prisoners"), in which the anti-fascists are portrayed as outsiders in the Soviet prison camps.

The status of former members of the *Nationalkomitee* as "resistance fighters" has remained a hotly contested issue in unified Germany. The inclusion of the *Nationalkomitee* in the permanent exhibition of the *Gedenkstätte deutscher Widerstand* opened in Berlin in 1989 was a symbolic act that sent a clear political message indicating official recognition of the *Nationalkomitee* as a resistance group. In subsequent years influential German newspapers have published articles by historians who argue that the *Nationalkomitee* should be recognized as a legitimate resistance group.[79] The reactions to this of some newspaper readers—in particular World War II veterans—nevertheless suggest ongoing unease and continuing resentment against former members of the *Nationalkomitee*.[80] Such resentment remains especially strong in the German armed forces.[81]

Conclusion

Conversion narratives by returnees from war captivity are complex narrative constructs. They serve an important function for the retrospective description and interpretation of the past, particularly for an individual's transition from wartime to the postwar period. In the GDR, the narrative pattern of an anti-fascist conversion during Soviet captivity provided a framework that allowed individual returnees to interpret their personal reorientation in a meaningful way that corresponded to ideologically legitimate narratives. It enabled them to integrate themselves more smoothly into a politically changed society and to create a postwar identity as GDR citizens. As the example of Bernt von Kügelgen shows, this did not simply mean following a precise, predetermined narrative pattern; rather, personal interests and anticipations about reader expectations, as well as requirements of the publisher, all influenced the ways in which returnees publicly remembered their past. Returnees adapted the transformation narrative and used it to serve their own ends and interests. By compiling and publishing their memories, they could actively contribute themselves to the existing discourse on anti-fascist memory and identity in East Germany.

The transition from a divided to a united Germany certainly varied in its impact on individual ways of reflecting on the past. For Kügelgen and other anti-fascist returnees, the transition marked a clear break that enabled them to become more actively engaged with their past in rethought, revised, and even more ambivalent ways. Public attention may have shifted away from anti-fascist returnees after reunification, but the anti-fascist conversion narrative remained an important way of remembering the past—especially for those returnees for whom this narrative had become an integral part of their postwar identity. For people such as Bernt von Kügelgen, the anti-fascist worldview was not only an "ideology of confession," but also a constituent part of their self-understanding both during the GDR and after it had ceased to exist.[82]

The anti-fascist conversion narrative helped individuals navigate the personal transition from Nazi Germany to postwar Socialist East Germany. But it also survived the transition from divided to unified Germany—though in an altered form: one that took account of the changed political circumstances following unification, that allowed for a rethinking of previous ideas and beliefs, and, last but not least, that demonstrated the individual agency and subjectivity of East Germans who dealt with and fashioned their own past for their own personal ends and interests.

Suggested Readings

Barck, Simone. *Antifa-Geschichte(n). Eine literarische Spurensuche in der DDR der 1950er und 1960er Jahre*. Cologne, 2003.
Behrends, Jan C. *Die erfundene Freundschaft. Propaganda für die Sowjetunion in Polen und in der DDR*. Cologne, 2006.
Biess, Frank. *Homecomings. Returning POWs and the Legacies of Defeat in Postwar Germany*. Princeton, N.J., 2006.
Danyel, Jürgen. "Die SED und die 'kleinen Pg's.' Zur politischen Integration der ehemaligen NSDAP-Mitglieder in der SBZ/DDR." In *Helden, Täter und Verräter. Studien zum DDR-Antifaschismus*, ed. Annette Leo and Peter Reif-Spirek, 177–96. Berlin, 1999.
McLellan, Josie. *Antifascism and Memory in East Germany. Remembering the International Brigades 1945-1989*. Oxford, 2004.
Morina, Christina. *Legacies of Stalingrad: Remembering the Eastern Front in Germany since 1945*. Cambridge, 2011.
Niemetz, Daniel. *Das feldgraue Erbe. Die Wehrmachtseinflüsse im Militär der SBZ/DDR*. Berlin, 2006.
Satjukow, Silke. *Befreiung? Die Ostdeutschen und 1945*. Leipzig, 2009.

Schwelling, Birgit. *Heimkehr—Erinnerung—Integration. Der Verband der Heimkehrer, die ehemaligen Kriegsgefangenen und die westdeutsche Nachkriegsgesellschaft.* Paderborn, 2010.

Ueberschär, Gerd R., ed. *Das Nationalkomitee "Freies Deutschland" und der Bund Deutscher Offiziere.* Frankfurt am Main, 1995.

Wienand, Christiane. "Performing Memory: Returned German Prisoners of War in Divided and Reunited Germany." Ph.D. diss., University College London, 2010.

Notes

1. Quotations from Herfried Münkler, "Antifaschismus und antifaschistischer Widerstand als politischer Gründungsmythos der DDR," *Aus Politik und Zeitgeschichte* 45 (1998): 16–29; Josie McLellan, *Antifascism and Memory in East Germany: Remembering the International Brigades 1945-1989* (Oxford, 2004), 10. According to McLellan, anti-fascism was a way to describe and interpret the past that, in turn, has also been used to legitimize the present. See McLellan, *Antifasciscm and Memory*, 75f. Danyel distinguishes between a historical and a legitimizing component of anti-fascism. See Danyel, "Gründungskonsens," 36f. The idea of describing anti-fascism as a political myth became popular after 1990. See the overview in Jürgen Danyel, "Die Opfer- und Verfolgtenperspektive als Gründungskonsens? Zum Umgang mit der Widerstandstradition und der Schuldfrage in der DDR," in *Die geteilte Vergangenheit. Zum Umgang mit Nationalsozialismus und Widerstand in beiden deutschen Staaten*, ed. Jürgen Danyel (Berlin, 1995), 40f.; Bill Niven, *The Buchenwald Child: Truth, Fiction and Propaganda* (Rochester, N.Y., 2007), 200.
2. See Rainer Gries, "Die Heldenbühne der DDR. Zur Einführung," in *Sozialistische Helden. Eine Kulturgeschichte der Propagandafiguren in Osteuropa und der DDR*, ed. Silke Satjukow and Rainer Gries (Berlin, 2002), 89.
3. For in-depth analyses of the conflicting ways in which Communist veterans were instrumentalized in official memory culture, see McLellan, *Antifascism and Memory*; Catherine Epstein, *The Last Revolutionaries: German Communists and Their Century* (Cambridge, M.A., 2003). On ways in which anti-fascist discourse about Communist resistance influenced GDR fiction, see Simone Barck, *Antifa-Geschichte(n). Eine literarische Spurensuche in der DDR der 1950er und 1960er Jahre* (Cologne, 2003).
4. On war captivity see the overview in Rüdiger Overmans, "Das Schicksal der deutschen Kriegsgefangenen des Zweiten Weltkriegs," in *Der Zusammenbruch des Deutschen Reiches 1945. Zweiter Halbband: Die Folgen des Zweiten Weltkrieges*, ed. Militärgeschichtliches Forschungsamt (Munich, 2008), 379–507. On returnees in the first postwar decade, see Frank Biess, *Homecomings. Returning POWs and the Legacies of Defeat in Postwar Germany* (Princeton, 2006); Robert Moeller, *War Stories: The Search for a Usable Past in the Federal Republic of Germany* (Berkeley, 2001); Arthur L. Smith, *Heimkehr aus dem Zweiten Weltkrieg. Die Entlassung der deutschen Kriegsgefangenen* (Stuttgart, 1985); Albrecht Lehmann, *Gefangenschaft und Heimkehr. Deutsche Kriegsgefangene in der Sowjetunion* (Munich, 1986); Annette Kaminsky, ed., *Heimkehr 1948. Geschichte und Schicksale deutscher Kriegsgefangener* (Munich, 1998). On memories of returnees beyond 1955 see Svenja Goltermann, *Die Gesellschaft der Überlebenden. Deutsche Kriegsheimkehrer und ihre Gewalterfahrungen im Zweiten Weltkrieg* (Munich, 2009); Birgit Schwelling, *Heimkehr—Erinnerung—Integration. Der Verband der Heimkehrer, die ehemaligen Kriegsgefangenen und die westdeutsche Nachkriegsgesellschaft*

(Paderborn, 2010); Christiane Wienand, "Performing Memory: Returned Germany Prisoners of War in Divided and Reunited Germany" (Ph.D. diss., University College London, 2010).
5. On the East German–Soviet friendship, see Jan C. Behrends, *Die erfundene Freundschaft. Propaganda für die Sowjetunion in Polen und in der DDR* (Cologne, 2006); Silke Satjukow, *Befreiung? Die Ostdeutschen und 1945* (Leipzig, 2009).
6. See Emil Jeschonnek, *Wo der Landser denken lernte. Die sowjetische Kriegsgefangenschaft im Spiegel der Zeitung "Nachrichten"* (Berlin, 1959).
7. See Jürgen Danyel, "Die SED und die 'kleinen Pg's.' Zur politischen Integration der ehemaligen NSDAP-Mitglieder in der SBZ/DDR," in *Helden, Täter und Verräter. Studien zum DDR-Antifaschismus*, ed. Annette Leo and Peter Reif-Spirek (Berlin, 1999).
8. See Biess, *Homecomings*, 126–42.
9. In fact, the anti-fascist conversion narrative appeared in letters and pamphlets written by individuals and groups of anti-fascist returnees immediately after their return. See, e.g., a letter written by young returnees to the Free German Youth in Erfurt in Thüringisches Hauptstaatsarchiv Weimar [THStAW], Land Thüringen/MdI, 3680, 50r.
10. See Biess, *Homecomings*, 142–45.
11. For the reeducation of German soldiers in Soviet war captivity see Arthur L. Smith, *The War for the German Mind: Re-educating Hitler's Soldiers* (Providence, 1996), 105–23; Kurt Libera, "Zur Entwicklung der antifaschistischen Bewegung unter den deutschen Kriegsgefangenen in der UdSSR nach dem Sieg über den Hitlerfaschismus 1945-1950" (Ph.D. diss., Berlin, Institut für Gesellschaftswissenschaften beim ZK der SED, 1968). Libera was himself an anti-fascist returnee.
12. GDR studies about the *Nationalkomitee* include Bruno Löwel, "Die Gründung des NKFD im Lichte der Entwicklung der Strategie und Taktik der KPD," *Beiträge zur Geschichte der Arbeiterbewegung* 5 (1963), 613–31; Gerald Diesener, "Geschichtspropaganda und Geschichtsdenken im Nationalkomitee 'Freies Deutschland'" (Ph.D. diss., Universität Leipzig, 1983). For a pathbreaking West German publication, see Bodo Scheurig, *Verrat hinter Stacheldraht? Das Nationalkomitee "Freies Deutschland" und der Bund Deutscher Offiziere in der Sowjetunion 1943—1945* (Munich, 1965); also see Gerd Ueberschär, ed., *Das Nationalkomitee "Freies Deutschland" und der Bund Deutscher Offiziere* (Frankfurt am Main, 1995).
13. See Daniel Niemetz, *Das feldgraue Erbe. Die Wehrmachtseinflüsse im Militär der SBZ/DDR* (Berlin, 2006), 27.
14. The total number of antifa school alumni was around 48,000. See Stefan Karner, *Im Archipel GUPVI. Kriegsgefangenschaft und Internierung in der Sowjetunion 1941-1956* (Vienna and Munich, 1995), 104.
15. On the impact of anti-fascist returnees on the East German military, see Niemetz, *Erbe*.
16. On this film and its reception, see Henning Wrage, *Die Zeit der Kunst. Literatur, Film und Fernsehen in der DDR der 1960er Jahre* (Heidelberg, 2008), 277–99; Wienand, "Performing Memory," 84–87.
17. *Heimkehr in ein fremdes Land* was a film adaptation of a popular autobiographical novel by Günter Görlich, *Heimkehr in ein fremdes Land* (Berlin, 1974).
18. On *Heimkehr in ein fremdes Land* and its reception, see Wienand, "Performing Memory," 87–90.

19. See Hermann Kant *Der Aufenthalt* (Neuwied, 1977); Franz Fühmann's *Vor Feuerschlünden: Erfahrungen mit Georg Trakls Gedicht* (Rostock, 1982). The *Wandlung* (change) from being a follower of the Nazi regime to being a Communist was the central theme of Fühmann's oeuvre—even if he took a critical stance toward the ideological indoctrination he had experienced during war captivity in his later works. See, e.g., Günther Rüther, "Franz Fühmann. Ein deutsches Dichterleben in zwei Diktaturen," *Aus Politik und Zeitgeschichte* 13 (2000), 11–19. On autobiographical novels about anti-fascist returnees as part of the renaissance in GDR literature of *Entwicklungsromane* (coming-of-age novels) depicting young German soldiers after World War II, see Martin Straub, "'Die Abenteuer des Werner Holt' oder die Sehnsucht nach dem gefährlichen Leben," in *Helden, Täter und Verräter: Studien zum DDR-Antifaschismus*, ed. Annette Leo and Peter Reif-Spirek (Berlin, 1999), 216.
20. See the manuscript *AG Wandlungsliteratur* in SAPMO-BArch, DY 17/3453.
21. See the documentation of the *Autorenberatungen* in SAPMO-BArch, DY 17/3454.
22. See Wilhelm Adam, *Der schwere Entschluss* (Berlin, 1965); Egbert von Frankenberg, *Tradition im Kreuzverhör. Meine Familie in der Geschichte* (Berlin, 1987); Egbert von Frankenberg, *Meine Entscheidung* (Berlin, 1963); Otto Rühle, *Genesung in Jelabuga*. (Berlin, 1967); Luitpold Steidle, *Entscheidung an der Wolga*, 3rd ed. (Berlin, 1972).
23. See SAPMO-BArch, NY 4583/4; Paul Heider, "Das NKFD und der BDO in der Historiographie der DDR und die 'Arbeitsgemeinschaft ehemaliger Offiziere,'" in *Das Nationalkomitee "Freies Deutschland" und der Bund Deutscher Offiziere*, ed. Gerd R. Ueberschär (Frankfurt am Main, 1995), 170.
24. Julia Warth, *Verräter oder Widerstandskämpfer? Wehrmachtgeneral Walther von Seydlitz-Kurzbach* (Munich, 2006), 281.
25. On the shift in literary production, see Barck, *Antifa-Geschichte(n)*; see also Heider, *NKFD*, 174f.; Warth, *Verräter*, 309.
26. See Christina Morina, *Legacies of Stalingrad: Remembering the Eastern Front in Germany Since 1945* (Cambridge, 2011), 93–100; Heider, *NKFD*, 165f.
27. See BA-Berlin, DR1/2411. A second edition was published in 1985 with a run of 9,500 copies; see SAPMO-BArch, NY 4583/13.
28. The book appeared under a slightly different title as *Nacht der Entscheidung. Der Weg eines deutschen Offiziers zum Nationalkomitee Freies Deutschland* (Cologne, 1984). The new title emphasized the political aspect of his autobiography, as did the cover of the West German edition, which shows a portrait of Kügelgen in his *Wehrmacht* uniform.
29. See in detail Wienand, "Performing Memory."
30. Dirk von Kügelgen kindly granted access to these papers.
31. See SAPMO-BArch, NY 4583/21. He received an honorary pension as a fighter against fascism, which he still received even after reunification. See the 1965 letters from the FDGB in SAPMO-BArch, NY 4583/15, and the April 2002 letters from the *Bundesversicherungsanstalt für Angestellte* in SAPMO-BArch, NY 4583/20.
32. For a reference to Kügelgen's Stasi file (BStU, ZA, AIM 8371/91), large parts of which were destroyed in December 1989, see Joachim Walther, *Sicherungsbereich Literatur. Schriftsteller und Staatssicherheit in der Deutschen Demokratischen Republik* (Berlin, 1996), 87.
33. See the documents in SAPMO-BArch NY 4583/4.
34. See Kügelgen's manuscript *Danach* in SAPMO-BArch, NY 4583/4, 17 and his disappointed remarks about the fortieth anniversary of the *Nationalkomitee* in SAPMO-BArch, NY 4583/19, letter to Ernst E, 21 September 1984.

35. See Harald Schmid, *Antifaschismus und Judenverfolgung. Die "Reichskristallnacht" als politischer Gedenktag in der DDR* (Göttingen, 2004), chaps. 7 and 8; Hans-Erich Volkmann, "Das verweigerte historische Erbe. Der Umgang der DDR mit militärischem Widerstand und Kriegsverbrechen im Zweiten Weltkrieg," in *Militär, Staat und Gesellschaft in der DDR. Forschungsfelder, Ergebnisse, Perspektiven*, ed. Hans Ehlert und Matthias Rogg (Berlin, 2004), 31–33.
36. See SAPMO-BArch, DY 17/3176, letter to *Verlag der Nation*, 7 April 1987.
37. See Bernt von Kügelgen. *Nacht der Entscheidung. Erinnerungen an Familie und Jugend*, 2nd ed. (Berlin, 1985), 334.
38. Kügelgen, *Nacht*, 126f.
39. Ibid., 149, 151, 256, 321.
40. Ibid., 361, 378, 443, 457.
41. See Kügelgen, *Nacht*, 133–36. He also dedicated his first leading article in the POW newspaper *Das freie Wort* to the oath of allegiance. See ibid., 366.
42. See Rühle, *Jelabuga*, 276–80.
43. Kügelgen, *Nacht*, 296.
44. See the manuscript of the working group *Autobiographien* presented at a meeting of the VdN in 1966 in SAPMO-BArch, DY 17/ 3454.
45. See SAPMO-BArch, NY 4583/2, Konzeption zu einem autobiographischen Buch. Erinnerungen (1914–49).
46. See Alan Nothnagle, *Building the East German Myth: Historical Mythology and Youth Propaganda in the GDR, 1945-1989* (Ann Arbor, 1999), chap. 2; Mary Fulbrook, *German National Identity after the Holocaust* (Cambridge, 1999), 87.
47. Kügelgen's account was not exceptional in this respect. Several other self-confessed anti-fascist returnees who later held leadership positions in the GDR shared Kügelgen's bourgeois background, and thus also offered opportunities for such an identification. This included the former *Wehrmacht* officers Egbert von Frankenberg, Arno von Lenski, Luitpold Steidle, and Bernhard Bechler. See Frankenberg, *Tradition*; Wenzke, *Arno von Lenski*, 94; Steidle, *Entscheidung*, 5f; Diedrich, *Bechler*, 61–62.
48. For similar examples of this style, see Rudolf Petershagen, *Gewissen in Aufruhr* (Berlin, 1957); Adam, *Entschluss*.
49. See, e.g., the interviews he gave after the publication of his book in *Mitteldeutsche Neueste Nachrichten Leipzig*, 24 September 1983; *Neue Deutsche Presse*, August 1983. On his efforts to use the experiences of war and anti-fascist conversion to create a historical consciousness among young East Germans, see SAPMO-BArch NY 4583/19, letter from Kügelgen to Artur Arndt, 9 February 1985.
50. See the reviews in *Neues Deutschland*, 11 February 1984; *Neue Deutsche Literatur* 5 (1985); *Beiträge zur Geschichte der Arbeiterbewegung* 26 (1984): 704; *Freiheit*, 29 September 1983; *Berliner Zeitung*, 6 March 1984.
51. See SAPMO-BArch, NY 4583/16, radio manuscript, 16 January 1986.
52. Kügelgen, *Nacht*, 488–89.
53. See SAPMO-BArch, NY 4583/13, statement by Kügelgen family, August 1987.
54. See the letters in SAPMO-BArch NY 4583/13 and 4583/19.
55. See "Schön war's im alten St. Petersburg," *Die Welt*, 15–16 June 1985. Additional manuscripts were published in *Die Zeit* (15 June 1984) and broadcast on *Deutschlandfunk*. See the broadcast manuscript from 16 January 1986 in SAPMO-BArch, NY 4583/16.

56. See, e.g., Birgit Schwelling, *Wege in die Demokratie. Eine Studie zum Wandel und zur Kontinuität von Mentalitäten nach dem Übergang vom Nationalsozialismus zur Bundesrepublik* (Opladen, 2001).
57. See Peter Steinbach, "Neuorientierung im Umbruch. Zum Wandel des Selbstverständnisses deutscher Kriegsgefangener in England und den USA," in *Doppelte Zeitgeschichte. Deutsch-deutsche Beziehungen,* ed. Martin Sabrow, Bernd Stöver, and Arnd Bauerkämper (Berlin, 1998), 234–50; Wienand, "Performing Memory," 168–71 and 174–82; Christiane Wienand, "Den Übergang vom Krieg in die Nachkriegszeit erzählen. Transformationserzählungen und Identitätskonstruktionen heimgekehrter Kriegsgefangener nach 1945," in *Kriegsenden, Nachkriegsordnungen, Folgekonflikte. Wege aus dem Krieg im 19. und 20. Jahrhundert,* ed. Jörg Echternkamp (Freiburg, 2012), 161–78.
58. The *Verband der Heimkehrer* inverted experiences in Soviet war captivity, regarding returnees from Soviet captivity as "avant-garde against communism." See *Der Heimkehrer,* 10 January 1964.
59. See my discussion of West German media and private memory accounts in Wienand, "Performing Memory," chaps. 1 and 3.
60. See Biess, *Homecomings,* 153ff.; Wienand, "Performing Memory," 46–50.
61. See "Verräter oder Widerstandskämpfer," *Der Spiegel* 36 (1977), 67f.
62. See Jesco von Puttkamer, *Irrtum und Schuld. Geschichte des Nationalkomitees Freies Deutschland* (Neuwied, 1948), 111ff. Despite his critical stance, Puttkamer declared in 1971 that he would still fully support the manifesto of the *Nationalkomitee*. See his interview in *deutschland-berichte,* 8 March 1971.
63. The West German media had already begun to approach this subject less emotionally in the 1970s. See the fictional documentary *Das Haus Lunjowo,* which was broadcast on television in 1970, as well as articles in *Der Spiegel,* 5 (1970), 140, 142; *Der Heimkehrer,* 15 February 1970. *Die Zeit* posthumously honored Walther von Seydlitz as a "general who followed his conscience." See *Die Zeit,* 7 May 1976.
64. These arguments surfaced in a television debate among *Wehrmacht* veterans on 16 July 1989; see also the VdH leaflet "*Gehört das Nationalkomitee Freies Deutschland in die Berliner Gedenkstätte für Widerstand*" (Bad Godesberg, 1989).
65. See the reader reports in SAPMO-Barch, DY 17/ 3663, as well as the edited manuscripts in SAPMO-BArch, DY 17/1800 and 1801.
66. See SAPMO-BArch, NY 4583/14, letter to Heinrich v. H, 4 October 1993.
67. See SAPMO-BArch, NY 4583/14, letter to Arthur L. Smith, 13 October 1991.
68. See SAPMO-BArch, NY 4583/14, letters to Bernd K, 8 February 1999; and to Heinrich v. H, 4 October 1993 and 23 August 1994.
69. See SAPMO-BArch, NY 4583/14, letters to Heribert S, 11 February 1999; and to Heinrich v. H, 23 August 1994.
70. See SAPMO-BArch, NY 4583/14, letter to Heribert S, 11 February 1999.
71. See SAPMO-BArch, NY 4583/14, letters to Bernd K, 8 February 1999, and Heinrich v. H, 23 August 1994.
72. See Hermann Kant and Gerhard Zwerenz, *Unendliche Wende. Ein Streitgespräch* (Querfurt, 1998), 12.
73. See Kant/Zwerenz, *Unendliche Wende,* 14.
74. See Wienand, "Performing Memory," chaps. 1 and 2.
75. See Schwelling, *Heimkehr,* 281–87; Wienand, "Performing Memory," 126–38; 165–67; 219–21.

76. See Wienand, "Performing Memory," 133.
77. See, e.g., Bill Niven, ed., *Germans as Victims: Remembering the Past in Contemporary Germany* (Basingstoke, 2006).
78. Media coverage of the film mentioned, but did not comment upon, the fact that the returnee appeared here as an anti-fascist returnee. See, e.g., "Deutsche Geschichte, von Giftstaub kontaminiert," *Süddeutsche Zeitung*, 7 December 2011; "Unverheilte Wunden," *Neues Deutschland*, 7 December 2011.
79. See Andreas Fischer, "Widerstand hinter Stacheldraht," *Frankfurter Allgemeine Zeitung*, 10 July 1993; Hans Mommsen, "Widerstand hat viele Namen," *Süddeutsche Zeitung—SZ am Wochenende*, 16 July 1994. In a public address in 2000, Wolfgang Thierse, the vice-president of the German parliament, explicitly named the *Nationalkomitee* along with other resistance groups. See http://www.20-juli-44.de/pdf/2000_thierse.pdf (accessed 25 August 2012).
80. See the letters to the editor in *Frankfurter Allgemeine Zeitung*, 17 and 19 July 1993, 1 September 1993, 27 June 1994, 7 July 1994, and 21 April 1998, and in *Süddeutsche Zeitung*, 29 July 1994 and 4 August 1994.
81. In 2003 the German Ministry of Defense refused to support the celebrations of the sixtieth anniversary of the *Nationalkomitee* organized by the *Verband Deutscher in der Résistance, in den Streitkräften der Antihitlerkoalition und der Bewegung "Freies Deutschland"* e.V., claiming that it was still controversial whether "real resistance" had been possible in Soviet war captivity. See Peter Rau, "Koalition des Gewissens," *Information DRAFD* (June 2003), 1.
82. Danyel has argued that a precondition for the relatively seamless integration of former NSDAP members and *Wehrmacht* soldiers in the GDR was a "transformation of antifascism from actual memory … towards a de-differentiated ideology of confession (*entdifferenzierte[n] Bekenntnisideologie*)." See Danyel, *Gründungskonsens*, 42. With respect to anti-fascist returnees, their conversion stories can be seen as an individual way to remember their anti-fascist conversion experiences, and as a confession, i.e., a political statement that helped them integrate after the war—or, in the case of Kügelgen, to emphasize their identity as GDR citizens.

PART II

Health, Food, and Embodied Citizens

CHAPTER 5

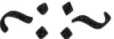

Perceptions of Health after World War II
Heart Disease and Risk Factors in East and West Germany, 1945–75

JEANNETTE MADARÁSZ-LEBENHAGEN

At the beginning of the twentieth century, infectious diseases such as typhus and cholera were on the retreat while chronic diseases were on the rise in Germany. Closely associated with industrialization and urbanization, rising living standards, and higher life expectancies, the epidemiological transition put chronic diseases of the cardiovascular system (i.e., heart disease), such as arteriosclerosis, hypertension, and myocardial infarct, at the forefront of an extensive critique of civilization.[1] Debates on the prevention of heart disease not only reflected medical and popular perceptions of health, but also linked chronic disease to social, cultural, and political constellations.

Looking at prevention practices in different European health-care systems between 1830 and 1930, Peter Baldwin has shown that social and political context shapes prevention practices. In particular, he has highlighted the links among political concepts and structures, as well as cultural settings, in the development of prevention programs.[2] Following Baldwin, this essay will examine the interaction between institutional settings and conceptual change after 1945 with respect to two different political systems built on the same cultural traditions in health care: that of the Federal Republic and that of the German Democratic Republic (GDR). It will also discuss the social and political conditions of epistemological change in East and West German health policies. Finally, it will draw on a variety of sources—ranging from newspaper articles, popular science publications, debates within the medical profession, and government sources—to trace the emergence of heart disease as a crucial public issue in the two postwar Germanys. The essay addresses three major questions: How did perceptions of heart disease as an illness change? In what ways did these changes affect prevention practices addressing heart disease? To what extent can shifting prevention practices be linked to broader sociopolitical changes?

The following analysis of shifting debates on the prevention of heart disease and related practices in postwar Germany highlights links between structural settings, political processes, and health policy. These debates closely engaged with public discussion about social and political values. In the context of German-German relations, this made them part of what Christoph Kleßmann has called an "asymmetrically intertwined parallel history" (*asymmetrisch verflochtene Parallelgeschichte*).[3]

But how exactly did the political and social context influence ideas about health? In the East German case, the Communist Party's insistence on collectively shared social responsibility underpinned social hygiene approaches to medical care and prevention. Social hygienists have traditionally aimed to improve working and living conditions to offset the negative effects of urbanization and industrialization.[4] Such an understanding of prevention corresponded to the collectivist and egalitarian aspects of Socialist ideology. In contrast, social hygiene was scorned in West Germany as statist interventionism and associated with Nazi Germany and the GDR. In an effort to distance the newly created democratic state from such unwanted associations, officials adopted an individualized approach to health care that, unlike centralized East German procedures, entrusted the field of prevention to private practitioners who dealt with individual patients. The focus on populations in the East and on the individual in the West shaped prevention programs. Over time, however, heart disease prevention programs shifted in both Germanys. This essay will demonstrate the links between these adjustments and social and political changes that slowly took place from 1945 to 1975.

That period saw major transitions in disease patterns and the epistemology applied to heart disease. Shortly after the end of World War II, morbidity and mortality from heart disease surged and, for the first time, this group of diseases was considered to be an urgent health problem in medical and public debates. In spite of dramatic political, economic, and technological changes in Germany after 1945, several competing prewar conceptions of heart disease dominated popular and medical discourse in the East and the West until the middle of the 1960s. A marked break with older understandings came about only with the rise of an immensely influential scientific model in the late 1960s: the risk factor model, which brought to an end a transitional era and led to a convergence of prevention programs in the two German states.

Statistical and probability calculations have been used since the nineteenth century to detect, describe, and assess health risks.[5] The risk factor model clearly demonstrates the potential medical uses of such knowledge. Based on the ongoing Framingham Study conducted in the United States since the 1940s, this large-scale epidemiological study investigates cardiovascular disease and its long-term causes.[6] An analysis over many years of the lifestyles of a large population—the citizens of the town of Framingham in Massachusetts—revealed various risk factors (such as high-fat diets and serum cholesterol, high blood pressure, smoking, a lack of physical activity) that statistically heighten an individual's risk of dying of a heart attack. As a result of this study, ideal values for body weight, blood pressure, and other risk factors were suggested. This process of standardization meant that even small anomalies led to medical treatment, even if the person in question showed no symptoms of heart disease.[7] But statistics on disease distribution apply to large populations and thus say little about individual risk. Such data neither give conclusive information on disease etiology nor provide a definite assessment of the effects of preventive measures. The ambivalent use of statistical data in the risk factor model gives the model a flexible quality, as physician and medical historian Robert Aronowitz has pointed out.[8] Moreover, because it focuses on lifestyle, the risk factor model accommodates a wide range of prevention programs, ranging from healthy eating to sports to the medical control of high blood pressure. This made the model attractive even to the very different health-care systems and prevention practices in use in East and West Germany.

Carsten Timmermann has compared the introduction of the risk factor model in the two German states. Showing that the data upon which it is based provides ample scope for varying medical approaches, Timmermann argues that the risk factor model's inherent flexibility is the major reason for its success in such different political systems.[9] Looking beyond those epistemological aspects, this essay looks at how changes in medical discourse and political circumstances also contributed to the risk factor model's positive reception in both German states.

The Evolution of Discourse about Heart Disease and Prevention Practices

In the 1920s, social hygienists addressed the consequences of poor living conditions by introducing higher standards of hygiene and distributing knowledge about the possible causes of various diseases. They were mostly interested in diseases affecting the lower social classes, especially infectious diseases. Although heart disease was discussed, arteriosclerosis in particular was primarily associated with the more abundant lifestyle of the middle and upper classes and consequently received little attention from social hygienists. They nevertheless provided advice on healthy living practices in general and, in this way, fed a growing public interest in the health aspects of lifestyle choices.[10] Since the mid 1920s in Germany (and elsewhere), general lifestyle advice became more nationalist in tone, instructing the individual to keep healthy and fit in the interest of national strength.[11] National Socialist health policy radicalized this broad approach to health care by combining lifestyle advice with racist ideology.[12]

After the end of World War II, when the threat of epidemics had receded and adequate food supplies been restored, heart disease came to the fore in an unprecedented way. As early as 1954, the East German Ministry of Health's Working Group for Questions on Heart Disease called for a statewide effort in heart disease prevention by appealing to a sense of collective responsibility.[13] Four years later, the same ministry stressed the need for concerted action by the entire population.[14] Such population-wide initiatives reflected the reintroduction of social hygiene traditions to the East German health-care system.

Alfred Grotjahn, the founder of the leftist social hygiene movement, had intended to address the medical consequences of social inequality.[15] The postwar Socialist state set its target even higher by aiming, in line with basic claims of Communist ideology, to prevent disease by achieving social equality.[16] Arguably then, the reintroduction of social hygiene in East Germany represented a strong political statement.[17] By reviving longstanding traditions in medical discourse and by claiming allegiance to the social hygiene movement of the interwar period, East German health professionals rejected any association with the political appropriation of medical discourse and practices during the Third Reich. Instead, officials polemically drew such connections between the Nazis and the capitalist West. East Germany's turn to social hygiene was paralleled in West Germany by breaking with past practices. Here, health care was built on a conglomerate of state and private insurance schemes, which ensured individual treatment by private practitioners. These, in contrast to East German initiatives, were unable—even unwilling—to support population-wide prevention programs. This bifurcation of German medical traditions was part and parcel of the constant rivalry between the two German states regarding their achievements in health care. As a result, both states constantly compared morbidity and mortality rates as an indication of general success or failure. More specifically, the East German Socialist Unity Party (SED) perceived the increase in heart disease as a political issue and as a serious obstacle on the path to building a Socialist society.

In West Germany, heart disease was treated in the early 1950s as a disease that primarily affected a specific professional group. Not only the medical profession but also politicians and the mass media (such as the weekly newsmagazine *Der Spiegel*) discussed the "Manager's Disease" (*Manager-Krankheit*), associating myocardial infarcts with male middle-class managers.[18] West German medical opinions ranged, on the one hand, from a focus on males in highly responsible professional positions who succumbed to the strains of building the economic miracle, to doubts, on the other hand, about the reality of an actual "heart disease epidemic."[19] In contrast, East German medical professionals believed that heart disease affected men and women of all social ranks.[20] In both states, nevertheless, physicians linked heart disease to eating habits, body weight, the level of physical activity, and the stress associated with modern lifestyles.[21]

Conceptually, however, the two Germanys addressed health risks and their prevention in different ways. While West Germany kept state involvement at a minimum and instead emphasized individual action, East Germany stood for the "primacy" of state control: "The responsibility of the society and the state for health care has to be seen in a dialectical relation to the citizens' individual responsibility. But the primacy of the responsibility of society and the state has to be ensured."[22] Contrasting sociopolitical concerns help account for conceptual differences. In West Germany, for example, health education was seen as crucial in enabling individuals to make responsible decisions regarding their lifestyle choices.[23] In contrast, the East German health-care system was designed to incorporate all of society into an all-embracing prevention drive, which included sanctions for those who refused to comply.[24] The aim of the health initiatives was similar in both states, namely, to reduce the incidence of disease. But the impacts of the various prevention programs were hard to ascertain.[25] Moreover, prevention practices rarely went beyond early detection and curative treatment in either East or West. The following section, which examines the institutional setting of health care in the two Germanys, helps explain the similarity in outcomes despite categorically different approaches to the prevention of heart disease.

The Postwar Institutional Setting: Two German Health-Care Systems

In East Germany, social hygienists who had returned from exile after the end of World War II began to set up a comprehensive health-care system stressing the sociopolitical relevance of health issues.[26] As we have seen, officials politically endorsed this revival of German leftist traditions in health care, which was one reason why the foremost protagonists of social hygiene—such as Hermann Redetzky, Erwin Marcusson, and Kurt Winter—all became influential actors in East German health policy.[27] At the same time, however, increasing bureaucratic centralization deprived the medical profession of its former political influence, especially since the Communist leadership scorned doctors as bourgeois enemies of the new state.[28] Educational campaigns were largely facilitated by the German Hygiene Museum in Dresden, which first became internationally known for its cutting-edge health education programs following the international hygiene exhibitions in 1911 and 1930. In addition, the National Committee for Health Education (*Nationales Komitee für Gesundheitserziehung*) developed guidelines for health education and published the journal *Deine Gesundheit* (Your Health).[29] This centralized and state-controlled health-care system easily accommodated population-wide prevention programs, such as obligatory vaccination schemes and checkups, screenings for pregnant women and infants, as well as dental care.[30]

In the early postwar years, when epidemics threatened the population, practical medicine and bacteriological research stood at the forefront of medical activity.[31] With respect to preventing infectious diseases, reducing infant mortality, and providing medical care for the working population, the East German health-care system proved more successful than the West German one in the 1950s and 1960s. Educational campaigns addressing lifestyle issues relevant to chronic diseases had little effect, however. The political elite's flexible approach to nutritional guidance further undermined the difficult task of health education, for it often declared foodstuffs healthy solely based on availability rather than scientific evidence.[32] Furthermore, official advice regarding physical activity had explicit ideological overtones that may have put off those segments of the population whose members rejected state intervention in lifestyle choices.[33]

West Germany re-created a decentralized system with a large number of health insurance companies. In addition, a constitutional measure was introduced that divided control over public welfare between the federal states (*Länder*) and the federal government. This meant that the former were in a position to decide on relevant initiatives, such as heart disease prevention programs, if there had been no prior initiative at the federal level. In fact, state officials usually treated recommendations from the federal level with great suspicion.[34] This not only led to differing health care initiatives in the various federal states, but also hindered the development of population-wide prevention programs at the federal level.

Two factors abetted this tendency in West Germany: the strong position of the medical profession and a 1955 law (*Kassenarztgesetz*) that restored its members' monopoly on ambulatory treatment. Partly in an attempt to distance the health-care system from approaches that seemed reminiscent of Nazi medical crimes, the medical profession continually insisted on its responsibility and foremost suitability for administering preventive measures to individual patients.[35] In addition, arguments against state involvement in medical care—derogatively referred to as "state medicine"—regularly appeared in *Deutsches Ärzteblatt*, the most important political forum for the West German medical profession.[36]

More to the point, West German legislation on health care was restricted to the treatment of diseases rather than keeping people healthy. Within this legislative framework, little attention was given to primary prevention practices that addressed disease prior to the appearance of initial symptoms. Chronic heart disease in particular fell into this grey zone, for neither its causes nor its etiology were clear, and the effectiveness of possible prevention practices was uncertain.[37] As a result of this difficult legislative constellation, the prevention of chronic diseases was conceived mainly in terms of early detection and individual treatment up to the middle of the 1960s.

With respect to the institutional setting in both states, the presumed division between "collectivism" in East Germany and "individualism" in West Germany seems to have indeed been the case. In fact, it had a noticeable impact on prevention practices. In West Germany, structural conditions, legal restrictions, and the peculiar constellation of protagonists—first and foremost the strong position of the organized medical profession—diminished the influence of public health-care services, which were responsible for central prevention initiatives covering the entire population rather than individual patients.[38] In contrast, centralized structures and a politically weak medical profession in East Germany allowed for strong government influence and a collective approach to the prevention of both infectious and chronic diseases. The East German approach, which accommodated population-wide prevention programs, was most successful in combatting the spread of infectious diseases and those preventable by central measures, such as the fluoridation of drinking water—measures that were, in fact, closely related to the traditional range of social hygiene activities. But lifestyle changes deemed relevant to heart disease prevention proved more difficult to implement, as we shall see in the next section. In both East and West Germany, early detection and treatment of heart disease were implemented effectively, while primary prevention programs consistently failed to reach those most at risk.

Shifting Concepts of Heart Disease Prevention in a Changing Political Climate (1965–75)

Since the 1950s, scientific research conducted in America on heart disease etiology stressed lifestyle factors. West Germany paid attention to this as well, beginning in the mid 1950s, but without adopting U.S. public health efforts, such as implementing a National Health Survey or establishing so-called Schools of Public Health.[39] The East German approach to chronic cardiovascular diseases was also shaped by American influences: Albert Wollenberger, a German doctor who returned from exile in the United States in the early 1950s, brought back with him the risk factor model that had been recently developed. Social hygienists—such as the prominent and politically influential Kurt Winter, who had returned from exile in 1946—opposed Wollenberger's efforts to introduce that model in East Germany. He was able to block this successfully for some time because of the political elite's reluctance to adopt Western approaches to health care at the height of Cold War animosity.[40]

Beginning in the late 1950s, technological progress produced a more optimistic view of the future in both West and East Germany, where advances in technology were applied to many areas, including politics and economics, as well as health care.[41] This focus on treatment using new technology detracted public attention from the potential benefits of prevention programs. Heart surgery, for example, began attracting immense publicity worldwide beginning in the late 1950s. A pacemaker was implanted for the first time on 8 October 1958, and, almost ten years later in 1967, the South African surgeon Christiaan Barnard performed the first heart transplant. Such successes undermined discussion about prevention practices, for a promising future seemed to lie ahead in which chronic disease would be healed and damaged hearts repaired by medical interventions based on technological advances.[42] The initial euphoria about the enormous progress in heart surgery diminished in the late 1960s, however, as medical problems appeared and moral objections grew.[43] At the same time, heart surgery was no longer seen as an easy fix for rising mortality rates.

As a result, lifestyle changes were once again discussed as a more effective way to deal with the heart disease epidemic. This trend was supported by the growing critique of technocracy and materialism, voiced by civil movements in West Germany. In the GDR, this found expression in popular discontent with, and the political backlash against, Walter Ulbricht's policies during his final years in power. Since the late 1960s, East and West Germany had both witnessed a revival of pre-1933 criticisms of civilization processes, including technological advances and supposedly unhealthy lifestyle changes. This new concern for individual well-being paved the way for the adoption of the risk factor model and, in the GDR in particular, overshadowed earlier collectivist thinking in health care by promoting, on the part of East Germans, a "heightened responsibility for their own personal health."[44]

In the 1970s, the risk paradigm replaced technocratic approaches in both German states, though in different ways. West German public perception of risk was shaped by the economic slowdown and student protest movement. Both events undermined the economic and political security achieved so painstakingly after the war, and ushered in major cultural changes.[45] In contrast, the East German population experienced political change and economic difficulties less distinctly that decade, for the change in leadership from Ulbricht to Honecker was presented to the public as an easy transition; moreover, Honecker's new emphasis on expanding social welfare policies helped improved working and living standards, at least initially. By self-definition, in fact, the East German Socialist state stood for social security. Even though this promise was often undermined, in practice, by the constant lack of resources, the government's acceptance of this responsibility reduced, at least in theory and to some extent, the immediate relevance of the risk paradigm for most East Germans.

The risk factor model enhanced the idea of individual responsibility for keeping healthy and, in the medical sector, gave new impetus to dealing with the heart disease epidemic that reached new heights in the 1970s. As we will see in the next section, international relations encouraged conceptual shifts in the two German health-care systems, while concerns for the international recognition of East German research on heart disease related directly to political goals.

Foreign Policy Meets Health Care: The Influence of International Cooperation and the World Health Organization (WHO)

The early epidemiological studies in Eastern bloc countries (such as Bulgaria since 1960) and initiatives by the WHO had an important formative impact on East German prevention practices.[46] In addition, early Soviet influences encouraged the introduction of registries for diabetes in 1960 and, since the early 1970s, for myocardial infarct and stroke, which provided information about the prevalence, treatment, and course of these diseases.[47] Such registries, which were crucial for epidemiological research, were introduced in West Germany only in the 1980s. Soviet influence on the development of prevention practices seems to have been restricted to these registries and the so-called dispensary system (discussed later). In spite of surging rates of heart disease mortality in the Soviet Union since the middle of the 1960s, there is no clear evidence of a Soviet-led initiative involving increased support for existing prevention efforts or encouragement of conceptual changes regarding heart disease prevention (except for the extension of the dispensary system to include heart disease).[48] Both this early engagement with epidemiological research and the surprisingly minimal influence of Soviet research on heart disease studies in the GDR indicated major trajectories in East German prevention programs, which eventually would evolve in response to Western epidemiological research programs.

The GDR's links to the WHO proved especially crucial. "Ten-day workshops" allowed for intensive international exchange, from which East German scientists were otherwise often excluded because of extensive censorship, as well as their government's restrictive traveling regulations.[49] The cardiologist and epidemiologist Lothar Heinemann, for example, coordinated the East German part of the WHO's MONICA (Multinational MONItoring of trends and determinants in CArdiovascular disease) study, which was established in the early 1980s to monitor trends in cardiovascular diseases, and to relate these to risk factor changes in the population over a ten-year period.[50] As a result of his involvement with the WHO, Heinemann was able to work with Rose and Jeremiah Stamler, both prominent American cardiologists, and Geoffrey Rose, an eminent British epidemiologist, who, in his own work, engaged intensively with the risk factor model and its application to prevention practices.[51] In addition to such personal networks of scientists, the East German government actively supported the establishment of international links. This included various research programs and specifically epidemiological studies that were conducted in close cooperation with the WHO, such as the European CANON/CINDI (Countrywide Integrated Noncommunicable Diseases Intervention) program. In short, then, the East German government cooperated with the WHO in an exemplary manner, with the clear intention of heightening its international reputation and acquiring some influence on global health debates.[52]

In spite of this strong political interest in heart disease prevention in East Germany, the short-term implementation and long-term maintenance of practical measures were hindered by a constant lack of resources. For example, the introduction of a dispensary system in the Soviet tradition provided ambulatory health care to sufferers of chronic diseases such as diabetes. This was hailed as a great step forward in dealing with chronic diseases, but East German efforts in the 1960s to set up a number of independent dispensaries for heart disease were hindered by organizational difficulties. In light of the new risk factor model and because of a lack of money and personnel, central administrators considered it inefficient to create different dispensaries for a variety of chronic diseases that were associated with the same risk factors.[53] While attempts to introduce prevention programs addressing myocardial infarct and high blood pressure proved similarly difficult to implement in the late 1970s, East German cardiologists closely cooperating with the WHO did succeed in building up an extensive program of epidemiological research.[54]

In West Germany, by contrast, epidemiological studies only took place sporadically in some federal states, with the sole support of communal money and local health insurance companies. In the late 1960s, for example, the Ministry of Work and Social Issues (*Ministerium für Arbeit und Soziales*) in Baden-Württemberg cooperated with regional health insurance groups and the local medical profession on some pilot studies to determine the possibility of prevention programs administered by private practitioners.[55] Such pilot studies were based on a model program for the early detection of heart disease that had been developed by a new working group of the German Medical Association. These studies were used by the medical profession to highlight the need to establish prevention programs in private practitioners' practices.[56] Within the heterogeneous West German structure balancing federal and state interests, the risk factor model offered the chance to bundle prevention efforts in a multifactorial approach. Because of its strong link to lifestyle issues, the model also enabled private practitioners to make a strong case that their special aptitude for conducting such prevention programs lay in their the one-to-one relationships with their patients. The risk factor model was employed successfully in this manner from the early 1970s in an effort to foster early detection and medical treatment of cardiovascular risks. For example, articles in the *Deutsche Ärzteblatt* repeatedly stressed the importance of requisitioning patients while ignoring other aspects of the risk factor model, such as epidemiological research, which aimed at interventionist prevention programs.[57]

From the early 1970s onward, West German politicians, the medical profession, and the public perceived the health-care system to be in crisis. It seemed structurally fragmented and not financially viable anymore because of its focus on technology-intensive therapeutic efforts rather than on keeping people healthy.[58] Debates about this further encouraged acceptance of the risk factor model, which promised effective prevention and, in the long term, a reduction in medical costs. This hope was bolstered by the WHO's support of the risk factor model. In turn, WHO programs strongly influenced the Federal Office of Health Education (*Bundeszentrale für gesundheitliche Aufklärung*).[59] In addition, successful initiatives in other European countries (such as the 1974 World Health Day on nutrition and the Swedish prevention program "Diet and Exercise") also encouraged activities in West Germany.[60] Responding to an international trend, in 1978 the West German government approved the program "Research and Technology in the Service of Health," which repeatedly referred to the risk factor model. It provided 450 million marks through 1981 for research on preventive health care and disease etiology. One specific outcome of the program, which was also intended to address the health-care system's structural problems, was the first large-scale epidemiological study in West Germany on heart disease: the so-called German Cardiovascular Prevention Study (*Deutsche-Herzkreislauf-Präventionsstudie*). In close alignment with North American studies (e.g., the Multiple Risk Factor Intervention Trial [MRFIT]), this study combined epidemiological surveillance with intervention trials and outcome analysis inspired by the risk factor model.[61] Finally, public health initiatives were given priority for funding at the end of the 1980s. The introduction of the "Checkup 35" program in 1989, which offered every person older then thirty-five a free medical checkup every two years, institutionalized heart disease prevention in private practices—one of the major goals of the West German medical profession since 1945.[62]

The adoption of the risk factor model in West Germany was supported by the institutional setting, then, as well as by a conceptual readjustment moving toward a multifactorial approach to heart disease prevention that suited the medical profession and the government. But the German-German rivalry in the international arena underpinned the participation of both states in WHO initiatives as well. In 1973, for example, West German government officials hoped to cooperate with the WHO in order to improve the standing of the

Federal Office of Health Education "in [its] competition with the DHMD [German Hygiene Museum in Dresden]."[63] The East German government, for its part, increasingly considered the improvement of German-German relations and international recognition more attractive than confrontation, especially in times of economic and political instability.[64] After Honecker replaced Ulbricht as head of state in 1971, German-German rapprochement—a result of Willy Brandt's *Ostpolitik*—allowed for greater openness toward West German and American science.

The conceptual change in health care was paved by a generational shift that gradually undermined the social hygiene approach. In the GDR, as we have seen, Wollenberger failed to introduce the risk factor model in the 1950s because of strong resistance by social hygienists. In 1965, however, Hermann Redetzky was given emeritus status; Erwin Marcusson left his position as the Director of the Institute of Social Hygiene in 1969; and Kurt Winter, who was given emeritus status in 1975, became the head of the Academy for Medical Training and Education (*Akademie für ärztliche Fortbildung*) and gradually developed an interest in WHO programs. New people with little attachment to social hygiene but a great interest in both epidemiological research and international exchange subsequently came into positions of influence. In the Ministry of Health, Horst Heine had begun promoting both the risk factor model and cooperation with the WHO since 1967. Heine and cardiologist Heinemann joined forces with Wollenberger at the newly founded Central Institute of Cardiovascular Research (*Zentralinstitut für Herz-Kreislaufforschung*). It actively fostered international cooperation and, in 1986, became a center that collaborated with the WHO. This generational shift corresponded to changing political priorities with respect to international affairs and German-German relations. It also established the risk factor model in East German cardiovascular research. Epidemiological research, health education, and the system of dispensaries characterized prevention practices and applied the risk factor model population-wide.[65] Within a decade, then, an environment emerged that proved accommodating to Western health concepts and, in particular, the new risk factor model.[66]

With respect to the adoption of the risk factor model, the importance of the WHO for both Germanys should not be underestimated in terms of political relevance and conceptual shifts in health care. At the latest, after both Germanys finally joined the WHO in 1973, perceptions about health care were shaped in both states by a global discussion of self-empowerment to deal with risk factors. More to the point, the risk factor model was flexible enough to suit both the collective approach to health care in East Germany and the individualized responsibility scheme in West Germany.

With the introduction of the risk factor model, perceptions of disease as preventable and as linked primarily to individual lifestyle choices grew and led to more coherent prevention practices. Despite all the systemic differences between East and West Germany, the risk factor model emphasized the duty of the individual to keep healthy in both health-care systems. In fact, physicians on both sides of the Berlin Wall called for financial penalties for those who refused to comply with this new insistence on self-responsibility.[67] In both German states, the risk factor model became the main medical approach to dealing with the prevention of heart disease, as well as other diseases such as cancer. In fact, it remains today the most influential conceptual model shaping prevention practices.[68]

Conclusion: Preventing Heart Disease in East and West Germany

Up to the late 1960s, East German health policy focused on the social hygiene tradition, which was successfully reestablished by returning émigrés. This comprehensive approach to health included strong government intervention programs that were unimaginable in West Germany at the time. In West Germany the traditional health-care system was basically restored after the end of World War II. But in an effort to dissociate the new West German state from both the Nazi past and Socialist East Germany, policymakers impeded state intervention in health care. In particular, population-wide prevention programs were obstructed in favor of individualized prevention in private practices. In addition, the German states used each other as reference points, not only in their continuing political rivalry, but also in the long scramble for international recognition.

In both countries, where political ideology clearly molded perceptions of health and prevention practices, heart disease was linked to lifestyle choices relatively early. But in line with their opposing collectivist and individualistic approaches, East German prevention practices included the entire population—while the West German media tended to focus on professional elites, e.g., discussing the so-called Managers' Disease. In this period, neither country was very successful in implementing practical measures for preventing cardiovascular disease.

Since the late 1960s, the adoption of the risk factor model moved prevention practices in the two Germanys closer together. Yet, the reasons for this convergence once again accentuated the two systems' differences. After World War II, the West German government had found it extremely difficult to introduce public health measures. In the late 1970s, however, the recession of that decade, along with a shifting conceptual approach to health care, made it possible to introduce a new approach toward population-wide prevention programs. Epitomized by the adaptation of the risk factor model to West German power structures—and especially to the interests of the medical profession and the federal system—this policy shift eventually prepared the ground for a cautious reestablishment of public health initiatives after the initial rejection of longstanding public health traditions in light of the medical crimes committed during the Third Reich.[69] East Germany's centralized structures made the health-care system more susceptible to the political desires of the SED. Accordingly, political changes in the early 1970s facilitated conceptual adjustments in health policy and also accommodated a generational change, which helped replace social hygiene traditions with a new emphasis on risk factor analysis. In the context of the changing political climate from the late 1960s, East German political and medical elites proved less reluctant to adopt a Western scientific model. A pronounced interest in international integration eventually allowed Western influences to promote an understanding of prevention practices linked to the risk factor approach. In West Germany, by contrast, this new approach fit into longer continuities in the health care system—while challenging the longstanding refusal to support population-wide prevention programs.

With the introduction of the risk factor model, both states conceived of the conceptual links between lifestyle, health, and relevant prevention practices in similar ways. First, large sections of the population were included in the discussion about disease prevention and categorized as potential patients. Second, both countries stressed individual responsibility for staying healthy. Third, East and West German prevention practices converged by combining a population-wide approach with individualized prevention practices—thus suggesting a parallel history with similar developments in both German states. At the same time, the use of the same scientific model in two vastly different political systems highlighted the flexibility of the risk factor model as one of the foremost causes of its success worldwide. Conceptual similarities prevailed in the long term, despite differences in the way in which the risk factor model was applied.

Prevention practices recommended by the risk factor model provide no guarantees about health. In both German countries, heart disease mortality rose through 1980, with statistical evidence suggesting slightly higher rates for East Germany.[70] In terms of measurable success, only a small difference in the effect of prevention practices in both states can be gleaned from available statistical evidence. From the early 1980s, however, mortality rates slowed down in both Germanys. Whether this can be linked to contemporary prevention practices remains unclear.[71] This very uncertainty about the potential benefits of the risk factor model suggests the importance of another issue not discussed in this chapter—though it often surfaces in the work of both private practitioners and public health experts: the difficulty and complexity of bringing about changes in individual behavior in specific sociocultural settings.

Selected Readings

Aronowitz, Robert A. *Making Sense of Illness: Science, Society, and Disease*. Cambridge, 1998.
Baldwin, Peter. *Contagion and the State in Europe, 1830-1930*. Cambridge, 1999.
Elkeles, Thomas, Jens-Uwe Niehoff, Rolf Rosenbrock, and Frank Schneider, eds. *Prävention und Prophylaxe. Theorie und Praxis eines gesundheitspolitischen Grundmotivs in zwei deutschen Staaten, 1949-1990*. Berlin, 1991.
Hong, Young-Sun. "Cigarette Butts and the Building of Socialism in East Germany." *Central European History* 35/3 (2002): 327–44.
Jarausch, Konrad. *Das Ende der Zuversicht? Die siebziger Jahre als Geschichte*. Göttingen, 2008.
Kleßmann, Christoph. "Spaltung und Verflechtung — Ein Konzept zur integrierten Nachkriegsgeschichte 1945 bis 1990." In *Teilung und Integration*, ed. Christoph Kleßmann and Peter Lautzas, 20–36. Schwalbach, 2006.
Kury, Patrick. "Zivilisationskrankheiten an der Schwelle zur Konsumgesellschaft. Das Beispiel der Managerkrankheit in den 1950er- und 1960er Jahren." In *Die vergangene Zukunft Europas. Bevölkerungsforschung und –prognosen im 20. und 21. Jahrhundert*, ed. Petra Overath, 185–210. Cologne, 2011.
Lengwiler, Martin and Jeannette Madarász, eds. *Das präventive Selbst. Eine Kulturgeschichte moderner Gesundheitspolitik*. Bielefeld, 2010.
Lindner, Ulrike. "Chronische Gesundheitsprobleme. Das deutsche Gesundheitssystem vom Kaiserreich bis in die Bundesrepublik." *Aus Politik und Zeitgeschichte* B33–34 (2003): 21–28.
Madarász, Jeannette. "Prävention chronischer Herzkreislauf-Krankheiten. BRD, DDR und Großbritannien im Vergleich, 1945-1990." *Prävention und Gesundheitsförderung* 5/4 (2010): 313–18.
Moser, Gabriele. *"Im Interesse der Volksgesundheit..." Sozialhygiene und öffentliches Gesundheitswesen in der Weimarer Republik und der frühen SBZ/DDR. Ein Beitrag zur Sozialgeschichte des deutschen Gesundheitswesens im 20. Jahrhundert*. Frankfurt am Main, 2002.
Rothstein, William G. *Public Health and the Risk Factor: A History of an Uneven Medical Revolution*. Rochester, N.Y., 2003.
Schagen, Udo and Sabine Schleiermacher, eds. *100 Jahre Sozialhygiene, Sozialmedizin und Public Health in Deutschland. Berichte und Dokumente zur Zeitgeschichte der Medizin*. Berlin, 2005.
Stöckel, Sigrid and Ulla Walter, eds. *Prävention im 20. Jahrhundert. Historische Grundlagen und aktuelle Entwicklungen in Deutschland*. Weinheim, 2002.
Timmermann, Carsten. "Appropriating Risk Factors: The Reception of an American Approach to Chronic Disease in the Two German States, c. 1950–1990." *Social History of Medicine* 25/1 (2012): 157–74.

Notes

1. See Florentine Fritzen, *Gesünder leben—Die Lebensreformbewegung im 20. Jahrhundert* (Stuttgart, 2006).
2. Peter Baldwin, *Contagion and the State in Europe, 1830-1930* (Cambridge, 1999).

3. Christoph Kleßmann, "Spaltung und Verflechtung—Ein Konzept zur integrierten Nachkriegsgeschichte 1945 bis 1990," in *Teilung und Integration*, ed. Christoph Kleßmann and Peter Lautzas (Schwalbach, 2006), 20–36.
4. Alfred Grotjahn, *Soziale Pathologie. Versuch einer Lehre von den sozialen Beziehungen der menschlichen Krankheiten als Grundlage der sozialen Medizin und der sozialen Hygiene* (Berlin, 1923).
5. In fact, it was the insurance industry that became concerned relatively early with the probabilities of sickness. This provided a strong impetus for the development of statistical and probability calculations. Theodore M. Porter, *Trust in Numbers: The Pursuit of Objectivity in Science and Public Life* (Princeton, 1995). See also J. Rosser Matthews, *Quantification and the Quest for Medical Certainty* (Princeton, 1995).
6. See http://www.framinghamheartstudy.org/ (accessed 18 November 2011).
7. On the background and reception of the risk factor model in the United States, see William G Rothstein, *Public Health and the Risk Factor: A History of an Uneven Medical Revolution* (Rochester, N.Y., 2003).
8. Robert Aronowitz, *Making Sense of Illness: Science, Society, and Disease* (Cambridge, 1998).
9. Carsten Timmermann, "Risikofaktoren. Der scheinbar unaufhaltsame Erfolg eines Ansatzes aus der amerikanischen Epidemiologie in der deutschen Nachkriegsmedizin," in *Das präventive Selbst. Eine Kulturgeschichte moderner Gesundheitspolitik*, ed. Martin Lengwiler and Jeannette Madarász (Bielefeld, 2010), 257.
10. Grotjahn, *Soziale Pathologie*.
11. This became apparent, for example, in the 1926 Düsseldorf exhibition GESOLEI, which celebrated the withdrawal of the French occupation forces. The acronym stands for "health care" (GEsundheitspflege), "social care" (SOziale Fürsorge), and "physical exercise" (LEibesübungen). See Hans Murchhauser, "Die Ernährung," and Ernst Wilms-Posen, "Leibesübungen," in *Gesolei. Grosse Ausstellung Düsseldorf 1926. Für Gesundheitspflege, Soziale Fürsorge und Leibesübungen*, vol. 2, ed. Arthur Schloßmann (Düsseldorf, 1927), 528, 536, 940f. See also Matthias Weipert, *"Mehrung der Volkskraft". Die Debatte über Bevölkerung, Modernisierung und Nation 1890-1933* (Paderborn, 2006), 139.
12. Heinrich Klepp, "Die deutsche Großstadtbevölkerung im Jahre 1933," *Deutsches Ärzteblatt* 64/1 (1934): 383, Also see Robert N. Proctor, *The Nazi War on Cancer* (Princeton, 1999). For the political use of metaphors of illness, see Susan Sontag, *Illness as Metaphor* (New York, 1978).
13. Timmermann, *Risikofaktoren*.
14. BArch DQ 1/15037, Hauptabteilung medizinische Forschung.
15. Grotjahn, *Soziale Pathologie*.
16. Erich Fischer, Lothar Rohland, and Dietrich Tutzke, *Für das Wohl des Menschen. 30 Jahre Gesundheitswesen der DDR* (Berlin, 1979), 9, 14f. See also Anna-Sabine Ernst, "Die beste Prophylaxe ist der Sozialismus". Ärzte und medizinische Hochschullehrer in der SBZ/DDR 1945-1961 (Munster, 1997), 36.
17. For more detail see Gabriele Moser, *"Im Interesse der Volksgesundheit..." Sozialhygiene und öffentliches Gesundheitswesen in der Weimarer Republik und der frühen SBZ/DDR. Ein Beitrag zur Sozialgeschichte des deutschen Gesundheitswesens im 20. Jahrhundert* (Frankfurt am Main, 2002).
18. "Das gefährliche Gerinnsel," *Der Spiegel* 42 (1955): 36–37.

19. Otto Graf, "Die Krankheit der Verantwortlichen," *Schriftenreihe des deutschen Gesundheitsmuseums* 1/3 (1953): 3–14. Cf. Herbert Immich, "Nehmen Herz- und Gefäßkrankheiten überall zu?" *Deutsches Ärzteblatt* 42/8 (1957): 220.
20. See Patrick Kury, "Zivilisationskrankheiten an der Schwelle zur Konsumgesellschaft. Das Beispiel der Managerkrankheit in den 1950er- und 1960er Jahren," in *Die vergangene Zukunft Europas. Bevölkerungsforschung und –prognosen im 20. und 21. Jahrhundert*, ed. Petra Overath, (Cologne, 2011), 190.
21. "Wen die Götter lieben," *Der Spiegel* 16 (1954): 34–37. Karl Kaiser, "Die 'Manager-Krankheit' ist vermeidbar," in *Schriftenreihe des deutschen Gesundheitsmuseums* 1/3 (1953): 15–29. For East Germany see BArch DQ 1/23962, HA II/3 HKL 1967–1970, vol. 2.
22. Klaus Gläß, and Werner Schmidt, eds., *Recht und Gesundheitsförderung unter besonderer Beachtung der Lebensweise. Eine vergleichende Forschungsstudie in Europa* (Dresden, 1986), 25 (p. 20 for the West German approach).
23. Ibid., 20f.
24. Ibid., 24f.
25. Ibid., 41.
26. Jens-Uwe Niehoff and Ralf-Raigo Schrader, "Gesundheitsbilder — Absichten und Realitäten in der Deutschen Demokratischen Republik," in *Prävention und Prophylaxe. Theorie und Praxis eines gesundheitspolitischen Grundmotivs in zwei deutschen Staaten, 1949-1990*, eds. Thomas Elkeles, Jens-Uwe Niehoff, Rolf Rosenbrock, and Frank Schneider (Berlin, 1991), 59f.
27. For more detailed information on Winter, Redetzky, and Marcusson, see Udo Schagen and Sabine Schleiermacher, eds., *100 Jahre Sozialhygiene, Sozialmedizin und Public Health in Deutschland. Berichte und Dokumente zur Zeitgeschichte der Medizin* (Berlin, 2005).
28. Ernst, *Die beste Prophylaxe*.
29. Günter Ewert, "Organisation und Praxis der Prävention in der Deutschen Demokratischen Republik," in Elkeles, *Prävention und Prophylaxe*, 109.
30. The latter involved adding fluorine to drinking water supplies. See Dieter Borgers, "Primärprävention durch biotechnischen Eingriff versus Gesundheitserziehung. Das Beispiel der Kariesprävention durch Fluoridierung," in *Präventionspolitik. Gesellschaftliche Strategien der Gesundheitssicherung*, ed. Rolf Rosenbrock, Hagen Kühn, and Barbara M. Köhler (Berlin, 1994), 83–95.
31. Moser, *Volksgesundheit*, 198f.
32. Patrice Poutrus and Burghard Ciesla, "Food Supply in a Planned Economy: SED Nutrition Policy Between Crisis Response and Popular Needs," in *Dictatorship as Experience: Towards a Socio-Cultural History of the GDR*, ed. Konrad Jarausch (New York and Oxford, 1999), 143–62.
33. Ewert, *Prävention*, 121. For a more detailed discussion, see Jeannette Madarász, "Prävention chronischer Herzkreislauf-Krankheiten. BRD, DDR und Großbritannien im Vergleich, 1945-1990," in *Prävention und Gesundheitsförderung* 5/4 (2010): 313–18.
34. See BArch B310/134, letter from Bernhard Zoller (Senior Governmental Official and Medical Officer in the Federal Ministry of the Interior) to Harald Petri (German Health Museum), 7 June 1956.
35. See, e.g., Josef Stockhausen, "Tätigkeitsbericht der Bundesärztekammer," *Deutsches Ärzteblatt* 63/20 (1966): 1320–27.

36. See "Mehrheit gegen Kompetenzverschiebung. Große Grundsatzdebatte des Deutschen Bundestages zur Gesundheitspolitik," *Deutsches Ärzteblatt* 65/28 (1968): 1571, 1580.
37. Rald Groven, "Bundesregierung will die Primärprävention noch stärker betonen," *Deutsches Ärzteblatt* 79/17 (1982): 23–24.
38. Wilhelm Ahrens, "Grundlagen einer sinnvollen Gesundheitspolitik," *Deutsches Ärzteblatt* 72/32 (1975): 2270. See also "Allgemeine Vorsorge—Probelauf mit 40000 Versicherten," *Deutsches Ärzteblatt* 66/39 (1969): 2647; Madarász, *Prävention*.
39. For American influences on German cardiology, see Bruno Kisch, *Die Geschichte der Organization der Kreislaufforschung in Deutschland* (Darmstadt, 1955).
40. Timmermann, *Risikofaktoren*.
41. For technocratic thinking in East Germany, see Peter Caldwell, *Dictatorship, State Planning, and Social Theory in the German Democratic Republic* (Cambridge, 2003). See also Peter Hübner, "Mensch-Macht-Maschinen. Technokratie in der DDR," in *Eliten im Sozialismus. Beiträge zur Sozialgeschichte der DDR*, ed. Peter Hübner (Cologne, 1999), 325–60.
42. See *Archiv für Hygiene und Bakteriologie*, esp. the years 1952–58. See also *Öffentlicher Gesundheitsdienst* from 1955 to 1956.
43. See "Herzverpflanzung. Grenzen verwischt," *Der Spiegel* 2 (1968): 72. See also Gerhard Jungmann, "Von der Fürsorge zur Vorsorge," *Deutsches Ärzteblatt* 69/14 (1972): 831–35.
44. Young-Sun Hong, "Cigarette Butts and the Building of Socialism in East Germany," *Central European History* 35/3 (2002): 342.
45. Konrad Jarausch, *Das Ende der Zuversicht? Die siebziger Jahre als Geschichte* (Göttingen, 2008).
46. Lothar AJ Heinemann, W. Barth, et al., *Chronik der Epidemiologie und Prävention chronischer Krankheiten in Ostdeutschland*, vol. 1 (Berlin, 2008), 10 (unpublished manuscript in possession of the author).
47. Ibid.
48. Richard Cooper, "Rising Death Rates in the Soviet Union: The Impact of Coronary Heart Disease," *The New England Journal of Medicine* 304/21 (1981): 1259–64.
49. The first of these workshops, which took place in Stockholm in 1971, offered the opportunity to discuss epidemiological research and practical issues. See Heinemann, *Chronik der Epidemiologie*, 13. For a more general overview see Dietrich Pfeiffer, "Herz-Kreislauf-Gesellschaft in der DDR," in *75 Jahre Deutsche Gesellschaft für Kardiologie—Herz- und Kreislaufforschung*, ed. Bernd Lüritz (Berlin, 2002), 74–117.
50. There were total of thirty-two MONICA Collaborating Centres in twenty-one countries. See http://www.ktl.fi/monica/ (accessed on 19 May 2011).
51. Heinemann, *Chronik der Epidemiologie*, 7.
52. Ibid., 8. See Gläß, Schmidt, *Recht und Gesundheitsförderung*.
53. Günter Ewert, *Dispensairebetreuung in der DDR. Ein Rückblick nach vorn* (Berlin, 2002), 30.
54. Heinemann, *Chronik der Epidemiologie*, 8.
55. "Allgemeine Vorsorge—Probelauf mit 40000 Versicherten," *Deutsches Ärzteblatt* 66/39 (1969): 2647. For pilot studies specifically discussing heart disease and the risk factor model, see Ahrens, „Grundlagen einer sinnvollen Gesundheitspolitik," 2270. Similar initiatives were started in North Rhein-Westphalia, Hamburg, and Rheinland-Palatinate, often under the guidance of major health insurance groups.

56. One example of this strategy was the political wrangling over the prevention program for mothers in the mid 1960s. See Ulrike Lindner, "Chronische Gesundheitsprobleme. Das deutsche Gesundheitssystem vom Kaiserreich bis in die Bundesrepublik," *Aus Politik und Zeitgeschichte* B33–34 (2003): 25f.
57. Herbert Czwikla, "Beispielhaftes Gesundheitsbewußtsein bei Ärzten," *Deutsches Ärzteblatt* 80/6 (1983): 49–50.
58. See, e.g., Ernst Berger, ed., *Krank. Zur Krise der Medizin* (Vienna, 1977).
59. The Federal Office of Health Education was founded as the counterpart to the East German Hygiene Museum in 1968. Its second International Seminar for Health Education, which took place in 1970 and was organized in close cooperation with the WHO, focused on heart disease prevention and the implications of the risk factor model for prevention practices. See Bundeszentrale für gesundheitliche Aufklärung, *Herz- und Kreislauf-Krankheiten. Die Rolle der Gesundheitserziehung in der Erst- und Zweitprävention. II. Internationales Seminar für Gesundheitserziehung in Höhenried, 5.-10-7.1970* (Cologne, 1973).
60. BArch B310/38. The German Society for Nutrition tried to make the Federal Ministry for Youth, Women, and Health aware of Swedish initiatives in this field, and encouraged their application in West Germany, where the Swedish example was, as a result, more influential than the internationally more prominent Finnish North Karelia Project.
61. For further information see Hansheinz Kreuter, Lothar Klaes, Hans Hoffmeister, and Ulrich Laaser, *Prävention von Herz- Kreislaufkrankheiten. Ergebnisse und Konsequenzen der Deutschen Herz-Kreislauf-Präventionsstudie (DHP)* (Weinheim, 1995).
62. BArch B189/16768, Jahresbericht der Bundesregierung (1976), Gesundheitspolitik, vol. 1, 21 December 1976; Diskussionsentwurf des Programms von BMJFG (Bundesministerium für Jugend, Frauen und Gesundheit) und BMFT (Bundesministerium für Forschung und Technologie), 28 April 1976.
63. BArch B310/56, Kontakte WHO, Referat 302 (BMJFG), Zusammenarbeit zwischen der BRD und der WHO auf dem Gebiet der Gesundheitserziehung, 9 October 1973.
64. The GDR became increasingly dependent on West German economic support, which may have also promoted greater openness toward Western concepts.
65. In fact, the Anglo-American origins of the risk factor model and related prevention practices emphasized the model's inherent public health components. See Rothstein, *Public Health and the Risk Factor*.
66. Niehoff, *Gesundheitsleitbilder*, 64. See also Jens-Uwe Niehoff, "Sozialepidemiologie in der DDR — Probleme und Fakten," *Kritische Medizin* 16 (1991): 53–83.
67. See Jens-Uwe Niehoff and Torsten Röding, "Steuerung und Regulierung von Prävention in der Deutschen Demokratischen Republik," in Elkeles, *Prävention und Prophylaxe*, 162. For a West German example, see Ferdinand Schmidt, "Stiefkind Prävention," *Deutsches Ärzteblatt* 76/17 (1979): 1190.
68. Jürgen von Troschke, "Das Risikofaktorenmodell als handlungsleitendes Paradigma der Prävention in Deutschland," in *Prävention im 20. Jahrhundert. Historische Grundlagen und aktuelle Entwicklungen in Deutschland*, ed. Sigrid Stöckel and Ulla Walter (Weinheim, 2002), 190–203.
69. Another prominent example was the government's support for self-help groups since the 1970s, when the health insurance companies were required by law to support financially forms of self-help. For a detailed discussion of self-help in East and West

Germany, see Annette Elisabeth Mund, *Ansprüche an gesundheitsbezogene Selbsthilfe im Vergleich West- und Ostdeutschland*, (Ph.D. diss., Cologne University, 2009).
70. There is no reliable data for heart disease mortality for the two Germanys before 1970. It should also be noted that statistical data on heart disease mortality can be misleading, especially when comparing data from different countries. See Rafael Lozano, Christopher JL Murray, Alan D. Lopez, and Toshi Satoh, "Miscoding and misclassification of ischaemic heart disease mortality," in *Global Programme on Evidence for Health Policy*, Working paper No. 12, WHO (2001) (http://cdrwww.who.int/healthinfo/paper12.pdf) (accessed on 19 September 2012). For this reason, it may suffice to indicate general trends rather than trying to construct a false impression of one country being more successful in dealing with heart disease than another.
71. East German rates remained slightly higher than West German ones, though differing methods of statistical calculation make this difficult to determine with any certainty.

CHAPTER 6

Socialism Fights the Proletarian Disease
East German Efforts to Overcome Tuberculosis in a Cold War Context

DONNA HARSCH

Tuberculosis (TB) resurged as a deadly contagion in Germany during and after World War II.¹ Especially likely to have or to contract TB were the thousands of former concentration camp inmates who lived in displaced persons camps in defeated Germany. Also particularly afflicted were the millions of refugees and expellees who flooded into Germany in the last months of the war and first years afterward.² The epidemic in the Soviet Zone of Occupation (SBZ) was worse than in the West because most German refugees and expellees from Poland and Czechoslovakia passed through the Eastern zone of occupation before moving further west. In 1947, tuberculosis killed 32,000 people in the SBZ.³ Soviet authorities and German officials took the TB epidemic seriously, not only because the situation was grave, but also because of the symbolic significance of tuberculosis for Communists and Socialists. Dubbed the "proletarian disease" early in the century by the Social Democratic social hygienist Alfred Grotjahn, tuberculosis was seen as the quintessential social disease—caused by a microbe but exacerbated by the inequities of capitalism.⁴

Confronted with a German capitalist rival, Communists in the German Democratic Republic (GDR) were eager to demonstrate the superiority of Socialist health care and believed that the conquest of TB would provide powerful confirmation of just that. In fact, health authorities made impressive progress in the fight against TB during the first ten to fifteen years after the founding of the GDR in 1949. TB morbidity and mortality rates declined dramatically—a result of TB policies, as well as improved social and economic conditions. One can disagree, though, about which policies and conditions contributed most to this decline. One can also debate the success of East German policies relative to those implemented by capitalist democracies that faced a postwar TB epidemic, such as the GDR's fellow German-speaking states, the Federal Republic and Austria. But this essay addresses different questions: What was the relationship between continuity and change in East German TB policy in the 1950s? What factors influenced the dynamic mix of tradition and innovation?

As we shall see, certain "inherited" practices and assumptions about TB and TB patients were tenacious. Moreover, East German health officials implemented new methods cautiously, despite what one might expect from a Socialist state with strong mechanisms of central control. Change certainly occurred in TB policy, but there was no rapid or thorough transformation. "Tried and true" methods were gradually discredited and erratically cast off; as new policies gained traction, they were carried out with greater authority and confidence.

The focus of this essay is on preventive measures because "prevention first" was the mantra of East German health care. A focus on prevention may seem odd, given the well-known revolution in TB treatment in the postwar era: the discovery of streptomycin and other drugs that ended TB's long reign as a mass killer in the West. But medical historians emphasize that the impact of those "wonder drugs" looks more sudden in hindsight than it actually was at the time. Only in the United States, where streptomycin was massively prescribed and where TB had long been in decline, did antibiotics produce dramatic effects—and even in the United States, sanatoriums were not completely shuttered until the late 1950s. In Europe, older treatments and preventive methods continued to play an important role in TB policy long into the postwar era.

Massive use of the new drugs was even more delayed in the GDR, not least because those new drugs were produced by Western pharmaceutical firms and were thus expensive for the GDR to buy. They were prescribed almost exclusively to patients in stationary care, i.e., in sanatoriums. The scarcity of antibiotics in the GDR became, as Melanie Arndt has shown, a hot potato in Cold War propaganda between East and West Germany. West German "charities" and the press made much of Communism's failures to produce and provide the new antibiotic drugs, while East German health officials denied the existence of shortages in penicillin, streptomycin, etc., and argued that preventive methods were better anyway.[5]

The "preventive" measures considered in this essay are compulsory institutionalization (*Zwangsasylierung*) of uncooperative TB patients who were presumed to be contagious, on the one hand, and vaccination against TB with Bacillus Calmette-Guérin (BCG), on the other. In the case of compulsory institutionalization, continuity with the past dominated in law and discourse, but was increasingly, if inconsistently, attenuated in practice by the late 1950s. BCG vaccination represented a break with traditional TB policy in Germany, but it was implemented unevenly and without force of law until 1961. Continuity and incomplete change were multiply determined: of major significance in both cases was the commitment of physicians and TB experts to older practices, ideas, and institutions that were, in part, specifically German and, in part, common in the wider world of medical practice during the first half of the twentieth century. Certainly, the failure to denazify the medical profession in either German state reinforced professional resistance to "new" methods in the first years after the defeat of National Socialism. In the case of state reluctance to make BCG vaccination obligatory, a significant factor was widespread popular suspicion of the vaccination.

Also working against change were, in all likelihood, political influences related to the introduction of "socialism" in East Germany. The struggle against TB occurred in parallel with the gradually accelerating socialization of the medical profession in the GDR in the 1950s. The temporal correspondence between the socialization of medicine, the considerable opposition of doctors in private practice to BCG vaccination, and, finally, state reluctance to enforce BCG vaccination suggest that Socialist health officials hesitantly introduced BCG vaccination before the later 1950s, at least in part, out of fear of driving up the already high rate of flight by private practice doctors to the West. If this supposition is correct, then German-German rivalry had the ironic effect of retarding innovation in East German health practices. In the case of continued resort to compulsory institutionalization, not German-German tensions but the guiding ideology of GDR health care—social hygiene—was an important factor. In the early postwar years, East German social hygiene was still dominated by prewar beliefs (not unique to social hygiene) that compulsory institutionalization was a legitimate "preventive" measure and that recalcitrant patients were "asocial."[6]

Compulsory Institutionalization (*Zwangsasylierung*)

Compulsory institutionalization was an ethically objectionable and medically questionable "preventive" measure in the fight against the spread of TB after 1945. But in postwar Germany, it was, paradoxically, the least contentious preventive measure among those used by either German state. It never became a political issue in German-German relations. Some health officials in both states had qualms about using force to institutionalize patients and, over time, fewer patients were unwillingly sent to TB institutions. Both states nonetheless retained the power to institutionalize TB patients against their will—and both states made use of that power. Given the convergence of theory, law, and practice, neither state even considered turning compulsory institutionalization into a Cold War issue. Health officials encountered only few and vague professional objections to the practice. In fact, TB specialists in both Germanys often lobbied for more, not fewer, restrictions on the rights of obstinate TB patients.[7]

The Third Reich had legalized compulsory institutionalization in 1938, and some states in the Federal Republic based their power to confine uncooperative patients on the Nazi law. The idea of forced confinement also had a left-wing intellectual and legal pedigree in Germany. Early in the century, Alfred Grotjahn had advocated compulsory institutionalization of supposedly irresponsible TB patients.[8] For its part, East German policy was modeled, in practice, on a Soviet decree: Order Nr. 297 of the Soviet Military Administration in Germany (SMAD), which empowered the "local police" to "observe" TB patients and to use "force" to isolate a TB patient—though "only with approval of the federal state (*Land*) or provincial health office," and only if the patient could not be secluded in his or her own home. In discussions with Soviet health officials, German health officers asked for clarification of the terms *police observation* and *force*. Their questions suggested unease with the Soviet order, but no one on the East German side made explicit objections.[9] In December 1946, the German health administration in the Soviet zone issued its own order that allowed for compulsory institutionalization of recalcitrant TB patients.[10] In reports on the acute postwar TB crisis, health officials noted practical skepticism about using "force" against patients who defied an order to enter or remain in a sanatorium.[11] In an account of anti-TB efforts in Chemnitz, Dr. Martin Fröhlich argued, "Only in cases in which...the sick person consciously endangers his environment should forced isolation be ruthlessly implemented." When these cases arose, he added, patients should be sent to a regular sanatorium, not an isolation ward.[12]

After almost ten years without mention in the files of the Ministry of Health, compulsory institutionalization comes up in correspondence between health officials and doctors in 1955 about how to handle "unregenerate" or "asocial" patients. The intervening practice can be gleaned from their letters and memoranda, if sparsely. Called in by health officials, the police often delivered an uncooperative patient to a sanatorium. As recommended earlier by Dr. Fröhlich, such patients lived without restraint among "voluntary" patients. The compulsory assignment of patients to a sanatorium had become "strikingly" less common, wrote Dr. Adolf Tegtmeier, director of the GDR's premier sanatorium at Bad Berka (in Thuringia). Tegtmeier offered no explicit clarification of this point, but additional remarks in the same letter suggested that he believed the new antibiotic treatments had contributed to the decline. Few patients remained "unregenerate," he noted, once they had received "first-class medical care." Indeed, he went on, their behavior usually became "irreproachable," a change that, he did not doubt, had provoked "embarrassment" among caregivers who had assumed the worst: "One has become, in sum, more careful about judging such patients."[13]

Rather than propose the abolition of special police powers over TB patients, Tegtmeier wanted to segregate completely those "few" patients whom he "would describe as asocial" because they had repeatedly refused to follow medical instructions, had escaped from (in his opinion) well-run TB institutions, and had "to be brought back by the police over and over again ... are aggressive ... steal, etc." For two years, Bad Berka conducted an experiment in "seclud[ing]" such patients. He judged the results as "not bad," and was therefore writing to Dr. Erwin Marcusson of the central health administration to recommend that the Ministry of Health open an official isolation ward for "asocial" TB patients inside a psychiatric asylum where, "under psychiatric guidance," "antisocial sick people ... would come under stricter conditions than is possible in a clinical sanatorium."[14]

The idea for a closed TB ward was pushed within the GDR's health system simultaneously from below and from above. The head administrator of the district health office in Erfurt, Dr. Kohlstock, had authority over the sanatorium at Bad Berka and had asked Tegtmeier to take the step of secluding "asocial" patients there.[15] Tegtmeier attempted, in turn, to convince Marcusson to create an official isolation ward in a more secure institution. Having heard "numerous complaints from our doctors" about contagious patients who refused to follow medical instructions, Marcusson had, on his own initiative, begun to query district administrators about the possibility of opening an isolation ward for "unregenerate" TB patients inside a psychiatric institution.[16]

Adolf Tegtmeier had joined the NSDAP in 1933 and remained in the party until 1945. His Nazi membership was not at all unusual among German physicians. His party membership might explain his notably free use of the term "asocial." In his reply to Tegtmeier, Marcusson used the less-freighted term "unregenerate." Marcusson was an "Old Communist" of Jewish background. He directed East Germany's Institute for Social Hygiene and served as Deputy Minister of Health from 1957 to 1958.[17] Yet, we should not assume that the concept of "asocial" sick people was simply a remnant of Nazi racial hygiene, for it had also been part of both Social Democratic and Soviet social hygienic language.[18] In the immediate postwar period, references to "asocial" sick people peppered East German reports that otherwise emphasized the TB epidemic's environmental causes.[19] In his correspondence, Marcusson employed the term as well, though less liberally than Tegtmeier did. Before condemning Communists and former Nazis as the only peas left in the eugenic pod, it should be noted that "asocial" was common parlance in official discourse about recalcitrant TB patients in all three German-speaking states after the war: the GDR, West Germany, and Austria.[20] And, if not the term, then the concept of "unregenerate" TB patients remained in use after 1945 in countries far from Central Europe. In the United States, for example, homeless alcoholic people with TB were often confined against their will into at least the mid 1950s—something not true of nonalcoholics.[21]

The stigmatization and forced confinement of noncompliant patients after 1945 was not, then, unique to East Germany. Still, Tegtmeier's plan to isolate difficult patients has to be considered in the framework of the recent Nazi past.

The institution that Tegtmeier, Kohlstock, and Marcusson all considered to be the best place for an isolation ward was the psychiatric asylum at Stadtroda—which, as they well knew, had been the Third Reich's "first and most well-known compulsory confinement ward."[22] In discussing the plan, only Marcusson hinted at slight discomfort with Stadtroda as the site of an isolation ward.[23]

As it turned out, the plan was not realized at Stadtroda or elsewhere. Every district health officer and every director of a psychiatric institute canvassed by the Ministry of Health refused to open such a ward. They allegedly declined because they did not want to assign scarce beds to TB patients. According to East German Minister of Health Luitpold Steidle, however, "no district wanted such a station" for "forcibly confined asocial sick people."[24] And Berlin did not insist. Faced with continued pressure from TB doctors to do something, the Ministry instead considered denying welfare payments to uncooperative patients—an idea rejected by the East German trade unions, which administered social welfare in the GDR.[25]

The Ministry was consequently unable to move forward with the plan. Marcusson blamed the murky legal regulation of TB for preventing the Ministry from taking decisive action. As he explained to the director of the TB sanatorium in Stralsund, "asocial TB sick people will be taken into forced confinement in limited numbers, but only after a TB-law has issued clear guidelines about the treatment of forced confinees."[26] In 1956, the health ministry again began to discuss the elements of a new TB law that would include a stipulation for "compulsory confinement of unregenerate TB patients."[27] Various committees deliberated intermittently for years. In 1965, the GDR passed a "law for the prevention and combating of contagious diseases," which provided for the trial and imprisonment for up to two years of a person with a contagious disease who had disobeyed a doctor's orders and thus potentially became the source of wider infection.[28]

East German officials knew that the FRG was caught in a similar medical and legal dilemma. Various federal states (*Bundesländer*) wanted a new, uniform national law to regulate the terms of compulsory confinement. It turned out to be impossible to negotiate such a law because of competing public interests in West Germany: while TB doctors called publicly for imprisonment of uncooperative patients in the mid 1950s, West German TB patients began to speak out around the same time about their right to "personal liberty."[29]

In both Germanys, then, influential physicians assumed that the state had the authority to enforce a doctor's orders against the patient's will, and that disobedient patients were willfully risking the health of the larger community. Officials in both states entertained the idea of introducing such a radical measure, but, in the end, did not insist on it. Legal qualms seem to have held them back—and that, too, was the case in both states. By the late 1950s, their ambivalence seemed also to reflect discomfort about applying the concept of "asociality" to uncooperative TB patients. In the Federal Republic, academics influenced by American sociological theory began to advocate a social-psychological understanding that considered the behavior of uncooperative patients within their family situation and social milieu.[30] In the GDR, the term "unregenerate" gradually replaced "asocial" in internal reports and correspondence about noncompliant TB patients. Based on available archival sources, it was not until 1963 that East German sanatoriums began to provide psychological counseling for sanatorium patients who did not follow their prescribed medical regimens.[31]

The Ministry of Health came around only slowly to either a social or a psychological perspective on patient behavior, perhaps because a social explanation of undesirable behavior might have suggested that Socialist conditions were less than ideal; at the same time, a psychological analysis would have been considered overly individualistic. Reflecting both a gradual and uneven process of destalinization and an increasing, if circumscribed, recognition of the complexity of Socialist society, sociopsychological explanations of a variety of undesired, but apolitical, behaviors finally became acceptable to the ruling Socialist Unity Party (SED) in the 1960s.[32]

Hesitant Implementation of the "New": BCG Vaccination

Questions about the efficacy of Bacillus Calmette-Guérin (BCG), a vaccine against TB that was developed in France in 1921, have prevented—and continue to prevent—BCG from finding universal support among doctors and public health officials. Some national public health services—e.g., in Sweden, the USSR, and the United Kingdom—have long insisted that BCG is effective, while others, especially in the United States, have refused to use it, pointing to evidence that it does not protect all recipients. It is now recognized as about 80 percent effective for fifteen years. BCG is nonetheless accepted today by the United Nations as a powerful preventive tool in the fight against TB, especially among infants in societies where its incidence is widespread.[33]

BCG became especially controversial in Germany due to a tragic mistake. In 1929, batches of the vaccine administered in Lübeck were contaminated by a virulent strain of the bovine bacillus (from which BCG is produced), causing the death of seventy-two infants. This catastrophe set back BCG vaccination all over the world and ended its use in Germany until after World War II. Although BCG was recognized as a very safe vaccine by 1945, memory of the Lübeck tragedy led postwar Germans, both physicians and the populace, to believe otherwise.[34] West German doctors were highly skeptical of BCG and communicated their doubts to parents. Into the late 1950s, as a result, the rate of infant vaccination was low in most, though not all, federal states.[35]

East German health authorities were well disposed toward BCG for a variety of reasons. In 1949, the influential Communist physician Rudolf Neumann argued for the introduction of obligatory BCG vaccination of children in the GDR. Its safety and efficacy were confirmed, he wrote, by "international journals," Soviet practical experience since 1925, and trials conducted in Schleswig-Holstein in 1947. "Cost-benefit" analysis spoke in favor of BCG, he concluded.[36] The GDR waited until 1961, however, to make BCG vaccination compulsory for all infants, despite the belief of the Socialist medical establishment in BCG as a major preventive tool against TB—and despite the example of required BCG vaccination in the USSR and in Sweden, which, in the mid 1950s, emerged as a major model for East German social and health policy.

Official sensitivity to popular recollection of the Lübeck disaster clearly influenced the Ministry of Health's delay in making BCG vaccination obligatory. Its hesitation also reflected the resistance to BCG on the part of doctors in private practice, who still comprised the vast majority of medical practitioners in the early 1950s. But in 1951, the Ministry did carry out the first of many mass voluntary vaccination campaigns at clinics and schools. Vaccination of infants and children was propagated for weeks beforehand by schoolteachers and by doctors who worked in state polyclinics. The huge campaign, a summary report concluded, resulted in "no cases of serious harm" and was judged to be a medical success.[37]

Doctors in private practice nevertheless continued to focus on the risks of BCG. Like BCG opponents in West Germany, East German skeptics highlighted individual cases in which BCG had been ineffective or seemed to have caused harm. These examples were spoken about in doctors' offices and elsewhere, stirring fears among parents.[38] Reports of scattered cases of (alleged) BCG-related damage also alarmed GDR health authorities, who investigated every incidence of alleged BCG inefficacy or harm.[39] In internal discussions among medical officials, two opposing opinions emerged about how to respond to alleged BCG damage: one side worried about the few instances of harm that seemed related to BCG and argued for greater caution in administering BCG to infants and children. The other side insisted that BCG was an "unusually well-prepared" vaccine whose risks were statistically insignificant.[40]

Official assurances did not convince fearful parents. A social worker reported that "rejection of the vaccination is strikingly high" among people who had heard about alleged BCG-induced eye ailments.[41] In Leipzig, another observer claimed, opponents of the vaccine not only attributed any illness of a vaccinated child to BCG, but also spread stories about imaginary post-vaccine ailments: "It has, in sum, to do with the usual rumor mill (*Es handelt sich also um die übliche Gerüchtsbildung*)," concluded this report.[42]

Health officials blamed anti-BCG physicians for intentional unpreparedness, foot-dragging, and fearmongering during the first mass voluntary vaccination drive.[43] Doctors in the town of Lübbenau reported several BCG-related injuries, but according to an official investigation, these very physicians had not adhered to the protocols for vaccinating children and, in some cases, had not attended any of the training sessions offered by the district. Doctors, Lübbenau's municipal authorities contended, had begun to denounce BCG before any vaccinations were administered. An anti-BCG doctor countered that personnel from local health services had threatened noncompliant parents with loss of health-care coverage or even prosecution: "[M]any children were involuntarily vaccinated," he claimed.[44]

Popular and medical resistance to BCG continued throughout the 1950s, though opposition grew increasingly scattered and intermittent later in the decade.[45] By the mid 1950s, the relationship between doctors and the state had evolved. Most doctors were not in full-time private practice anymore and, thus, had at least some professional ties to state-run health services. Many vociferously anti-Socialist doctors had moved to the West by the mid 1950s, though the number of physicians fleeing the GDR reached a new peak in 1959 to 1960 following the "Second Berlin Crisis." While the relationship between many physicians and the East German state remained tense, BCG vaccination was no longer a major bone of contention, presumably because it had proved to be very safe. As in West Germany, ever fewer doctors were strongly opposed to its use. For their part, health officials felt ever less need to discredit the remaining pockets of opposition, given the Ministry of Health's considerable success in getting newborns vaccinated.

In 1957, 80 percent of East German newborns were vaccinated, though regional variations were considerable.[46] Asked by the Ministry of Health to explain their own district's "score," local officials noted that the rate of vaccination positively correlated with the level of urbanization. They sometimes highlighted cultural factors as well, including, most specifically, memory of the Lübeck disaster of 1929. In a rural county with an especially low rate of vaccination, for example, a medical officer explained: "Recollection of the Calmette-disaster in nearby Lübeck is still strongly rooted in the people of the county of Grevesmühlen and every vaccination is looked upon with the greatest mistrust."[47]

Health administrators used a variety of tactics to pressure parents to have their babies and children vaccinated. From 1954 on, school children who refused vaccination were required not only to present a letter of exemption from their parents, but also from a physician.[48] At prenatal checkups, pregnant women encountered "lively propaganda" in favor of BCG. Almost 95 percent of babies born in maternity hospitals were vaccinated. The rate was much lower for home births. Rural doctors collaborated with the local police to "catch" (*erfassen*) home births in rural areas. Social workers visited isolated villages, where they "use[d] persuasion (lectures and announcements) to change skeptical attitudes."[49] Pushed from above to raise their quotas, district officials asked Berlin why it did not simply require vaccination: central health administrators replied that a law was unnecessary to attain 100 percent coverage of children.[50]

Berlin administrators were determined, above all, to avoid any hint of force in the case of BCG vaccination. The minutes of a meeting held in 1954 insisted that the terms "compulsory vaccination" (*Zwangsimpfung*) and "obligatory vaccination" (*Pflichtimpfung*) must be "retired."[51] This stood in sharp contrast to authorities' willingness not only to force TB patients into a sanatorium, but also to consider isolating a subgroup of them in a psychiatric ward. The contradiction presumably expressed the genuinely different attitudes of health officials toward two target sets of East Germans: noncompliant, contagious patients, on the one hand, and "ordinary" East German parents whose suspicion of BCG might have been justified, on the other. The inconsistency was probably opportunistic as well: no one in East or West Germany—Communist or not, doctor or lay person—was likely to stand up for the rights of noncompliant TB patients, though plenty of people in both states were likely to squawk if BCG vaccination of healthy infants was compelled.

In 1957, the head of the GDR's "tuberculosis department" did call for an ordinance that would make BCG "a duty." Its "formulation," he emphasized, "must be so cleverly chosen that the citizen does not get the feeling of acting under compulsion. Something like a "conscience-clause" (*Gewissensklausel*) should make it as difficult as possible to refuse the required vaccination."[52] He presumably wanted to tap into East Germans' sense of moral obligation to maintain a healthy community, but his recommendation was not followed, in the end. Nor did authorities initially heed the recommendation from a "vaccination committee" for an outright vaccination requirement. It members had pointed to the example of Sweden, where BCG vaccination was a "duty" (*Pflicht*). The director of the GDR's TB research center at Berlin-Buch called for a legal requirement in 1960.[53]

Despite ever more calls from district health officials and prominent TB experts to consolidate and revise TB policy, the GDR passed no comprehensive ordinance until October 1961. The new law made it obligatory for newborns to be vaccinated and for all citizens to get an annual x-ray to check for TB. Passed two months after the construction of the Berlin Wall, the law's timing was certainly not coincidental. BCG opponents could not simply leave the GDR.[54] State officials could also predict that opposition to compulsory vaccination would be minimal, given the years of voluntary campaigns and propaganda that had brought the vast majority of babies and children into a vaccination program that had proven to be extremely safe.

Conclusion

Seen from the perspective of the social history of medicine, the practice and discourse of "preventive" East German TB policy in the 1950s overlapped with similar trends in the GDR's rival state, the Federal Republic of Germany, as well as in other industrialized nations, including the United States. Yet, as Ulrike Lindner argues, tuberculosis was one of "the important problems of all-German politics" in the early postwar era.[55] Consequently, the political context of TB policy in East Germany should also be considered—in particular, within the Cold War framework of the German-German rivalry. Cold War considerations influenced specific policies such as the availability of, and competitive discourse about, streptomycin and other new anti-TB drugs. On the preventive side of the ledger, the division of Germany shaped, above all, the ups and downs of BCG vaccination policy in the GDR. Anxiety about how West Germany might exploit a program of "forced" vaccination of East Germans with the historically tainted BCG vaccine almost certainly contributed to the prolonged hesitation to enforce universally a measure that fit so well with the Socialist emphasis on preventive health.

TB policy and discourse were influenced not only by postwar political divisions, but also by culture and historical circumstance shared by the two Germanys. The past hung over TB policy in the young GDR in many guises: memory of the Lübeck tragedy; the high number of older doctors, many of them former Nazis; vestiges of "racial-hygiene" theory; and a "social-hygiene" ideology suffused with a dated understanding of the relationship between medicine and human behavior. The relevant carry-overs were not equivalent to those in the Federal Republic, but they intersected at significant points, especially medical and popular anxiety about BCG, doctors' commitment to the sanatorium as a venue of prevention as well as of treatment, and the dominant interpretation of medical noncompliance. In both Germanys, official rhetoric about TB patients (and other issues) shifted in the later 1950s away from the earlier emphasis on defiance, willfulness, and anti-social attitudes and toward sociological and psychological explanations of uncooperative behavior. As in the case of the evolving discourse about the dangerous influence of Americanization on youth, TB policy and discourse reflected not only Cold War distinctions, but also cultural commonalities between the two postwar Germanys.[56]

TB policies and attitudes toward uncooperative patients interacted as well with the ideology and politics of the "Socialist" present. Prejudicial assumptions about and restrictive measures toward uncooperative TB patients corresponded to a broader discourse about "asociality" in the GDR and to policies that, especially in the early 1950s, socially isolated and/or actually confined East Germans who, for whatever reason, did not march to the beat of the Communist program.[57] After the mass strikes of June 1953 and especially in line with fitful "destalinization" after 1956, academic, including medical, interpretations of social behavior, as well as SED social and economic policies, grew gradually more conscious of (and less fearful of acknowledging) the existence of social problems in the GDR, including the situation of TB patients.

The dynamic interplay between continuity and change in TB policy in the GDR, was, finally, a structural process of negotiation among central health authorities, local medical professionals, TB patients, and the general population. This process resulted in a gradual acceleration of the "new" in TB policy—not only because of changes "from above" in the Cold War context, SED policies, and Socialist health-care ideology, but also due to a generational turnover in medical personnel and among young parents that seems to have enhanced the standing of Socialist health policies. By the early 1960s, most practicing physicians were employed in state service and, more important, had been trained in Socialist medical schools. Moreover, the medical profession had begun to "feminize," meaning that increasing numbers of young doctors were also mothers who could presumably communicate sympathetically with lay mothers about state vaccination policy.[58] The young average age of first-time mothers (twenty-two years old in 1960) meant that most of them had come of age and been socialized in the GDR. They had not only been indoctrinated about the benefits of universal health care, but also experienced its impressive accomplishments in prenatal, neonatal, and young-child care.[59] Whatever their political stance toward the regime, they nevertheless had many reasons to trust state health policies.

Suggested Readings

Arndt, Melanie. *Gesundheitspolitik im geteilten Berlin 1948 bis 1961*. Cologne, 2009.
Dinter, Andreas. *Seuchenalarm in Berlin. Seuchengeschehen und Seuchenbekämpfung in Berlin nach dem II. Weltkrieg*. Berlin, 1999.
Elkeles, Thomas, Jens-Uwe Niehoff, and Rolf Rosenbrock, eds. *Prävention und Prophylaxe. Theorie und Praxis eines gesundheitspolitischen Grundmotivs in zwei deutschen Staaten 1949-1990*. Berlin, 1991.
Hähner-Rombach, Sylvelyn. *Sozialgeschichte der Tuberkulose. Vom Kaiserreich bis zum Ende des Zweiten Weltkriegs unter besonderer Berücksichtigung Württembergs*. Stuttgart, 2000.
Manow, Philip. "Entwicklungslinien ost- und westdeutscher Gesundheitspolitik zwischen doppelter Staatsgruendung, deutscher Einigung und Europäischer Integration." *Zeitschrift für Sozialreform* 43 (1997): 101-31.
Moser, Gabriele. "*Im Interesse der Volksgesundheit...*" *Sozialhygiene und öffentliches Gesundheitswesen in der Weimarer Republik und der frühen SBZ/DDR. Ein Beitrag zur Sozialgeschichte des deutschen Gesundheitswesens im 20. Jahrhundert*. Frankfurt am Main, 2002.
Niehoff, Jens-Uwe and Frank Schneider. "Sozialhygiene — das Ende einer akademischen Disziplin? Reflexionen zur Geschichte der Sozialhygiene in der DDR." *Jahrbuch für kritische Medizin* 18 (1992): 54–81.
Proctor, R.N. *Medicine Under the Nazis*. Cambridge, M.A., 1988.
Stöckel, Sigrid and Ulla Walter, eds. *Prävention im 20. Jahrhundert. Historische Grundlagen und aktuelle Entwicklungen in Deutschland*. Weinheim, 2002.

Süß, Walter. "Gesundheitspolitik." In *Drei Wege deutscher Sozialstaatlichkeit. NS-Diktatur, Bundesrepublik und DDR im Vergleich*, edited by Hans Günther Hockerts, 55–100. Munich, 1998.
Wilson, Leonard G. "The Historical Decline of Tuberculosis in Europe and America: Its Causes and Significance." *Journal of the History of Medicine* 45 (1990): 366–96.
Woelk, Wolfgang and Jörg Vögele, eds. *Geschichte der Gesundheitspolitik in Deutschland. Von der Weimarer Republik bis in die Frühgeschichte der doppelten Staatsgründung*. Berlin, 2002.

Notes

1. Dirk Blasius, "Tuberkulose: Signalkrankheit deutscher Geschichte," *Geschichtswissenschaft und Unterricht* 47 (1996): 323; Ute Frevert, *Krankheit als politisches Problem. Soziale Unterschichten in Preussen zwischen medizinischer Polizei und staatlicher Sozialversicherung* (Göttingen, 1984), 240; Bundesarchiv Berlin (BArch), DQ1/ 930, Todesfälle an TB berechnet auf 10 000 Einwohner in Sachsen und Chemnitz 1900 bis 1945 (n.d. [1946]); DQ1/ 930, Dr. Martin Fröhlich, "Die Tuberkulose in Chemnitz in den Jahren 1929-1944," January 1946.
2. Klaus-Dieter Müller, "Die Ärzteschaft im staatlichen Gesundheitswesen der SBZ und der DDR 1945-1989," in Robert Jütte, *Geschichte der deutschen Ärzteschaft. Organisierte Berufs- und Gesundheitspolitik im 19.und 20. Jahrhundert* (Cologne, 1997), 247; Anna-Sabine Ernst, *"Die beste Prophylaxe ist der Sozialismus." Ärzte und medizinische Hochschullehrer in der SBZ/DDR 1945-1961* (Muenster, 1997), 171–72.
3. Müller, "Ätzeschaft," 247; Thomas Dormandy, *The White Death: A History of Tuberculosis* (New York, 2000), 348; BArch DQ 1/939, Tuberkulose 1946-1948, Ausbreitung und Bekämpfung der Tuberkulose in der SBZ, 3 July 1946.
4. Sylvelyn Hähner-Rombach, *Sozialgeschichte der Tuberkulose. Vom Kaiserreich bis zum Ende des Zweiten Weltkriegs unter besonderer Berücksichtigung Württembergs* (Stuttgart, 2000), 32.
5. Melanie Arndt, *Gesundheitspolitik im geteilten Berlin, 1948 bis 1961* (Cologne, 2009), 201, 204–6, 210–11. Also see BArch DQ 1 /939, Tuberkulose 1946-1948, Ausbreitung und Bekämpfung der Tuberkulose in der SBZ, Anlage 1, 3 July 1946; Ernst, *Prophylaxe*, 171–72.
6. For an elaborated version of the argument about social hygiene, which also incorporates analysis of TB treatment in the GDR, see Donna Harsch, "Medicalized Social Hygiene? Tuberculosis Policy in the German Democratic Republic," *Bulletin of the History of Medicine* 86/3 (Fall 2012): 394–423.
7. On the Federal Republic, see Ulrike Lindner, *Gesundheitspolitik in der Nachkriegszeit. Grossbritannien und die Bundesrepublik Deutschland im Vergleich* (Munich, 2004), 170–71.
8. Elisabeth Dietrich-Daum, *Die "Wiener Krankheit." Eine Sozialgeschichte der Tuberkulose in Österreich* (Munich, 2007), 295.
9. BArch DQ 1/173, Besprechung Tuberkulose SMA Befehl 278, n.d. (Order 278 provided for better conditions in sanatoriums and hospitals); BArch DQ 1 /939, Entwurf, Befehl des obersten Chefs der SMA...Nr. 297, 3 October 1946. Until 1949, German officials operated under the occupational authority of the Soviet Military Administration (SMA or SMAD). In cases involving contradictory policies, SMAD orders overruled German legal provisions until the creation of the GDR in 1949.

10. Barch DQ 1/20663, Anweisung der D[eutsche] Z[entral]V[erwaltung] für das Gesundheitswesen in der SBZ, 9. December 1946.
11. BArch DQ 1 /939, Ausbreitung und Bekämpfung der Tuberkulose in der SBZ, Anlage 1, 3 July 1946.
12. BArch DQ 1/930, Fröhlich, "Die Tuberkulose in Chemnitz in den Jahren 1929-1944," January 1946.
13. BArch DQ 1/2950, Chefarzt Professor Dr. Adolf Tegtmeier, Heilstätten Bad Berka, an Professor Dr. Marcusson, Ministerium für Gesundheitswesen, 2 September 1955.
14. Ibid.
15. BArch DQ 1/2950, Dr. Kohlstock, Bezirkarzt Bezirk Erfurt Gesundheitswesen an Rat des Bezirkes Gera Zentralstelle zur Bekämpfung der Tbk, 4 September 1955.
16. BArch DQ 1/2950, Dr. Marcusson, Tbk Referat HA Heilwesen an Rat Gera Abt. Gesundheitswesen, Zwangsasylierung, 25 September 1955; BArch DQ 1 /20663, Ministerium für Gesundheitswesen Hauptabteilung Heilwesen an Minister Steidl, Betr: Zwangsasylierung von asozialen TB-Kranken, 10 October 1956.
17. For biographical information on Tegtmeier, see DQ 1/1888, Tbc Heilstätte Bad Berka. On Marcusson, see http://berlin.kauperts.de/Strassen/Hildegard-Marcusson-Strasse-10317-Berlin (accessed 15 July 2010).
18. See Diane B. Paul, "Eugenics and the Left," *Journal of the History of Ideas*, 45 (1984): 567–90; Alberto Spektorowski, "The Eugenic Temptation in Socialism: Sweden, Germany, and the Soviet Union," *Comparative Studies in Society and History* 46 (2004): 84–106 (esp. 92, 96). American progressive ideas about health and hygiene were characterized by a comparable mix of social critique and moral and/or biological prejudice, but developed in the framework of "public health" as opposed to that of "social hygiene," which had a strong "communalist" strain. See Sheila Rothman, *Living in the Shadow of Death: Tuberculosis and the Social Experience of Illness in American History* (Baltimore, 1994), 184, 186.
19. See, e.g., BArch DQ 1 /939 TB 1946-1948, Ausbreitung und Bekämpfung der Tuberkulose in der SBZ, Anlage 1, 3 July 1946.
20. On the Federal Republic, see Lindner, *Gesundheitspolitik*, 171. On Austria, see Daum-Dietrich, '*Wiener Krankheit*', 346.
21. Barron H. Lerner, "From Careless Consumptives to Recalcitrant Patients: The Historical Construction of Non-Compliance," *Social Science Medicine* 45/9 (1997): 1424–26.
22. See BArch DQ 1/2950, Bl.435, Chefarzt Professor Dr. Adolf Tegtmeier, Heilstätten Bad Berka, an Professor Dr. Marcusson, Ministerium für Gesundheitswesen, 4 September 1955; Dr. Kohlstock, Bezirkarzt Bezirk Erfurt Gesundheitswesen an Rat des Bezirkes Gera Zentralstelle zur Bekämpfung der Tbk, Dr. Marcusson, Tbk Referat HA Heilwesen an Rat Gera Abt. Gesundheitswesen, Zwangsasylierung, 25 September 1955. The quote is from Hähner-Rombach, *Sozialgeschichte der Tuberkulose*, 272. Also see Christine Wolters, *Tuberkulose und Menschenversuche im Nationalsozialismus. Das Netzwerk hinter den Tbc-Experimenten im Konzentrationslater Sachsenhausen* (Stuttgart, 2011), esp. 68–72.
23. Marcusson suggested that Stadtroda's ward would eventually be replaced by a ward at a different asylum. See BArch DQ 1/2950, Dr. Marcusson, Tbk Referat HA Heilwesen an Rat Gera Abt. Gesundheitswesen, Zwangsasylierung, 25 September 1955.
24. BArch DQ 1/2950, Dr. Marcusson Tbk Referat HA Heilwesen an Rat Gera Abt. Gesundheitswesen, Zwangsasylierung, 25 September 1955; BArch DQ 1/ 20663, Bl.

430 Mf G HA Heilwesen an Minister Steidl, Betr: Zwangsasylierung von asozialen TB-Kranken, 10 October 1956.
25. BArch DQ 1/2950, Bl. 437, Abt. Volkskrankung, Entwurf für die Verfugungen und Mitteilungen des Ministeriums für Gesundheitswesen, 6 November 1956; BArch DQ 1/20663, Uneinsichtigkeit von TB-Kranken, (n.d. [1956]); BArch DQ 1/4388, Bl. 922, Aktenvermerk. Meine Dienstreise nach Stralsund-Heringsdorf, 20 Oct. 1956; BArch DQ 1/20663 Bl. 437.7, Anweisung über Massnahmen bei Uneinsichtigkeit von TB-Kranken, vom 6., November 1956; BArch DQ 1/20663, Bl. 437.2, FDGB Bundesvorstandverwaltung Sozialversicherung, 5 September 1956.
26. BArch DQ 1/4388, Bl. 922/06, An das Heilwesen, Betr: Reisebericht über eine Dienstreise in die Bezirke Rostock und Schwerin am 3. und 4. April 1956, 12 April 1956.
27. BArch DQ1/5963, Dr. Gehring Abt. Volkskrankheiten, MfG an HA Mutter und Kind, Frau Dr. Sturmhoefel, 25 January 1957.
28. BArch DQ 1/5026, Gesetz zur Verhütung und Bekämpfung übertragbarer Krankheiten beim Menschen, pars. 47–48.
29. BArch DQ 1/20663, Bl. 432, Tuberkulosereferat, Berlin, Aktenvermerk! Betr: Zwangsasylierung; (Copy of West German) Mitteilung Nr. 65 (1956), 13 December 1956. Also see Lindner, *Gesundheitspolitik,* 170–71.
30. See, e.g., G. Baumert and R. Hoppe, "Untersuchungen über den Einfluss sozialer Faktoren in der Tuberkulose-Therapie," *Kölner Zeitschrift für Soziologie und Sozialpyschologie* Sonderheft 3 (1958): 221–24, 232–33.
31. BArch DQ109/214, Sitzung der Arbeitsgruppe zur Prüfung des Einsatzes von Diplom-Psychologen in Tuberkulosen-Heilstätten, 17 December 1963.
32. On the gendered societal and economic developments that contributed to the new interest in sociological studies, see Donna Harsch, *Revenge of the Domestic: Women, the Family and Communism in the German Democratic Republic* (Princeton, N.J., 2006), 4–7, 237–41.
33. Dormandy, *White Death,* 348–49; Georgina D. Feldberg, *Disease and Class: Tuberculosis and the Shaping of Modern North American Society* (New Brunswick, N.J., 1995), 2–3, 24, 182; Linda Bryder, "'We Shall Not Find Salvation in Inoculation': BCG Vaccination in Scandinavia, Britain and the USA, 1921-1960," *Social Science and Medicine* 49 (1999): 1157–67; Thomas M. Daniel, *Captain of Death: The Story of Tuberculosis* (Rochester, N.Y., 1997), 141; Dietrich-Daum, '*Wiener Krankheit*', 351.
34. For a direct reference to the Lübeck disaster, see BArch DQ1/4756, V.2, Deutscher Tuberkulose-Kongress 3. Verhandlungstag,, Stenographische Niederschrift nach Tonband, Prof. Dr. Kathe, 16 December 1951.
35. Lindner, *Gesundheitspolitik,* 161–62.
36. Dr. Rudolf Neumann, "Zur Tuberkuloseschutzimpfung," *Zeitschrift für ärztliche Fortbildung* 43 Nr. 13/14 (1949): 371–76 (see offprint in BArch DQ1/6417, Bl. 221).
37. BArch DQ1/1374, Tuberkulose 1951, Bericht über die Erfahrungen mit der Calmette-Impfung [1951].
38. Lindner, *Gesundheitspolitik,* 161–62.
39. See files in DQ1/4884, BCG Schäden 1952, e.g., Tbc Referat an den Chefarzt des Krankenhauses Feldberg, 22 October 1953; DQ1/4884, Augenschaden nach BCG, Universität Augenklinik Leipzig, An das Ministerium für Gesundheitswesen, Berlin, 13 May 1952; DQ1/4884, Universität Augenklinik Jena, 17 May 1952; DQ1/4884, Hygienisches Institut der Universität Rostock an das Ministerium für Gesundheits-

wesen, Tuberkulose Referat Berlin, Betr: Tuberkulöse Meningitis nach BCG Impfung, 24 September 1953. Most serious were at least five cases in which a recently vaccinated child had contracted TB meningitis. TB meningitis is a fast developing and, at that time, usually fatal, form of TB, especially in children. The affected children were treated with streptomycin and penicillin, but at least two of them still died. The only archival references to alleged BCG-related TB meningitis and eye damage are in files from the years 1952 and 1953.

40. BArch DQ 1/4730, Protokoll zur Arbeitsbesprechung am 10.5.52 über Augenschaden nach BCG Impfung oder Testung, 10 May 1952.
41. Ibid.
42. BArch DQ1/4884, Universität Augenklink Leipzig, An das Ministerium für Gesundheitswesen, Berlin, 13 May 1952.
43. BArch DQ1/1374, Tuberkulose 1951, Bericht über die Erfahrungen mit der Calmette-Impfung [1951].
44. BArch DQ1/4884, Dr. Järisch an Professor Kathe; 14.2.52, Landesregierung Brandenburg an MfG Berlin, 26 January 1952; Dr. Järisch an Professor Kathe, 15 February 1952; An Herrn Dr. Järisch in Lübbenau und die Landesregierung, Brandenburg, Ministerium für Gesundheitswesen, von Herrn Dr. Herrmann, Potsdam, Betr.: Beschwerde des Herrn Dr. Järisch über angebliche Schädigungen durch BCG Impfung, 28 March 1952; Bericht über den in Lübbenau gehaltenen Nachschau der schutzgeimpften Kinder (Nachprüfung der Angaben des Dr. Järisch, Lübbenau, von Dr. Herrmann) [1952], esp. 3-4. For more evidence of irritation about the ignorance of doctors, see BArch DQ1/4884, Institut für Mikrobiologie, Jena an Herrn Landesbezirksarzt Dr. Kallabis, Sachsen, 15 February 1952. For evidence that doubts about BCG also existed among medical professors at state-run institutes, see BArch DQ1/1374, Akten Vermerk Berlin, HA Mutter und Kind, Dr. N/. Betr: Rücksprache mit Prof. Holtz von Pharmakologischem Institut, Halle, 7 May 1951.
45. BArch DQ 1/20435, Institut für Mikrobiologie und experimentalle Therapie Jena an die Regierung der DDR, 10 September 1954.
46. BArch DQ1/1928, Futtig Bezirk Arzt an Ministerium für Gesundheitswesen, 21 April 1959.
47. BArch DQ1/1928, Warnke, Rat des Bezirkes Rostock, der Vorsitzende an MfG. Betr.: Massnahmen zur TBK-Bekämpfung bis zum Inkrafttreten des Tuberkulosegesetzes, 17 April 1959.
48. See, e.g., BArch DQ 1/20435, Institut für Mikrobiologie und experimentalle Therapie Jena an Regierung der DDR, 10 September 1954; BArch DQ1/1928, Poser, Rat des Bezirks Gera Land Thüringen, an Sefrin, MfG, 17 March 1959.
49. BArch DQ 1/1928, Rat des Bezirkes Rostock an MfG, Betr: Massnahmen zur Tuberkulosenbekämpfung bis zum Inkrafttreten des Tuberkulosengesetzes, 17 April 1959.
50. BArch DQ 1/1928, Sefrin an Rat des Bezirkes…Herrn Vorsitzden… Betr: Massnahmen zur TBK-Bekämpfung bis zum Inkrafttreten des Tuberkulosegesetzes, 26 January 1959.
51. BArch DQ 1/20435, BCG 1954-55, Abschrift. Sektion für Hygiene. Protokoll der Sitzung vom 13.10.54, 2-3.
52. BArch DQ1/1928, Dr. Bauer, Abt. Volkskrankheiten Tbk-Referat. Tuberkulosenverordnung—BCG Schutzimpfung Pflichtimpfung, 21 March 1957.
53. BArch DQ1/20435, Dr. Steinbrück, Tuberkulose Forschungsinstitut Berlin-Buch an Dr.Gehring MfG, 23 December 1960, 1-2.

54. After the construction of the Wall, a wide range of state policies shifted more or less rapidly, often in a more "Socialist" direction, sometimes promoting greater coercion, but other times promoting more progressive measures. See, e.g., Andrew I. Port, *Conflict and Stability in the German Democratic Republic* (New York, 2006), 272; Harsch, *Revenge of the Domestic*, 236–44.
55. Lindner, *Gesundheitspolitik*, 170.
56. On anxiety about the Americanization of youth, see Uta Poiger *Jazz, Rock and Rebels: Cold War Politics and American Culture in a Divided Germany* (Berkeley, 2000).
57. On the legal history of "asociality" in the GDR, see Sven Korzilius, *"Asoziale" und "Parasiten" im Recht der SBZ/DDR. Randgruppen im Sozialismus zwischen Repression und Ausgrenzung* (Cologne, 2005). On political uses of "asociality" in the early 1950s to stigmatize, relocate, and/or confine uranium miners and others who did not behave according to SED standards, see Port, *Conflict and Stability*, 65–68.
58. On the generational changeover and beginning of feminization of the medical field, see Harsch, *Revenge of the Domestic*, 269.
59. On the age of first-time mothers and the GDR's very solid showing in reducing infant mortality, in part through good prenatal care for young, single women, see Harsch, *Revenge of the Domestic*, 134–43.

CHAPTER 7

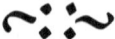

The Slim Imperative
Discourses and Cultures of Dieting in the German Democratic Republic, 1949–90

NEULA KERR-BOYLE

In 1987 Jutta N, a resident of Berlin, wrote the following to the daily *Berliner Zeitung*: "Recently, two words have been spiriting through the press: 'Get thinner!' Now, I have nothing against a good and thereby healthy figure. However, I do have something against the fact that suddenly we fatties (*Dickerchen*) are being so demonized."[1] She went on to lament that she and her husband felt embarrassed to finish their plates when dining out and that they were aware of the smirks of work colleagues when they heartily tucked into their breakfasts in the factory canteen.

That Jutta N felt compelled to write a letter to the *Berliner Zeitung* suggests that she, for one, perceived an intensification in calls in the East German media to diet, accompanied by an increasing stigmatization of "fatness" in the late 1980s. This raises a number of interesting questions about changing attitudes toward the body in the German Democratic Republic (GDR). First, what other evidence is there to suggest an intensification of incitements to diet in the 1980s? Second, if there was such an intensification, how can it be explained? Were these incitements driven primarily by official propaganda, or did they represent East Germans' participation in global cultural trends? Or was there another reason? Third, was there also a concomitant intensification of dieting practices? Fourth, and most important, what light does this shed on wider aspects of life in the GDR, such as the constructions and experiences of class and gender?

This essay begins by tracing the reemergence of discourses and practices of dieting after the postwar hunger years, arguing that it was a "return to normality" after the recent period of violence and deprivation.[2] It then shows how, starting in the early 1970s—and, as Jutta N perceived, continuing throughout the 1980s—there was an intensification of such discourses and practices. The essay will also argue that the topic of dieting represented an area in which state authorities sought to discipline the bodies of the East German population. Furthermore, by highlighting the tensions between official discourses and popular practices of dieting, it will highlight the limit of the state's reach into everyday life in the GDR.

The Reemergence of Dieting Discourses in the 1950s and 1960s

In the context of the serious food shortages of the immediate postwar period, dieting was obviously not an issue in public discourse. Basic rations in the Soviet Zone of Occupation (SBZ) in the winter of 1945 provided only 750 to 1,200 calories per day, and thousands consequently died from malnutrition and lowered resistance to epidemic diseases.[3] It is true that during this period, East Germans took a very real interest in that staple practice of modern dieting: calorie counting. But as pointed out in an article in the women's magazine *Die Frau von heute* in 1947, whereas the practice of calorie counting used to be driven by the desire to meet fashion's demands for a slim waistline, it was now borne out of empty stomachs and the urgent need to ensure that one consumed sufficient calories in order to maintain one's health and ability to work.[4] The worst of the food shortages were over by 1947 and rations slowly increased in the coming years, yet problems with food supply were particularly long-lasting in the SBZ and later in the GDR. It was only in 1958 that rationing was abolished (it had ended in the Federal Republic in 1951). What is striking, then, is that less than a decade after the postwar hunger years, discourses of dieting had begun to reemerge and the practice of calorie counting had begun to resume its prewar function.

The reemergence of discourses of dieting from the mid 1950s manifested itself in the return of magazine advertisements for slimming aids, such as teas and pills.[5] Articles about dieting also began to appear in popular East German magazines. For example, in 1954 the popular East German magazine *Das Magazin* published an article entitled, "Help! I'm becoming too fat."[6] The advice given in this article echoed prewar dieting advice, such as the adoption of a weekly "fruit day" and an occasional "milk day," on which, apart from a warm meal, only fruit or milk and a few slices of crisp bread were to be consumed. Weight-loss guides were also published.[7]

The reemergence of dieting discourses was driven in part by state authorities, particularly the Ministry of Health and the National Committee for Health Education. As Harsch's and Madarász-Lebenhagen's contributions to this volume make clear, in the 1950s the East German Ministry of Health became interested in tackling chronic diseases, such as tuberculosis (TB) and cardiovascular disease. This led to a focus on East Germans' eating habits, body weight, and physical activity. It was within this context that, by the late 1950s, East German health authorities were becoming increasingly alarmed by reports of rising rates of obesity in the GDR.[8] It was feared that the GDR was following the United States and West Germany into a future characterized by fatness and diet-related ill health. At a 1959 conference entitled "Nutrition and Health," it was claimed that "the GDR [was] perhaps ten years behind the USA and five years behind the Federal Republic of Germany" in terms of obesity (*Fettleibigkeit*) and its attendant diseases.[9] As stated at the conference, the GDR did not want to follow down this path. Thus, from the late 1950s on, healthy eating campaigns and dieting advice sought to tackle the GDR's expanding waistline by encouraging East Germans to maintain or regain "normal weight."[10]

The Ministry of Health and the National Committee for Health Education, aided by the Institute of Health Education of the German Hygiene Museum in Dresden, sought to create Socialist ways of consuming that emphasized health and moderation. This was a key part of the authorities' plan to promote a "healthy way of life," which, if successfully implemented, would boost socialism's legitimacy as a superior social system in which everyone could lead healthy, happy lives.[11] One of the central aims was to change traditional eating habits and combat *longue durée* models of desirable foods. As stated by a Ministry of Health report, "It must not be understood that '[t]he higher the consumption of fat, meat, white flour, and sugar, the higher our living standard', but rather: 'the more wholegrain bread, fruit, vegetables, and milk products we use, the quicker there will be an improvement in health conditions.'"[12] Pre-Socialist notions of a luxurious, rich diet were blamed for the GDR's expanding waistline, an idea promoted in healthy eating campaigns and dieting advice literature. A commonly used illustration was a cross-section cartoon showing the contents in the stomach of an "overweight" individual. Within the large stomach were "luxurious" foods such as cake, meat, lobster, and exotic fruits. The viewer was invited to regard this "overweight" individual as gluttonous, and, by implication, not a "Socialist" consumer. As we shall see, the authorities not only sought to create a Socialist "way of eating," but also a Socialist "way of dieting."

In order to understand the authorities' approach toward dieting, and toward health issues more generally, it is necessary to recognize the importance of two central concepts: *Leistungsfähigkeit* (productive capacities) and *Volksgesundheit* (the health of the nation), both of which stood at the heart of GDR health policy. From the late 1950s on, pronouncements by the ruling Socialist Unity Party (SED) asserted that it was the Socialist duty of every East German to maintain a healthy, productive body. In this way, each GDR citizen would play his or her role in furthering the *Volksgesundheit*. The focus of health-care policy at this time was very much on the health of the worker's body in particular—in order to ensure a high proportion of fit, able-bodied workers who could contribute productively to the building of Socialist society. Indeed, maintaining a "healthy" body by following a "healthy lifestyle" became a fundamental expectation of the "new Socialist person" whom East German authorities sought to create, one who maintained one's own individual health in the interest of society as a whole. This was motivated by pragmatic as well as ideological concerns. Beginning in the late 1950s, a focus on "healthy lifestyles" was acknowledged to be a less expensive means of securing the *Volksgesundheit* than a sole focus on public health initiatives (such as tackling venereal disease and TB) and the social causes of illnesses.[13]

The duty to maintain one's *Leistungsfähigkeit* played a key role in health propaganda, then, and this included official advice on how and how *not* to diet. From the 1960s on, East German dieting advice literature was often at pains to warn against extreme forms of dieting. Many articles explicitly warned against *Hungerkuren* (the practice of starving oneself for limited periods of time) because of the detrimental effect on *Leistungsfähigkeit*. Instead, East Germans were encouraged to change their long-term eating habits so that individual consumption levels ultimately met, rather than exceeded, personal energy requirements. In order to achieve this, East Germans were urged to show self-discipline and to monitor their calorie intake with the help of calorie tables which, from the 1960s on, appeared in magazines and were also available from bookshops and from the District Offices for Health Education (*Kreiskabinetten für Gesundheitserziehung*). In this way, East Germans were expected to embody the "constant striving to be economical" that Walter Ulbricht, first secretary of the SED, had stipulated in his "Ten Commandments for the New Socialist Person" in 1958.

As well as an emphasis on the importance of dieting in such a way as to maintain one's "productive capacities," beginning in the 1950s official dieting advice was also characterized by efforts to discredit Western dieting methods as faddish, ineffective, and contrary to the current nutritional scientific evidence supplied by the Institute for Nutrition in Potsdam-Rebrücke near Berlin.[14] For example, a cartoon appearing in a 1958 issue of the East German women's magazine *Die Frau von Heute* poked fun at Western slimming pills. It showed an "overweight" woman saying to her friend, "Yes, you're amazed, aren't you?! I have only the Western slimming pill to thank for my ideal figure."[15] Not all condemnations of Western dieting methods were this lighthearted. From the late 1960s on, the East German media regularly published didactic articles attacking Western diets.[16] For example, while the *Pünkte-Diät* ("points diet") was being hailed as a dieting miracle in Western Europe toward the end of the 1960s, East Germans were repeatedly told that it was scientifically unsound and therefore not recommended.[17]

Appeals to the wisdom of Socialist science were a particularly striking feature of official East German dieting advice, which was usually wholly didactic in its presentation and often given by an eminent East German nutritionist, such as Professor Helmut Haenel, director of the Central Institute for Nutrition. This style of presentation remained a constant feature of East German dieting advice throughout the remaining decades of the GDR. Whereas the West German women's magazine *Brigitte* often featured the personal dieting stories of West German women (and sometimes men), replete with "before" and "after" photos, the East German women's magazine *Für Dich* contained turgid advice from the "experts," occasionally accompanied by a simple illustration, such as a drawing of a woman standing on a pair of scales.

The Gendering of Dieting Discourses in the 1950s and 1960s

In order to understand fully the dieting culture of the GDR and what it revealed about wider cultural norms and values, it is necessary to explore the gendered nature of dieting discourses. What is striking about dieting articles from the 1950s is that they were directed exclusively at women. In some of the articles this is merely implied, through, for instance, the exclusive use of images of the female body to illustrate the text. Other articles addressed the gendered nature of the topic more directly. The 1956 article "Around the Waist," which appeared in *Das Magazin*, claimed that a famous leader of a GDR dance orchestra particularly liked "pretty" women to have a waist so narrow that he could wrap his hands around it. This, the article explained, was a desire shared by many men. Rather than challenge these expectations, the article championed them by exhorting women to monitor their waistline constantly in case their "own, future, or longed-for man also values the delicate waist."[18] Female readers were advised to take action—through dieting and exercise—if their waists were not the "correct" circumference for their height. The double standards applied to male and female body expectations were again made explicit in another article from 1956. Here a female author, recounting her own failed attempts to lose weight, ruefully reflected on how lucky men were that they did not have to worry about their waistline and would be loved regardless of their shape. This point was driven home by the illustration of an "overweight" man receiving the loving attentions of two slim women.[19]

What these examples revealed was that despite official policies calling for sexual equality (*Gleichberechtigung*), traditional attitudes toward gender remained, not only in the popular imagination, but also in the state-controlled media.[20] Female beauty continued to be equated with slenderness, and women were expected to discipline their bodies in accordance with male desires. Thus, East German women received conflicting messages: they were expected to embody the "new Socialist woman," who was fully engaged in the public sphere, and yet they were also expected to embody traditional, pre-Socialist ideals of femininity.

Dieting advice in the 1960s did increasingly allude to the idea that men should also be interested in dieting, but the link between dieting and *female* beauty remained strong. According to a 1969 article that addressed the issue of "overweight" males, men were much more prone to overeating and thus to obesity than women because women were more conscious of the need to maintain a slim figure.²¹ The article made no suggestion that "excess" body weight reduced male attractiveness. Men were expected to want to lose weight purely because of the purported health benefits. Other dieting advice, supposedly aimed at both men and women, often similarly omitted to say anything about the link between fat and male attractiveness—but made it abundantly clear that slenderness was crucial to female beauty. For example, in the introduction to a 1961 publication entitled *Slim Through Correct Nutrition*, the reader was told that the advice in this booklet provided the woman who was serious about her beauty and health with practical and effective tips on how to regulate weight through diet.²² Similarly, a 1967 publication declared that "our layers of fat take away our young, fresh look and destroy women's lovely appearance."²³ Some publications, such as Lisa Mrose's *Slim Through Correct Nutrition*, did acknowledge that the dieting advice they gave was also suitable for men, but the target audience was declared to be primarily female.

Thus, despite evidence suggesting that the topic of dieting had been coopted into state efforts to create a "new Socialist person," official dieting advice also revealed the continuation of traditional, pre-Socialist beauty ideals and gendered body expectations. And despite the official policy of *Gleichberechtigung*, the appearance of women continued to be deemed more important than that of men. Furthermore, the appearance for which women were encouraged to strive was the same graceful slenderness promoted in the prewar years as essential to female beauty. This ideal was propagated not only in dieting advice, but also in the use of slim models in the pages of women's magazines and in fashion shows.²⁴ These continuities with pre-Socialist ideals can be conceived of as a "return to normality" after the disruption of the immediate postwar years—and as what Ernst Bloch derided as the GDR's "dictatorship of petit-bourgeois taste in the name of the proletariat."²⁵

The Intensification of Dieting Discourses in the 1970s and 1980s

By the start of the 1970s, then, dieting had clearly been reestablished as a topic of discussion in the East German public sphere. Why, then, did discourses and cultures of dieting intensify during the 1970s and 1980s, and what evidence supports this claim? One indicator was the increased number of dieting articles that appeared in the women's magazine *Für Dich* at the time.²⁶ Furthermore, whereas such articles were published as occasional "one-offs" in the 1950s and

1960s, they were often published in the 1970s and 1980s as series running over many months.[27] Other official forums for the propagation of dieting discourses in these later decades included the popular health magazine *Deine Gesundheit*, as well as newspapers, health propaganda films, and radio. For example, "Radio DDR" broadcast the series "Slim for the holidays—a radio program to lose weight" in 1987.[28]

Another aspect of the intensification of dieting discourses was the way in which the tyranny of calorie counting tightened its grip. Calorie tables were regularly published alongside dieting articles, and it became common for recipes to include caloric content. Posters, booklets, and films produced by the German Hygiene Museum also regularly enjoined people to count their calories. For example, a 1974 film entitled *Calories* showed two slim people happily eating cake. Both used to be "overweight," the narrator explains, but they now remain slim by counting their calories and not exceeding their daily requirement. The narrator then recommends that viewers should always have a calorie table at hand to ensure that they, too, keep within their daily calorie limit.[29]

The publication of calorie tables was supported by the Central Institute for Nutrition, which recommended in a 1987 report that such tables be made even more readily available for the whole population.[30] Furthermore, beginning in the 1970s, East German teenagers were also told to pay attention to the number of calories they consumed. In fact, a 1974 report by the Central Institute for Youth Research concluded that the education of young people about healthy eating needed to focus on their ability to estimate the calorie content and nutritional value of foods.[31] This type of recommendation was publicized in articles such as "Good Advice: First Chubby (*pummelig*), then Fat (*dick*)," which stated that "larger children and adolescents should be made familiar with their calorie requirements and the caloric content of foodstuffs."[32]

This was just one aspect of the expansion of dieting discourses to include "overweight" children and teenagers in the 1970s. East German women had long been held responsible for ensuring that their families ate healthy, low-fat, low-calorie meals at home. However, during the 1970s and 1980s the East German press frequently told parents, particularly mothers, to monitor closely their children's body weight. At the first sign of "excess" kilograms, they were to implement a weight-loss program. Such vigilance was to begin during infancy. A 1974 article told mothers of the importance of not giving their babies more than the prescribed amount of nutrition.[33] This was particularly important if their baby had "a too pronounced layer of fat." The advice given to mothers for their "overweight" children echoed the advice given to "overweight" adults: meal sizes were to be reduced, sweeteners were to be used instead of sugar, low-fat margarine was to replace butter. It was even recommended that "overweight" children have a "fasting day" one or two times a week. Another option was to enroll them in a weight-loss course.[34] Teenagers were also targeted, as articles such as "15 Years Old and Too Many Kilos" made clear.[35] Suggested weapons in the battle to get the "overweight" child and teenager to diet included mirrors and scales which were to be used to strengthen resolve. Parents, teachers, and friends were also advised to play up the benefits weight loss would have for an "overweight" young person's appearance and athletic ability.[36]

All of the above evidence strongly indicates that incitements to diet strengthened and widened in scope in the 1970s. What, then, explains increased state interest in East Germans' body weight at this time? As noted earlier, there were official concerns already in the 1950s about rising rates of obesity. But starting in the early 1970s, the Central Institute for Nutrition began to devote greater resources to the study of body weight and obesity. This shift was justified by the figures. At the Fourth National Conference for Health Promotion, held in Berlin in November 1971, Professor Haenel announced that between 10 and 15 percent of East German children, 20 percent of East German men, and 40 percent of East German women were at least 20 percent overweight.[37] These figures were then regularly quoted in the East German media and health propaganda. They were, no doubt, intended to shock the population into action. But it is interesting to note that authorities could not resist putting a subtly positive spin on them as well, claiming that such statistics were typical of a highly industrialized, modern society such as the GDR.

It is difficult to know how accurate the cited figures were. Indeed, there was some dispute about them among East German scientists and medical professionals themselves.[38] But what can be said with certainty is that, despite the GDR being a "shortage economy" in which scarcity was a distinguishing feature of daily life, there was no overall shortage of food. It is true that there were periods in which supplies of certain consumables dwindled—potatoes in 1970–71, for example, and coffee in the late 1970s and early 1980s. Furthermore, obtaining certain products could often mean an arduous search involving long waits standing in line. That said, food was generally in plentiful supply and cheaply available thanks to state subsidies. Consumption climbed as a result—particularly the consumption of fatty foods, such as pork and butter. As noted by Paul Freedman in this volume, the East German diet was a high-calorie one. In addition, food played an important role at social gatherings, where "tables groaned under breads, cheeses, butter, sausages, cold meats, schnapps, and beer."[39] In such a context, it is perhaps unsurprising that there were reports of large numbers of "overweight" East Germans.

Heightened interest in obesity and its impact on health was not specific to the GDR. This was a trend on both sides of the Iron Curtain, leading in the 1970s to many conferences on this topic, in which delegates from both East and West participated. One important reason for this heightened interest was the adoption of the "risk factor model" as the key explanatory model for disease, as discussed in the chapter by Jeannette Madarász-Lebenhagen. In the

United States, the concept of risk factors, such as being "overweight" or consuming "excess" fat, had come to dominate scientific approaches to chronic diseases, particularly heart disease, in the 1960s. Since the founding of the GDR, East German medicine had been dominated by social hygienists who focused on living conditions and the economics of health, rather than on risk factors associated with patterns of behavior or physical characteristics of groups of individuals. This changed in the late 1960s when the risk factor model was embraced.[40] Although there had been an emphasis on "lifestyle" choices since the 1950s, the adoption of the risk factor model placed a new onus on the purported links between "overconsumption" and specific illnesses, such as diabetes and heart disease.

In an effort to reduce risk factors by helping East Germans to lose "excess" weight, new reduced-calorie and weight-loss products were brought onto the market. One weight-loss aid launched in the 1970s was *Redukal*, which many former East Germans remember as being utterly foul-tasting[41]—despite being advertised in magazines such as *Für Dich* and *Deine Gesundheit* as an almost tasteless powdered soup that contained 1,000 calories, plus the recommended daily amount of protein, carbohydrates, and fat.[42] The 1970s also witnessed the introduction of products with the label "ON-Calorie reduced." These were products, such as salad dressing and margarine, with a reduced fat and calorie content.[43] This marked the first time that a standardized range of calorie-reduced products had been mass produced and marketed in the GDR. Dieting literature now advised the consumption of such calorie-reduced products, thus adding a new dimension to dieting discourses.

Dieting Practices in the 1970s and 1980s

All of the above developments suggested a widening in scope and an intensification of official discourses on the subject of dieting. But what evidence was there to suggest that issues of body weight and dieting had, by the end of the 1980s, come to play an important role in the everyday lives of many East Germans, as Jutta N suggested in her letter to the *Berliner Zeitung*? The many surveys carried out by various East German institutions, such as the Central Institute for Youth Research and the Central Institute for Nutrition, provide insight into this aspect of life in the GDR. Unfortunately, no relevant surveys were conducted in the 1950s and 1960s about dieting practices and attitudes toward body weight, so no direct comparisons can be made between these earlier decades and the 1970s and 1980s. But surveys from the 1980s strongly suggested that by the final decade of the GDR's existence, dieting discourses were being taken up and engaged with by many East Germans. For example, a 1987 study conducted by the Central Institute for Nutrition suggested that many East Germans were "figure-conscious."[44] Of the 439 participants, taken from the working adult population between the ages of 18 and 65, over 50 percent agreed to the statement that they regularly paid attention to ensuring that they did not put on weight.[45] It was also reported that around 60,000 people took part in the 1987 Radio DDR slimming series, "Slim for the Holidays."[46] Weight and dieting also appear to have been popular topics of everyday conversation, as implied by a letter published in *Für Dich* in 1987, in which Bärbel K from Borsdorf stated that "weight is also the number one topic of conversation in my work collective and in my circle of friends and acquaintances."[47]

Dieting practices and popular discourses about weight loss occurred in the context of health propaganda about maintaining or regaining "normal weight." But it would be simplistic to argue that they were being driven and controlled solely by the pronouncements of the state authorities. As we shall see, much of the evidence suggested that East Germans were dieting in ways deemed "inappropriate" by the authorities—both in terms of the methods used and in terms of those who actually dieted, many of whom were not regarded as having been "overweight" to begin with. All of this suggested that a culture of dieting was being driven by factors that included, but were not limited to, official campaigns and literature.

Perhaps the most important factor accounting for cultures of dieting in East Germany in the 1970s and 1980s was the gradual process of increasing individualism identified by a number of scholars. Mary Fulbrook, for example, points out that, over time, a pattern of individualism emerged that could be observed in virtually every area of society.[48] This was linked to wider trends of consumerism, materialism, and the globalization of culture that began to take hold in the GDR in the 1960s, but really gained momentum in the 1970s and 1980s. The "consumer socialism" ushered in by Honecker's "unity of social and economic policy" fostered new private aspirations that focused on the satisfaction of individual desires, rather than on the collectivist goals championed by the state. At the same time, East Germans gained greater access to Western culture. By the 1960s the vast majority of households listened to Western radio stations. This was followed in the 1970s by increased viewing of Western television, particularly once this was finally permitted by the state in 1972.[49] With the introduction of the five-day workweek in 1967, East Germans also had more leisure time, which contributed to a gradual "withdrawal into the private sphere" in what Western observers referred to as the "niche society."[50] It was in this context that East Germans became increasingly preoccupied with individual identity and the pursuit of personal goals for private happiness.[51] Much of this was expressed in practices such as the purchasing of consumer goods and the tending of private agricultural allotments.

Another important site for the expression of this new individualism was the human body. As Josie McLellan has shown, there was a shift in the "bodily iconography of the Socialist state" in the 1970s, as Socialist bodies ceased to be presented primarily as agents of work and reproduction, but were instead increasingly presented as sites of pleasure, consumption, and leisure.[52] This involved a boom in commercialized sexuality, such as the advent in the 1980s of soft porn on late night television and striptease shows; it also found expression in the new sex manuals of the 1970s, which emphasized that the main purpose of sex was "pleasure and delight."[53] As this suggests, East Germans were made more aware of their bodies' potential in the pursuit of personal happiness and the expression of individual identity. Mike Featherstone has argued that in Western consumer capitalism's culture of narcissistic individualism, people are constantly bombarded with the message that "the body is the passport to all that is good in life. Health, youth, beauty, sex, fitness are the positive attributes which body care can achieve and preserve."[54] In the absence of powerful dieting, advertising, and fashion industries, East Germans were not subjected to this message as intensely as their Western counterparts, but the attractions of "body care" were coming ever more to the fore in this increasingly individualist society. As in the West, one of the chief aspects of "body care," particularly for women, was, of course, dieting.

What is most striking about the evidence regarding dieting practices in the GDR in the 1970s and 1980s is how clearly it revealed continuities in the traditionally gendered nature of such practices. Of the 60,000 participants in the aforementioned radio series "Slim for the Holidays," 78 percent were female.[55] A report published in 1987 by the Central Institute for Nutrition also highlighted differences between the sexes with respect to dieting. Significantly larger numbers of female than male participants agreed to the following statements: "I regularly pay attention to ensuring that I do not put on weight," "I feel better in myself when I do not eat too much," and "When choosing meals I think about my health or my weight."[56] Other reports highlighted the extent to which East German schoolgirls engaged in dieting practices. A 1990 report from the Central Institute for Nutrition described how "the modern fashion for slimness" drove "some young girls, out of fear of too much, in the direction of too little." It went on to claim that "they only think of themselves as attractive when they are super slim or stick-thin (*klapperdürr*). Around 40 percent of the surveyed 15- to 17-year-old girls want to lose weight, although only around 4 percent are overweight. Similar results are not found with boys."[57] Such reports were not new: in 1984, an investigation by the Central Institute for Youth Research of the habits of Leipzig schoolchildren in grades seven to ten had reported that "girls are not seldom practising inappropriate fasting diets—even when they are of normal weight."[58] Ten years earlier, another investigation had similarly reported on the pronounced wish among "normal-weight" girls and young women to lose weight.[59]

The extent of "unnecessary" dieting among girls was perceived by the authorities as being so great that health propaganda films and press articles were produced to try to dissuade "normal-weight" girls from pursuing this course of action. For example, a health propaganda film from 1978, entitled "Healthy Nutrition for Those Aged 16-20," pointed out that "all those aged between 16 and 20, particularly girls, are fully aware that skipping meals and even forcible *Hungerkuren* (fasting diets) are not the exception, but are, unfortunately, instead a part of everyday behaviour."[60] The film went on to warn of the health risks involved in such practices—a message not only delivered in health propaganda films. Medical professionals from the Charité Hospital in East Berlin were also invited to schools to discuss issues of dieting with teenage girls.[61] There was a vast array of other dieting methods besides *Hungerkuren* that "experts" warned against, including the use of laxatives and appetite suppressants, as well as an overreliance on *Redukal*.[62] But despite the propagation of these concerns, there was no significant public discourse about the eating disorders known as anorexia and bulimia nervosa. It was only after the fall of the Berlin Wall that such a discourse emerged, even though both had already existed in East Germany.[63]

Female university students also seem to have been particularly active in the culture of dieting in the 1970s and 1980s. In a presentation delivered in 1986 to a working group for nutrition set up by the National Committee for Health Education, it was noted that "among female students, even among those who are underweight, a striving toward weight loss for fashion reasons prevails."[64] An earlier report about youth and body culture had highlighted the fact that female students were the only section of the study population with an average body weight under the "ideal": whereas the average female student weighed 1.5 kg less than the "ideal weight," their male counterparts weighed 8 kg too much.[65] Another report found that female students were not the only group within the 16- to 35-year age range that displayed a tendency toward being "underweight." Female *Angestellte* (white-collar workers) and female members of the intelligentsia also displayed this tendency. Conversely, the group containing the highest percentage of "overweight" people was the male intelligentsia, followed by male *Angestellte* and female blue-collar workers.[66]

The results of these surveys raise some interesting questions about how the intersection of gender and class affected East German eating and dieting practices. The surveys suggested that women who would have belonged to the middle class in Western societies (by virtue of their high level of education or professional position) tended to be slimmer than blue-collar women, as well as men of all "classes." These findings echoed surveys conducted in the United States between 1971 and 1974 and in the United Kingdom between 1986 and 1987, which found that affluent, educated women had lower BMI (Body Mass

Index) scores than men, poor women, and women with little education.[67] This suggests that the intersection of gender and class operated in similar ways on both sides of the Iron Curtain—despite the very different social, economic, and political systems—in terms of eating and dieting practices.

Much has been written about the "cult of slenderness" in Western societies and many theories have been advanced to explain its tenacious grip on the lives of women in the twentieth and twenty-first centuries. These theories have focused on a range of cultural ideas and social processes, such as dominant beauty ideals and the rise of a powerful dieting industry. This essay has shown that, as in the West, beauty ideals in the GDR also prescribed female slenderness and that, while this ideal was not promoted by a commercial dieting industry, there were strong social and cultural imperatives to retain or regain a slim figure. But why, as in the West, was it well-educated, white-collar women who were particularly successful at maintaining a slim figure?

Even if it is impossible to answer this question definitively, any attempt must consider the role of gender and class. The importance of gender is obviously suggested by the fact that female students and white-collar women were slimmer than their male counterparts. As already noted, in the GDR, as in the West, the gendered aspect of this issue was explained with reference to women's propensity to "follow fashion." But there is another explanation, one that takes fuller account of the gendered values and systems that were integral to the social and cultural structures of both East Germany and contemporaneous Western democracies. This involved key similarities in cultural ideas and social processes that manifested themselves in women's attitudes toward their bodies on both sides of the Iron Curtain.

Feminist philosopher Susan Bordo has argued that in Western societies, the slender female body serves as the locus where "the traditional construction of femininity intersects with the new requirement for women to embody the 'masculine' values of the public arena."[68] In other words, many women desire to be slim not only because a slender body corresponds to dominant ideals about female beauty, but also because it symbolizes highly prized values, such as self-control and self-discipline, which, in Western capitalist societies, are coded as "masculine." According to this feminist argument, women perceive that their success in the public arena of education and the workplace will be made easier if they embody these values.[69]

Is it legitimate to apply this argument to the GDR? The values of self-control and self-discipline were indeed promoted as virtues by official East German health discourses, and, as this essay has shown, these values were associated with a slim body. At the same time, the slender body was strongly associated with female attractiveness. But despite these similarities with Western values and ideals, the GDR also prided itself on its policy of sexual equality and on the high numbers of women in education and employment.[70] One might therefore assume that, in such a context, women were accepted as social equals in public and in private. If this had been the case, there would have been no need for East German women to use their bodies to symbolize certain values any more than East German men would have.

But sexual equality remained elusive in the GDR despite official rhetoric about *Gleichberechtigung*. Many women undoubtedly benefited from certain aspects of the GDR welfare state, such as state-run childcare. Yet, the East German system also displayed the inherent sexism and double standards typical of a patriarchal society in which almost all key positions in politics, industry, and the professions were occupied by men.[71] Women continued to be positioned as the female "other," and traditional expectations about "sex-appropriate" ways of behaving continued to be culturally embedded. According to Irene Dölling, "women were supposed to behave in a traditionally 'female' manner while neither 'femininity' in the customary sense, nor the insistence on gender difference, was recognized or honoured—women were supposed to work, think, develop their abilities 'like men.'"[72] It is thus feasible that, as in the West, many East German women felt the (often unacknowledged) need to use their bodies to prove their own worth, e.g., by embracing and embodying values of self-control and self-discipline. The impetus to do this was bolstered by prevailing beauty ideals and health propaganda that favored the slender body.

This explanation focuses on explaining why East German women engaged in dieting practices more than East German men did. It is even more difficult to explain why educated, white-collar East German women were more successful at keeping down their weight than their less educated, blue-collar counterparts were. Here it is worth considering the way in which class and gender systems operated and their impact on women's lives. To be sure, all East German women, regardless of the color of their collar, bore the "triple burden" of paid work, housework, and sociopolitical activities.[73] Almost all had to deal as well with being positioned as the female "other" in the "masculine" GDR. That highly educated East German women laid particular emphasis on maintaining a slim figure could reflect the importance of the values of self-discipline and self-control among the GDR's intelligentsia. It is feasible that, faced with the inherent sexism of the patriarchal GDR, women who sought to enter, or who were already employed in, highly skilled professional jobs in typically male-dominated environs felt under particular pressure to "prove" themselves by embodying these values. Certainly, there is evidence that, by the 1980s and in comparison to their blue-collar counterparts, it was more common for white-collar East German women to perceive sex-specific disadvantages in their professional lives. For example, in 1986 the Central Institute for Youth Research conducted a survey of 2,188 men and women with an average age of twenty-four. It found that 93 percent of female workers fully agreed with the statement that women could be successful in positions of leadership—significantly higher than the 85 percent of women with advanced degrees, who also agreed with this statement. The survey revealed a similar disparity in response to the statement: "at work I feel that I am taken seriously in comparison to my equally-qualified male work colleagues." Of the female workers, 50 percent fully agreed with this statement, compared to only 40 percent of female *Hochschulkader*.[74]

Conclusion: East German Discourses and Cultures of Dieting in a Global Perspective

The foregoing exploration of discourses and cultures of dieting in the GDR between 1949 and 1990 highlights some of the ways in which the GDR participated in wider global developments. Like those in all modern states, East German authorities sought to achieve specific sociopolitical goals through efforts to discipline the bodies of the populace. From the 1950s, many of these efforts focused on persuading individuals to maintain or regain "normal weight"—something that held true on both sides of the Iron Curtain. The adoption of the Western risk factor model and reports of significant numbers of "overweight" citizens fueled an already existing interest in the topic of obesity, as well as an intensification of state-sponsored dieting discourses in the 1970s and 1980s.

But despite such similarities in state-sponsored efforts to control citizens' body weights, there existed significant differences between East German dieting discourses and those produced in Western democracies. The most obvious and significant difference was that in the West, dieting discourses were produced by state authorities *and* representatives of the private sector; the absence in East Germany of a free press, as well as of powerful dieting and advertising industries, meant that dieting discourses in the GDR—which were promoted by the state-controlled media—*originated* almost exclusively from the ruling party and state. This led to a distinctive form of Socialist dieting discourse that was didactic, dominated by "expert" advice, and largely impersonal. The Socialist inflection of dieting discourses can also be seen in the frequent references to the concept of *Leistungsfähigkeit* and in the criticism of Western dieting methods, which gained publicity in the GDR via Western media.

This meant, in turn, that the context in which many East Germans adopted dieting practices was also significantly different. Official dieting discourses in the GDR sought to persuade East Germans of the benefits of "normal weight," but authorities did not have the same vested (financial) interests as Western advertising and dieting industries in creating "a world in which individuals are made to become emotionally vulnerable, constantly monitoring themselves for bodily imperfections which could no longer be regarded as natural."[75] In such a context, the topic of dieting did not become as prominent or as all-pervasive in everyday life in the GDR as it did in the postwar West. There were, for instance, no giant advertising billboards in the GDR with slim models advertising dieting products.

Beginning in the late 1950s, slenderness was nevertheless officially propagated in the East German media as a health and beauty ideal and, as a result, a culture of dieting did emerge and grow in the GDR. The dieting discourses from the 1950s and 1960s exhibited continuities with prewar trends, such as the marketing of slimming aids and the focus on the female body. There were new developments in the 1970s and 1980s, such as the introduction of calorie-reduced products. Yet, the developments in these later decades are best described as an intensification of already existing trends and features.

The intensification of dieting culture in the 1970s and 1980s may have been in step with official incitements to diet, but this essay has shown that popular dieting practices in the GDR underscored the limits of the East German state's ability to discipline and control the population. East Germans who dieted were not simply responding to state propaganda about appropriate, "Socialist" ways of consuming and dieting. Rather, their behavior was influenced by cultural, political, and economic trends and structures—both within and outside the GDR. Discourses and cultures of dieting can thus be regarded as sites of struggle for control and agency at both the macro and micro levels of East German society, within the context of Cold War rivalry, as well as global developments in health, science, and consumption.

Suggested Readings

Betts, Paul. *Within Walls: Private Life in the German Democratic Republic.* Oxford, 2010.
Fulbrook, Mary. *The People's State: East German Society from Hitler to Honecker.* New Haven, C.T., 2005.
———. "The Concept of 'Normalisation' and the GDR in Comparative Perspective." In *Power and Society in the GDR, 1961-1979: The 'Normalisation of Rule'?* ed. Mary Fulbrook, 1–30. New York, 2009.
Harsch, Donna. *Revenge of the Domestic: Women, the Family and Communism in the German Democratic Republic.* Princeton, N.J., 2007.
Herzog, Dagmar. *Sex after Fascism: Memory and Morality in Twentieth-Century Germany.* Princeton, N.J., 2005.
McLellan, Josie. *Love in the Time of Communism: Intimacy and Sexuality in the GDR.* Cambridge, 2011.
———. "State Socialist Bodies: East German Nudism from Ban to Boom." *Journal of Modern History* 79 (2007): 48–79.
Merta, Sabine. *Wege und Irrwege zum modernen Schlankheitskult. Diätkost und Körperkultur als Suche nach neuen Lebensstilformen 1880-1930.* Stuttgart, 2003.
Stitziel, Judd. *Fashioning Socialism: Clothing, Politics and Consumer Culture in East Germany.* Oxford, 2005.
———. "On the Seam between Socialist and Capitalism: East German Fashion Shows." In *Consuming Germany in the Cold War,* ed. David Crew, 51–85. Oxford, 2003.

Thoms, Ulrike. "Separated, but Sharing a Health Problem: Obesity in East and West Germany, 1945-1989." In *The Rise of Obesity in Europe*, ed. Derek J. Oddy, Peter J. Atkins, and Virginie Amelien, 207–22. Farnham, 2009.

Notes

1. "Kampagne gegen die Dicken?" *Berliner Zeitung*, 10/11 October 1987.
2. See Mary Fulbrook, "The Concept of 'Normalisation' and the GDR in Comparative Perspective," in *Power and Society in the GDR, 1961-1979: The 'Normalisation of Rule'?*, ed. Mary Fulbrook (New York, 2009), 11.
3. See Mary Fulbrook, *The People's State: East German Society from Hitler to Honecker* (New Haven and London, 2005), 89.
4. "Kalorien im Kochtopft," *Die Frau von heute* 21 (1947).
5. Advertisements for slimming aids had appeared in magazines in Weimar and Nazi Germany, including in the Nazi Party's women's magazine, *NS-Frauenwarte*.
6. "Hilfe! Ich werde zu dick," *Das Magazin*, December 1954.
7. See, e.g., Dorothea Schmidt and Jutta Schicht, *Kost zur Gewichtsverminderung* (Berlin, 1959). For an overview of prewar dieting cultures in the German context, see Sabine Merta, *Wege und Irrwege zum modernen Schlankheitskult. Diätkost und Körperkultur als Suche nach neuen Lebensstilformen 1880-1930* (Stuttgart, 2003).
8. Concerns about rising rates of obesity were emerging in other countries on both sides of the Iron Curtain at this time. See, e.g., Martin Franc, "Socialism and the Overweight Nation: Questions of Ideology, Science and Obesity in Czechoslovakia, 1950-1970," in *The Rise of Obesity in Europe*, ed. Derek Oddy, Peter Atkins, and Virginie Amelien (Farnham and Burlington, 2009), 193–205; Ulrike Thoms, "Separated, but Sharing a Health Problem: Obesity in East and West Germany, 1945-1989," in Oddy, Atkins, and Amelien, *Rise of Obesity*, 207–22.
9. SAPMO-BArch, DQ1/22303: "Ernährung und Gesundheit," 18 December 1959.
10. A number of different indices and formulas were used in the GDR to calculate "normal weight." One of the most popular was the Broca-Index, invented by the French surgeon Paul Broca in 1871. It held that "normal weight" in kilograms was equal to height in centimeters minus 100.
11. In 1960 the Medical Commission of the Central Committee of the SED agreed that a "healthy way of life" (*gesunde Lebensführung*) for the whole population was to be the basic guiding principle for the development of medicine and public health in the GDR. See Young-Sun Hong, "Cigarette Butts and the Building of Socialism in East Germany," *Central European History* 3 (2002): 327–44.
12. SAPMO-BArch, DQ1/22303, "Jeder 10. isst sich krank," n.d. (probably late 1950s). Similar advice was propagated in West Germany at this time, and had been promoted by the Nazi regime. See Corinna Treitel, "Nature and the Nazi Diet," *Food and Foodways* 17 (2009): 139–58; Nancy Reagin, "*Marktordnung* and Autarkic Houskeeping: Housewives and Private Consumption under the Four-Year Plan, 1936-1939," *German History* 2 (2001): 162–84.
13. See Annette F. Timm, "Guarding the Health of Worker Families in the GDR: Socialist Health Care, *Bevölkerungspolitik* and Marriage Counselling, 1945-1970," in *Arbeiter in der SBZ—DDR*, ed. Peter Hübner and Klaus Tenfelde (Essen, 1999), 463–95.

14. In 1969, this body became the Central Institute for Nutrition. It was the GDR's leading research institute for matters concerning nutrition and diet. It played a key role in attempts to educate the public about these matters and thereby influence eating practices.
15. *Die Frau von Heute*, 42, 1958.
16. See, e.g., "Gut essen, gut trinken und trotzdem abnehmen," *Wochenpost*, 19 September 1969; "Sich gesund ernähren—aber wie?" *Presse Information*, 15 December 1975; "Kontra Punkte-Diät," *Neue Berliner Illustrierte*, December 1984; "Dicker werden ist nicht schwer...," *Neue Berliner Illustrierte*, February 1988.
17. Official criticism of Western diets was also common in other socialist countries. See, e.g., Franc, "Socialism and the Overweight Nation."
18. "Rund um die Taille," *Das Magazin*, June 1956.
19. "Schlanke Linie mit dickem Fragezeichen. Eine melancholische Betrachtung von Berta Waterstradt," *Das Magazin*, September 1956.
20. For further discussion of continuities in traditional attitudes toward gender, see Fulbrook, *The People's State*, chap. 7; Ina Merkel, *...Und Du, Frau an der Werkbank: Die DDR in den 50er Jahren* (Berlin, 1990); Irene Dölling, "Between Hope and Helplessness: Women in the GDR after the "Turning Point,"" *Feminist Review* 39 (1991): 3–15.
21. "Sprechstunde Für Dich bei Dr. med. Rolf Gerlach. Hinweise und Ratschläge zur Hygiene des Mannes," *Für Dich* 44 (1969).
22. Lisa Mrose, *Schlank durch richtige Ernährung. Eine Schlankheitskost auf laktovegetabilischer Ernährungsbasis* (Berlin, 1961), 3.
23. Eugen Baunach, *Das Geheimnis der schlanken Linie. Vom Wesen der Fettsucht Wege zu ihre Überwindung* (Berlin, 1967), 37.
24. For an analysis of discourses of body weight and size in relation to East German fashion, see Judd Stitziel, *Fashioning Socialism: Clothing, Politics and Consumer Culture in East Germany* (Oxford and New York, 2005); idem, "On the Seam between Socialism and Capitalism: East German Fashion Shows," in *Consuming Germany in the Cold War*, ed. David Crew (Oxford and New York, 2003), 51–85.
25. Paul Betts uses this quote to support his argument about the content of manners manuals, which were popular in the GDR in the 1950s and 1960s. See Paul Betts, *Within Walls: Private Life in the German Democratic Republic* (Oxford, 2010), 136–39.
26. No statistics for the number of dieting articles are available, but anyone perusing issues of the women's magazine *Für Dich* (and its predecessor *Die Frau von heute*) from the 1950s to the 1980s will be struck by the increasing frequency of articles addressing the topic of body weight and dieting. For more on *Für Dich*, see Martha Wörsching, "*Für Dich* and the *Wende*: Women's Weekly between Plan and Market," in *Women and the Wende: Social Effects and Cultural Reflections of the German Unification Process*, ed. Elizabeth Boa and Janet Wharton (Amsterdam and Atlanta, 1994), 139–54.
27. Examples of series of dieting articles published in *Für Dich* in the 1970s and 1980s include "Ich wiege zu viel" (1976); "Schlank werden und schlank bleiben" (1979); "Schlank wie eine Tanne" (1983); "Iß Dich schlank mit Für Dich" (1985); "Mit Spaß nach Maß" (1987).
28. See "Nach der Kur geht's nun 'Schlank in den Urlaub,'" *Berliner Zeitung*, 31 July 1987; Hans-Albrecht Ketz and Hans Eichhorn, *Eine Radio Kur zum Abnehmen. Schlank in den Urlaub* (1987).
29. *Kalorien* (1974).

30. Deutsches Institut für Ernährungsforschung, Box 91, "Psychologische Grundlagen des Ernährungsverhaltens und Möglichkeiten seiner Beeinflussung," Zentralinstitut für Ernährung, 1987.
31. SAPMO-BArch DC 4/2100, "Jugend und Gesundheit: Forschungsbericht," Zentralinstitut für Jugendforschung, 1974.
32. "Guter Rat. Erst pummelig, dann dick," *Für Dich* 40 (1986).
33. "Das raten wir Ihnen," *Deine Gesundheit*, April 1974.
34. Weight-loss courses for children were held by the Advice Bureau for Children and Young People's Health Protection (*Beratungsstelle für Kinder- und Jugengesundheitsschutz*) in Weimar, which ran thirteen courses over a two-year period during the 1970s. In 1983, groups of overweight youngsters spent three weeks during the summer holidays at the Berlin Children's Hospital (*Berliner Kinderklinik*) in Friedrichshain, where a weight-loss program was overseen by doctors, psychologists, nurses, and dieticians. Similar courses were also run in Potsdam and Brandenburg.
35. "15 Jahre und zu viele Kilo," *Guter Rat* 2 (1987).
36. See "'Speck' kann auf die Seele drücken," *Für Dich* 40 (1986).
37. SAPMO-BArch, DQ113/12, Stenografisches Protokoll, IV. Nationale Konferenz für Gesundheitserziehung, "Erziehung zur gesundheitsfördernden Ernährung," 1971.
38. For example, an article appeared in 1976 in the East German medical magazine *Humanitas* that questioned claims that such high percentages of East German men, women, and children were "overweight." In response, the director of the Central Institute for Nutrition, wrote to one of the coauthors to express his regret that such a debate about "facts" had taken place in public. See Neula Kerr-Boyle, "Orders of Eating and Eating Disorders: Food, Bodies and Anorexia Nervosa in the German Democratic Republic, 1949-1990" (Ph.D. diss., University College London, 2012), 73–74.
39. Donna Harsch, *Revenge of the Domestic: Women, the Family and Communism in the German Democratic Republic* (Princeton, 2007), 278. See also Jutta Voigt, *Der Geschmack des Ostens. Vom Essen, Trinken und Leben in der DDR* (Berlin, 2008).
40. See Madarász-Lebenhagen's essay in this volume. See also Carsten Timmermann, "Americans and Pavlovians: The Central Institute for Cardiovascular Research at the East German Academy of Sciences and Its Precursor Institutions as a Case Study of Biomedical Research in a Country of the Soviet Bloc (c. 1950-80)," in *Medicine, the Market and the Mass Media: Producing Health in the 20th Century*, ed. Virginia Berridge and Kelly Loughlin (London and New York, 2005), 244–65.
41. Based on interviews about eating and dieting in the GDR that the author conducted in Berlin, Dresden, and Leipzig in 2009 and 2010.
42. For example, "Redukal," *Deine Gesundheit*, April 1974; "Iss Dich gesund. Dazu diesen ärztlichen Ratschlag," *Für Dich* 13 (1975).
43. "ON" stood for *optimierte Nahrung* (optimized nutrition). The "ON" line included not only calorie-reduced products, but also products suitable for diabetics and babies. A color-coding system was used to differentiate products: a green dot indicated a calorie-reduced product, a red dot a product suitable for diabetics, and a yellow dot a product suitable for babies.
44. Deutsches Institut für Ernährungsforschung, Box 91, "Psychologische Grundlagen des Ernährungsverhaltens und Möglichkeiten seiner Beeinflussung," Zentralinstitut für Ernährung, 1987.

45. This could, of course, simply reflect what participants thought was the "correct" answer. But the result does not seem implausible when read in conjunction with other evidence about dieting cultures in the 1970s and 1980s.
46. Deutsches Institut für Ernährungsforschung, Box 232, *Psychological Aspects of Nutrition Information and Counselling in Respect to Nutrition Programmes*, June 1988. The report does not make clear whether this number of people simply listened to the program or whether they got actively engaged with it (e.g., by entering its weight-loss competition whereby, in order to win a trip to Berlin, Dresden, or Warnemünde, participants had to send in details of their weight before and after the series). See "Nach der Kur geht's nun 'Schlank in den Urlaub,'" *Berliner Zeitung*, 31 July 1987.
47. "Ich kenne meine Schwachstelle," *Für Dich* 42 (1987).
48. Fulbrook, *The People's State*, 15. Not all scholars agree with this assessment. For example, Andrew Port argues that high levels of individualism existed in East German society beginning in the late 1940s. See Andrew I. Port, *Conflict and Stability in the German Democratic Republic* (New York, 2007).
49. Fulbrook, *The People's State*, 135.
50. See Günter Gaus, *Wo Deutschland liegt. Eine Ortsbestimmung* (Hamburg, 1983).
51. See Betts, *Within Walls*.
52. Josie McLellan, "State Socialist Bodies: East German Nudism from Ban to Boom," *Journal of Modern History* 79 (2007): 48–79.
53. Dagmar Herzog, *Sex after Fascism: Memory and Morality in Twentieth-Century Germany* (Princeton, 2005), chap. 5. See also Josie McLellan, *Love in the Time of Communism: Intimacy and Sexuality in the GDR* (Cambridge, 2011), chap. 7.
54. Mike Featherstone, "The Body in Consumer Culture," *Theory, Culture and Society* 1 (1982): 18–33.
55. Deutsches Institut für Ernährungsforschung, Box 232, "Psychological Aspects," 1988.
56. Deutsches Institut für Ernährungsforschung, Box 91, "Psychologische Grundlagen," 1987.
57. Helmut Haenel, Dieter Johnsen, and Manfred Möhr, "Aufgaben und Probleme bei der Durchsetzung von Ernährungsempfehlungen bei Jugendlichen im Schulalter," *Ernährungsforschung* 2 (1990): B5–7.
58. SAPMO-BArch DC4/736, Monika Reißig, *Kurzbericht: Zum Gesundheitsverhalten Leipziger Schüler 7.—10. Klassen*, Zentralinstitut für Jugendforschung, 1984.
59. SAPMO-BArch DC4/210, *Jugend und Gesundheit. Forschungsberich*, Zentralinstitut für Jugendforschung, 1974.
60. *Gesunde Ernährung im Alter von 16-20 Jahre* (1978).
61. Thank you to Klaus-Jürgen and Ursula Neumärker for bringing this to my attention.
62. For examples of official advice against various dieting methods, see the series "Zurück zur Figur," *Deine Gesundheit* (1982).
63. See Kerr-Boyle, "Orders of Eating."
64. SAPMO-BArch DQ113/105, "Ernährung—Gesundheit—Genuß: Praxis und Wissenschaft," 1986.
65. SAPMO-BArch DC4/650, "Das Verhältnis Jugendlicher zu Körperkultur und Sport sowie Formen, Bedingungen und Probleme seiner Realisierung," n.d. (probably late 1970s).
66. SAPMO-BArch DC4/738d, "Zum Gesundheitsverhalten Jugendlicher: Ernährungsverhalten und Genußmittelkonsum," Zentralinstitut für Jugendforschung, 1988.

67. See Avner Offer, "Body Weight and Self-Control in the United States and Britain since the 1950s," *Social History of Medicine* 14 (2001): 79–106.
68. Susan Bordo, *Unbearable Weight: Feminism, Western Culture and the Body* (Berkeley and Los Angeles, 1993), 173.
69. Some social psychologists advance this argument. See, e.g., Richard Stein and Carol Nemeroff, "Moral Overtones of Food: Judgments of Others Based on What they Eat," *Personality and Social Psychology* 21 (1995): 480–90.
70. In the mid 1980s, 50 percent of all students in higher education were women. In 1989 around 90 percent of East German women were employed outside the home. See Rachel Alsop, *A Reversal of Fortunes? Women, Work and Change in East Germany* (New York and Oxford, 2000), 30–34.
71. For statistics of women in leadership positions, see Fulbrook, *The People's State*, 160–63.
72. Dölling, "Between Hope and Helplessness," 13. There is a rich literature discussing the ways in which East German women continued to be positioned as the female "other" and the continuation of sexist stereotyping and systemic disadvantage which this entailed. See, e.g., Alsop, *A Reversal of Fortunes?*; Merkel, *Frau an der Werkbank*; Harsch, *Revenge of the Domestic*.
73. On the "triple burden," see Port, *Conflict and Stability*, 210.
74. SAPMO-BArch, DC4/522, "Leistung und Lebensweise junger Frauen. Hauptforschungsbericht zur Studie. Leistung und Lebensweise junger Frauen in der DDR," Zentralinstitut für Jugendforschung, 1989.
75. See Featherstone, "The Body in Consumer Culture."

CHAPTER 8

Luxury Dining in the Later Years of the German Democratic Republic

PAUL FREEDMAN

Two aspects of privileged dining in the German Democratic Republic (GDR) during the 1970s and 1980s are discussed in this essay: state dinners given for visiting foreign dignitaries and meals served on vacation cruise ships run by the Freier Deutscher Gewerkschaftsbund (FDGB), the umbrella union organization. The guests at the official occasions were members of the ruling elite, but their experience of gastronomic luxury was similar to that of the guests on the cruise vessels. In fact, such boat trips represented a modest but significant level of social distinction. What was served to the fortunate workers and other loyalists picked for these voyages resembled the selections that were presented to foreign leaders as exemplary of the culinary ambitions of the GDR. Despite the notorious shortages and food supply problems of East Germany, there was a general aspiration for gracious, varied, and interesting dining. This was reflected in the growth of restaurants and in the changes in recipes proposed to the majority of East Germans, who usually cooked at home.

Food and Memory

There is a considerable amount of memoir literature about dining in the GDR, but historical studies tend to focus on durable consumer products, living standards, and differential access to apartments, automobiles, and appliances. Eating is ubiquitous, but once the basic necessities for survival are procured, it tends to be less interesting to historians, perhaps because of that very ubiquity. Yet, the repetition of meals and the consequent pleasures and frustrations of eating in a difficult but not exactly poor economy give dining out great significance in evaluating the everyday life of the vanished world of the GDR. Eating outside the home is a particular kind of consumerism, largely because its physical satisfaction and the possibilities for demonstrating taste and sophistication are at once powerful and short-lived. The world of culinary consumerism is also important because of the well-known power of taste and smell to evoke the past in a way that even the most iconic apartment furniture or washing machines do not.

A screenwriter recalls his youth in the former GDR thus: "How we wolfed down *Kasslerrollen* (smoked pork rolls) and how we laughed!"[1] The closeness of friends in adversity is remembered in association with not necessarily very good food. Elsewhere, too, adults look back on adolescent good times that were accompanied by mediocre dining. East German food-related recollections have a particular emotional power, however, because of the sudden break represented by the extinction of the regime, rather than a gentle decline of earlier ways of life. What Hungarians or Poles ate in 1993 was not as dramatically different from their diet in 1989 because their food supply networks (formal and informal) tended to function better than East Germany's. They also were not taken over immediately by a Western polity and economic system.[2]

The GDR has left a considerable and durable legacy of food nostalgia tinged with rueful humor. After the 1950s there was a more than adequate supply in general, but food remained hard to acquire and often of poor quality, while service in stores and restaurants was, for the most part, dreadful. Basic items such as butter or sugar were in constant danger of disappearing and so were hoarded. There were periodic crises like the sausage shortage of 1963, the unavailability of coffee in 1977, and butter and cheese problems in the fall of 1982. Except for apples and red cabbage, fresh produce was difficult to buy in decent condition because the transport and storage systems could not effectively handle perishable goods. As Jutta Voigt wryly notes in her memoir *Der Geschmack des Ostens* (The Taste of the East), fruit and vegetables were, in effect, "class enemies" that "sabotaged the building of socialism as much as they could."[3]

Variety and freshness were certainly not among the virtues of the GDR food regime, but per capita consumption was impressive. In 1986 the average citizen went through 96 kilos of meat, 43 kilos of sugar, 15.7 kilos of butter, and 307 eggs, all elevated numbers by international standards.[4] This high-calorie diet was obtained only with considerable effort because of shortages, chronic labor supply problems, and the aforementioned distribution deficiencies. In the later decades of the GDR, it was not so much an absolute dearth of food as the physical and mental costs of acquiring it that were most burdensome. For that reason, an important indication of high status was the steady availability of fairly nice food rather than the enjoyment of rarified products.

Buying major consumer goods such as washing machines, refrigerators, or, most notoriously, automobiles was always difficult and the ability to ease or speed up this process defined those who enjoyed a measure of privilege. The 1980s saw an increase in social differentiation, as well as in its disturbing visibility.[5] Apparent political stability coincided with the waning credibility of a future Socialist triumph—what has been termed "The Erosion of a Goal-Oriented Culture" (*Die Erosion der Zielkultur*).[6] Social distinction was linked to a scandalously obvious dependence on capitalism in general, and on the Federal Republic in particular, by differential access to West German marks. The ability to acquire hard currency became a key measure of status and made possible the purchase of small luxuries and comforts, including better kinds of food.[7]

The proliferation of the *Intershops*—which accepted only hard currency for the purchase of Western goods—increased social differentiation based not so much on job title or rank as on the possession of connections necessary to acquire West German marks. There were attempts to offset the threat to official equality represented by the *Intershops*, notably through the creation of *Exquisit* and *Delikat* stores (the latter dealing primarily in luxury—or at least sought-after—foods). Both accepted GDR marks, but these efforts failed as the desperation of the regime for foreign currency in the face of gradual but inexorable bankruptcy tied it to policies exalting the West German mark: hence the expansion of the *Intershops*.[8] By the 1980s distinctions based on access to hard currency were obvious, unavoidable, and resented by those consequently shut off from the enjoyment of even minor indulgences. At a luxurious but officially egalitarian French restaurant located within the Palace of the Republic complex, the seat of the GDR parliament, East German currency was usually accepted, but even here special offerings such as the "Pfeffersteak à la Toulouse-Lautrec," flambéed in Calvados, had to be paid for with West German marks. At issue in this instance was the expense of the imported Calvados.[9]

Outside of Germany the living standards of the GDR are best known through the film *Good Bye, Lenin!*, which depicts the overnight abandonment of old forms of material culture. Spreewaldgurken (pickles) and Mokka-Fix Gold coffee appear here as symbols of the abrupt shift from the comfortingly routine to the suddenly unobtainable.[10] Many food items of everyday use were shoved aside after 1989: "Goldbroilers" (industrially produced chickens sold for take-out), KUKO-Reis (preseasoned, instant rice), Erwa-Speisewürze (a seasoning mixture for cooking), or the emblematic Tempolinsen (chemically treated, quick-cooking lentils)—a whole category of things once considered "not beautiful, but usable."[11] Following the unification of Germany, however, a certain regret for a (putatively) quieter and more leisurely way of life set in, one whose backwardness and predictable tastes and smells were remembered with affection, albeit ironic affection.[12] Of course the struggle to assure adequate food and basic consumer goods, as well as the omnipresence of official propaganda, hardly made for a tranquil life in a literal sense. Yet, collectively experienced obligations and routines, along with limited media stimulation, were recalled as peaceful, much in the way that many older Western Europeans recollect the distant 1950s.[13] The GDR became an extinct civilization within a few months after the fall of the Berlin Wall, but preoccupation with the cuisine of the East still continues, almost twenty-five years after reunification, and some of the best work on food in the GDR has appeared only recently.[14] The culinary artifacts of the GDR obviously evoke complex and enduring responses.

Some aspects of East German food supply and consumption remained the same over the life of the regime: shortages (especially of fruit and vegetables), attempts to industrialize production. In fact, there were considerable changes and fluctuations between 1949 and 1989. The struggle to achieve an adequate diet in the 1950s gave way to an improvement in living standards that was especially notable in the late 1960s and early 1970s. The popular television chefs Kurt Drummer and Rudolf Kroboth popularized chicken, eggs, Eastern European recipes (in the case of Drummer) and fish (Kroboth's specialty). The first Goldbroiler shop opened in November 1967.[15] The 1960s also saw so much consumption of herring and other fish that stocks were depleted and the boom was over by the mid 1970s.[16]

The 1970s and 1980s witnessed a turn toward a more eclectic and international style, something that did not happen in the USSR: Arab, Cuban, and Vietnamese recipes proliferated—thanks, in part, to the influx of migrants from allied Socialist states. Curry, pizza, and fondue were popular, a delayed response to their diffusion throughout Western Europe. Authenticity was not vitally important: "Soy sauce? No problem! Erwa-Speisewürze tastes the same: you only need faith."[17] A 1979 menu from the main restaurant of the Palace of the Republic featured *nasi goreng*, an Indonesian rice dish.[18] On the inserted menu of the day (*Tageskarte*) for the week of 13–19 February 1979 was an intimidating Double Rumpsteak Mexican Style (for two persons), accompanied by pepper strips, tomatoes, pickles, artichoke hearts, beef marrow, and peas, all in a potato nest, along with anchovy butter and French-fried potatoes. Slightly more convincing Mexican cuisine was available at places like the Tampico, a restaurant in the Chemnitzer Hof Hotel, where an undated menu (likely from the 1980s) included chili con carne and the "Tampico Mixed Grill" with tortillas.[19]

Some attempt was made to jazz up the taste of food available to ordinary people. One method was to suggest the use of sharp or spicy flavorings, much as Americans have used Tabasco or steak sauces to overcome the industrial blandness of their modern processed food. "Koche mit Liebe, würze mit Bino" (Cook with love; season with Bino) was a 1950s advertising slogan for a concentrated soup cube of the Maggi type, recommended to add "a piquant note"—and, indeed, *pikante* was a favorite word in GDR cookbooks and menus. Then again, *pikante* appeared almost as frequently as *schnell* (quick) and *gesund* (healthy) in the recipes found in West German women's magazines.[20] For purposes of variety, as well as to promote Socialist solidarity, there was also an effort to feature products and recipes from fraternal Warsaw Pact countries. Russian and Ukrainian *soljanka* (a sweet and sour soup with sausage and vegetables), Bulgarian sausages or pepper salad, and Hungarian goulash and *letscho* were ubiquitous.[21]

Beyond comfortable generalizations about East German dining and the everyday diet and desires evoked by culinary memoirs, it is worth looking at what the privileged sectors of GDR society ate and what someone of only middling status might enjoy by special or temporary favor. How radically did the food in elite government institutions or settings differ from the plain style of the country's food as a whole? To what degree was there an attempt to assert an "East German identity," something difficult given the artificial circumstances of the GDR as half of a divided nation?

Luxury Dining in the German Workers' and Farmers' State: Official Occasions

Because access to any sort of food remained difficult in the early years of the GDR, the hierarchical distinction was more starkly drawn at this time between those with an adequate diet and those without one than would later be the case, when degrees of privilege involved nicer, fresher, or more refined food. Notwithstanding rising living standards or anxiety over the rapid growth of the Federal Republic's consumer culture, there was no strongly expressed "culture of gourmandise"; nor were there obvious culinary distinctions similar to those that obtained for electronic goods, apartments, or automobiles. SED General Secretary Erich Honecker himself did not display a fondness for cuisine, and those elite cadres who did have *Feinschmecker* proclivities practiced them discreetly. Honecker's personal chef Jürgen Krause has described the gastronomic tastes of the East German leader as modest and uninteresting. Honecker did not use his powerful position to eat in a radically different manner from that of his fellow citizens. He adored macaroni with tomato sauce, as well as schnitzel with potatoes and a vegetable medley (included only for health reasons). Honecker's favorite dish was *Kassler* with sauerkraut or potatoes. He had no liking for fish other than marinated herring.[22] This is not to say that Honecker was in all respects austere, but that his self-indulgence lay outside the realm of gastronomy. Though an enthusiastic hunter, Honecker did not like to eat game or, for that matter, other forest products such as berries or mushrooms.[23] His real enthusiasm and abuse of privilege were applied to fancy automobiles and what might politely be called "womanizing."[24]

Several members of the GDR inner circle were more serious connoisseurs. Albert Norden and Kurt Hager tried to institute greater variety in the gastronomic offerings at the Politburo's elite residential compound in Wandlitz north of Berlin, but even in the seemingly innocuous matter of using foreign terms in menus, little innovation was allowed beyond the ever-present *soljanka*. Honecker's chef recalled an incident in which he served "Steak Westmoreland," something he describes as "an age-old dish." This provoked consternation because the commander of the U.S. forces in Vietnam at that time was General William Westmoreland. So much for pretentious English or French menu descriptions.[25]

The Wende Museum in Los Angeles, which is dedicated to the material culture of former East Germany, has a collection of about 300 menus. Notable among them is a group of 12 menus from the 1980s for dinners given for visiting dignitaries hosted by Honecker and other high-level officials.[26] In addition, 27 menus from state occasions are presented (along with selected recipes) in *Essen wie Erich*, a humorous but thorough study of the general secretary's table. This begins with a June 1972 dinner for Soviet Foreign Minister Andrei Gromyko and ends with the Belshazzar's feast of 7 October 1989 in honor of the fortieth anniversary of the founding of the GDR, an event attended by Mikhail Gorbachev, Daniel Ortega, Yasser Arafat, and Nicolae Ceaușescu. There is also in the Bundesarchiv in Berlin a menu for a dinner given by Honecker in 1980 for the Cambodian head of state Heng Samrin.[27]

Visits by foreign leaders were favorable signs of what seemed to be the GDR's coming of age after more than two decades of international isolation. As a result of Willy Brandt's *Ostpolitik*, the idea of two German states was finally accepted in the West, and in 1973, the United Nations admitted both East Germany and the Federal Republic. The GDR had earlier established full diplomatic relations only with the Warsaw Pact nations and a few other more-or-less Socialist states, but by 1975, East Germany was recognized by eighty countries.[28] Despite their banal formality, the official meals served as opportunities to demonstrate East German political and cultural integrity, and the menus were meant to reflect a combination of national accomplishment and a muted ostentation suitable for a Socialist society with a gastronomically unadventurous leader.

Official dinners, which usually consisted of four courses, displayed a cautious sophistication, something between ordinary East German specialties and international taste. The menus of the cruise ships, like those of the nicer resort hotels in East Germany, included the best that was available to persons of modest but temporarily privileged status. These two types of menus represented different forms of elite dining, but, as indicated, the offerings were very similar. State banquets took place at the Palais Unter den Linden, which was rebuilt in 1969. Originally erected in 1663, it was the residence of the Hohenzollern Crown-Prince during the nineteenth century and part of the National Gallery from 1918 until its destruction in World War II. The menus for the dinners at the Palais followed an unwavering order of hors d'oeuvre, soup, main course, and dessert. The hors d'oeuvre was accompanied by vodka (usually from the East German town Wilthen) or Nordhäuser "Feiner alter Korn," a schnapps whose origins go back to the early sixteenth century. The wines were most often from the two small recognized East German wine regions: Saale-Unstrut and the tiny Saxon *terroir* on the Elbe near Meissen and Dresden. The ability to enjoy these was itself a mark of substantial distinction because their exiguous production made them virtually unknown to ordinary East German citizens. Dessert was occasionally accompanied by sparkling wine (*Sekt*) from Freyburg, often of the Rotkäppchen label, a celebratory beverage whose resurgent popularity since unification has practically effaced its former reputation as a symbol of the GDR's gustatory mediocrity.[29] Brandy (usually from Wilthen as well) was served with coffee after the meal.

The dinners were given in honor of a curious assortment of guests. The Wende collection in Los Angeles contains menus from occasions with West German dignitaries such as SPD leaders Oskar Lafontaine in 1987, when he was minister-president of the Saar, and Björn Engholm, who, at the time of his visit to East Berlin in early 1989, was the minister-president of Schleswig-Holstein and president of the Bundesrat. Also in the Wende Museum are menus for dinners given for President Daniel Ortega of Nicaragua in 1984, for U.N. Secretary General Javier Pérez de Cuéllar in 1987, for Prime Minister Andreas Papandreou of Greece in 1988, and for Tariq Aziz, the Iraqi foreign minister, also in 1988. The book *Essen wie Erich* features gastronomic records of visits from international leaders from other Socialist lands (Fidel Castro of Cuba, Todor Zhikov of Bulgaria, Janos Kadar of Hungary), from "peoples' democracies" in the developing world such as Yemen, Laos, and the Democratic Republic of the Congo, and from Western countries such as Greece (a visit by Papandreou in 1984 and by his successor Christos Sartzetakis in 1986) and Italy (Bettino Craxi in 1984). Preserved in these two sources are additional records of larger occasions, such as one commemorating the twenty-fifth anniversary of the erection of the "Anti-fascist Protective Wall" on 13 August 1986, another on 2 October 1984 honoring veterans who had founded the GDR, as well as a 6 May 1985 dinner with Soviet friends and German anti-fascist activists (menu no. 19 in *Essen wie Erich*).

There is not much variety in the style of these menus: an hors d'oeuvre often served with toast (such as the crab cocktail served to Pérez de Cuéllar), soup (oxtail, beef, curried chicken), and then a hearty meat course and finally some sort of sweet-cream dessert. One assumes that political leaders are accustomed to official banquets and bored by the offerings, but one still wonders what Andreas Papandreou might have made of *Kalbsrücken* und *Rinderspökelzunge* (saddle of veal and cured ox tongue) served in Burgundy sauce and accompanied by Brussels sprouts, asparagus (which must have been canned or frozen, given that the meal took place in January 1988), carrots, and potatoes. This had been preceded by stuffed pork tenderloin with "piquant" anise sauce (served with toast and rose-shaped butter), and double-strength beef tea with quail's egg. Dessert was orange mousse with chocolate cream. Of course he had been prepared by an earlier visit that had also featured beef broth (this time with liver dumplings) and stuffed pork filet in cream sauce.[30]

In June 1984, Daniel Ortega was served a slightly lighter meal beginning with what was translated into Spanish as merely "little veal salad with toasts" (*ensaladilla de ternera, tostadas*)—which misses the all-important adjective *pikanter* in the original German: "Pikanter Kalbfleischsalat, Toast." This was served with Nordhäuser "Feiner alter Korn." The soup was once again *Doppelte Rinderkraftbrühe* (given in Spanish as simply "*consomé*"), but this time without the quail egg. Chicken fried in spicy egg batter with mushrooms, peas, grilled tomatoes, and potato croquettes constituted the main course, and the meal finished with lemon cream and sour cherries. Meissener Weissburgunder was served with the main course, Rotkäppchen-Sekt with the dessert, and Weinbrand "Grande Reserve" from Wilthen, with coffee.[31]

The dinners in honor of West German dignitaries seemed a little less self-conscious with regard to food, perhaps indicating greater confidence that the guests would feel gastronomically at home. The menus still betrayed, however, an eagerness not to appear inferior to perceived Western sophistication. The main course at Oskar Lafontaine's dinner was a lavish Berlin-style platter that included beef roulade, veal shank, and pork tenderloin with baked onion puree, beans with *Speck* (meat fat, or bacon), carrots, and potato dumplings. A 1983 Ruländer Meissen was offered with this course. First came glazed quail breast with apple and celery salad, sour cherry sauce, and toast (served with German vodka), followed by game-bird soup with herb custard. Dessert was a confection of bilberries with cream. The sparkling wine was described as "Deutscher Sekt Lindenpalais trocken, Weinkellerei Berlin" (Rotkäppchen was not served at meals for West German visitors or other Western guests).[32]

Luxury Dining: Vacation Cruise Ships

When it comes to the meals of the moderately privileged, one must keep in mind that there was often a discrepancy between what menus listed and what was really available. An impressive menu from the historic Thüringer Hof in Leipzig listed two kinds of trout and two kinds of venison, for example. Since the menu has a specific date (23 September 1986), it is at least possible that these really were on offer.[33] A more generic Leipzig menu from the Hotel Astoria near the central train station listed fourteen hearty steak, pork, sausage, and chicken dishes, along with thirteen cold platters. Those who dined in East German hotel restaurants recall, however, that items on the elaborate menus were not all available at the same time.[34] The state-run restaurant Jägerhütte in Rostock featured venison and wild boar dishes, but here, too, it is impossible to say what customers might actually have been able to order.[35]

There were many elegant restaurants in the GDR by the 1980s, and some attention was now given to local specialties and historic atmosphere.[36] Manfred Otto's *Gastronomische Entdeckungen in der DDR*, published in 1984, listed 100 restaurants and offered recipes from each of them. The book was organized by historic region rather than—as in the more down-market *Restaurants und Gaställen der DDR*—by administrative district (*Bezirk*).[37] *Gastronomische Entdeckungen* seems to have been directed to foreign (i.e., West German) tourists, however. Even if almost anything was available for a price by the 1980s, it is not clear which GDR citizens could afford it.

An advantage of considering menus from the three vacation vessels run by the FDGB is that they included precise dates and offered a limited number of choices, which means that there was a likely match between claim and reality.[38] The first FDGB vacation cruise vessel, the *Völkerfreundschaft* (Friendship of Peoples), was acquired in 1959: it had previously been the Swedish ship *Stockholm*, built in 1948 and involved in the 1956 sinking of the *Andrea Doria* after a collision near the island of Nantucket. The *Völkerfreundschaft* made its first trip in January 1960 in honor of East German President Wilhelm Pieck's eighty-fourth birthday.[39] The *Fritz Heckert* was built in Rostock and completed in 1961; the *Arkona* was built in 1981 for a West German cruise line that later went bankrupt. The East German government bought it in 1985 and sold the *Völkerfreundschaft*.[40]

Because the ships were part of the FDBG vacation service's system of resorts and leisure activities, their passengers were principally from the GDR. The company most commonly offered weeklong Baltic cruises from the port of Warnemünde to Riga, Gdansk, Tallinn, and Leningrad.[41] There were occasionally more ambitious voyages, notably to Cuba and to the Black Sea. The long trips had to include a considerable amount of on-board entertainment because the geopolitical restrictions placed on the movement of East German citizens limited the number of places it was considered safe to stop. A Black Sea cruise of the *Fritz Heckert* in 1964 departed Warnemünde on 30 September and made its first landing at Sochi on the Soviet Black Sea coast on 11 October. The ship passed by Algeria, Tunisia, Italy, and Greece, and the menus noted some of the things worth seeing from the boat, but there was no opportunity to disembark anywhere except Sochi, Yalta, and Constanta in Romania. There were lectures, films, dancing, exercises, volleyball, and other games on board ("Kennen Sie Shufflebord?").[42]

One of the earliest cruise ship menus is from the *Völkerfreundschaft* and is dated 26 February 1961. The *Fritz Heckert* menus are from 1964 and 1965 (the latter a North Atlantic trip that went as far as Iceland but with no foreign stops). The *Völkerfreundschaft* seems to have had more elaborate food than the *Fritz Heckert*, and its menus for welcome-aboard meals (*Begrüssungsessen*) or farewell dinners (*Abschiedsessen*) indicated especially elegant affairs. During the 1960s voyages, lunch was a serious occasion while the evening meal tended to be lighter: a selection of cold meat, tinned fish, cheese, and salad, served with bread, butter, and tea. In 1961 the midday main meal started with meat broth with peas, or noodle soup. One could then choose among pork cutlet (with mixed vegetables and potatoes), escalope with paprika (*Paprikaschnitzel*) with spaghetti and salad, roast beef with remoulade sauce (and roasted potatoes and salad), or Labskaus mit Setzei (a corned beef and herring hash, served with a fried egg on top and beets on the side). Fruit ices with cream were served for dessert.[43] By contrast, the first meal on board the *Fritz Heckert* leaving Warnemünde en route to Cuba in 1964 offered only Bratwusrt as a lunch entrée—although later there would be a choice among such dishes as marinated liver, *Kassler*, Szeged-style pork goulash, and Serbian meat with rice.[44]

The elaborate meals on board the *Völkerfreundschaft* that marked the beginning and end of voyages resembled official dinners except that there was a fish course (usually halibut). On 12 October 1981, the *Begrüssungsessen* menu noted that the ship had fifteen cooks, two butchers, two bakers, two pastry chefs and eleven assistants. The guests were served "Alexandra" broth, halibut *Weinhändler Art* with dill potatoes, baked pork steak with vegetables and French-fried potatoes, and a strawberry ice confection. A vermouth cocktail accompanied the soup, and Bulgarian wines were presented with the fish and meat courses.[45]

In its few years of service for the GDR, the *Arkona* appears to have been even more elegant in its overall atmosphere than the *Völkerfreundschaft*. Most of its surviving menus, with unusually well-designed colors and graphics, are from just after the fall of the Berlin Wall and thus, in a slightly surreal fashion, memorialize a world in the process of disappearing. For a trip to Cuba at the beginning of 1990, the first menu is from January 10, when the ship was already in Havana Harbor. The farewell dinner was on 27 January, so the entire journey would probably have run for nearly an entire month. A celebratory dinner on 20 January 1990 offered dishes from Spain, Mexico, Norway, Turkey, and the USSR.[46] The farewell dinner menu from 29 November 1989 for another trip (to an unknown destination) included an appetizer of Norwegian smoked salmon, a second course of shrimp and Asian vegetables sautéed in garlic butter, a main course of beef filet with Cognac sauce and Roquefort cheese, and, for dessert, "Omelette Arkona," which was described as an "iced surprise."[47]

Other Dining Opportunities

The vacation ships were privileged zones, even if ones of restrained dimensions. The GDR did have other dining establishments that were exceptional, to a greater or lesser extent, because they were well-run, had carefully cooked food, or featured otherwise unavailable ingredients. For example, the restaurant of the Palace of the Republic in Berlin seems often to have had pheasant and trout in the late 1970s and early 1980s.[48] Six restaurants were opened in 1978 in an annex behind the ultraluxurious Hotel Neptun in Warnemünde, which had been built in 1971. The whole complex was known as the "Spezialitäten Restaurant Schillerstrasse 14." One of these served local Warnemünde seafood, while others featured exotic offerings: a Cuban *Bodega* and a Hungarian *Czarda*, for instance.[49] A more unusual anomaly was the Waffenschmied in Suhl, established in 1966 by the visionary chef Rolf Anschütz, who managed to cook Japanese food of surprising authenticity and quality. For many years, in fact, the Waffenschmied was considered the best Japanese restaurant in Europe.[50] Such establishments were remote islands of luxury, though more accessible to those with West German marks: there was a two-year wait for a reservation at the Waffenschmied for those paying with GDR marks if they did not have some sort of Party association.[51] At the Neptun restaurants, guests could pay with GDR marks, but the wait for a reservation was usually several weeks—unless hard currency was used.

Fine Dining and Food Nostalgia

The menus examined in this essay suggest a modest level of luxury with respect to what privileged people ate. The official occasions represented what was deemed appropriate for the public face of the German workers' and farmers' state, and were often supplemented by foreign specialties from other Socialist countries. To find a richer, more grandiose style beyond the quotidian round of hors d'oeuvres with toast, meat broth, beef, pork, or veal entrées, one would have needed an invitation to Politburo retreats such as Wandlitz. Here game, caviar, and Western imports were enjoyed by the inner circle in a more intimate setting than the official meals served to dozens, if not hundreds, of guests. Yet, even in such private, "unmarked" spaces, the distinctions did not seem to be radical: they amounted to a more assured supply and better quality—rather than to a cuisine completely different from what ordinary people ate.

The elite habits of dining put into relief the everyday experience of East Germans under "real-existing socialism." Some of the most enduring recollection of this time is not so much of the food itself, but rather constitutes a memory of private hospitality in an economy that provided limited consumer goods but plentiful opportunities for evading work. Combined with the lack of extensive travel possibilities, this tedious leisure could often mean a close social life with friends and neighbors. In the GDR a common saying was that in the West, the shop windows were full and the table at home was empty, while in the East, the shops windows were empty and the table was bedecked with food. With all the wealth of beautiful things for sale, West Germans were reputed to buy ham in misanthropic 50-gram units.[52] Whether or not any of this was true was less important than the sense of a close Eastern community, defined not by official socialism but by private celebration. People of a certain age remember paradoxical good times, the laughter rather than the dubious *Kasslerrollen*—or rather the laughter for which the *Kasslerrollen* were as much the accompaniment as the popular songs of the day. To some extent these are simply memories of youth.

Food nostalgia has a real content, nevertheless. There was indeed a *Geschmack des Ostens*, but it is not easy to describe or even to distinguish clearly from the *Geschmack des Westens*. The difference was more of a temporal nature, with the East lagging, than in a fixed aesthetic bifurcation. In the 1950s West Germany experienced a boom in frozen foods, canned fruit, soup mixes, soft drinks, and processed cheese.[53] These tastes antedated similar developments in the East, but were not particularly distinct in content.[54] To be sure, food in the GDR tended to be stronger, sharper, more direct—more "working class" than that in the FRG.[55] This did not necessarily reflect a difference based on contrasting political systems, however, since the same distinction could be drawn between regions forming parts of the same state and economy—e.g., between the food preferences of the gritty industrial North of England and the affluent, trendier tastes of the South. Some characteristics often trotted out as pathetically typical of East German delicacies were shared with richer societies—West Germany, Britain, or the United States—none of which was internationally famous for its sophisticated good taste in the Cold War era. Ersatz food was not limited to the benighted Warsaw Pact: many Americans in the 1960s abandoned orange juice as a breakfast drink in favor of Tang (an artificially flavored powder stirred in water); instant coffee took the United States by storm that same decade. Attempts to market mass-produced industrial food as gourmet were a feature of both Eastern and Western bloc countries. American women's magazines in the 1950s recommended adding canned pineapple to everything; Jell-O was fashionable for salads made to entertain company; Swiss Knight processed cheese triangles were offered to guests as well, along with cocktail frankfurters that came in a jar—in short, anything that could be served with toothpicks. Pseudo-foreign dishes that characterized East Germany were matched, if not inspired, by the once-ubiquitous "Polynesian" restaurants of the Trader Vic's type, or American Chinese restaurants with their shrimp toast of the 1950s, sweet and sour pork of the 1960s, or General Tso's

Chicken of the 1970s. The popularity of tableside flambé dishes transcended the international ideological divide in the 1960s and 1970s.

While there is some nostalgia for bygone food in the United States, it is only marginally significant as a cultural symbol and has produced little in the way of exploration of personal memories linked to social and gastronomic culture.[56] Crêpes Suzette at the high end, or TV dinners at the low, are associated with particular years, but do not evoke a way of life that has vanished entirely.

Already before 1989 the GDR was regarded by outsiders as living in the past, which meant that there was, in some sense, an anticipatory nostalgia even before the collapse of the regime. The GDR lagged behind the West more obviously in the relatively prosperous last two decades of its existence than during the "economic miracle" years of the Federal Republic in the 1950s and 1960s. Or it could just be that the lag seemed permanent by 1980, as the utopian future receded and dreams of catching up with the West became increasingly laughable.

The GDR did not participate in certain key consumer changes that affected Western Europe in the 1970s: a decline in the consumption of meat, the rise of supermarkets, and the impact of mass, long-distance tourism that created a space for the expansion of ethnic restaurants and home experimentation. In the West the 1970s also saw the beginning of a reaction against mass production of food in the form of nouvelle cuisine, with its emphasis on quality and minimalism. Attempts to revive and preserve local foodways, regional identity, and artisanal techniques began in the 1980s and would eventually crystallize as the international Slow Food movement.[57]

These developments either passed by the GDR entirely or were only dimly relevant, but the chronological gap was no more than about a decade. It is wrong to think that East Germany was a time warp, where the 1950s were frozen and perpetuated with respect to culinary taste and options. Such an impression is born of forgetfulness about what people in the West had thought was sophisticated in the 1950s, 1960s, and 1970s. East German food was not so alien or so scarce—certainly not on the order of that in the Soviet Union itself, or that in the deliberately impoverished realms of Romania and Albania. It was, above all, simply "old fashioned."[58]

As Stefan Wolle recollects, the smell of homemade plum cake wafted over the GDR and endless conversations took place accompanied by low-quality but comforting coffee.[59] There is a paradoxical sense of the East German past as less frenetic with regard to work and the drive for success—while at the same time more demanding and time-consuming in terms of one's daily existence, including the search for food. Some food nostalgia is related to the troublesome hunt to find it. Not that waiting on lines, struggling with the personnel of the state-run Handelsorganisation (HO) stores, special trips to Berlin, differential access to West German marks, or complicated barter improvisations conjure up pleasant memories, but the goods themselves attained vivid significance because of the very difficulty of acquisition. What is remembered is a contest, but not an extreme Darwinian one—not wartime privation, but rather monotony punctuated by sudden opportunities and windfalls: a struggle for nice and interesting food, not for survival.

Under such conditions, privilege was defined not so much as the ability to consume culinary luxuries unknown to the masses, but to be assured of supply, of not having to worry about how food was to be obtained. Naturally the political leaders were exempt from this preoccupation, and that was enough to distinguish their meals—even if these were otherwise pedestrian, with their toast and butter hors d'oeuvres and schnitzel entrées. For outstanding workers and functionaries, the *Völkerfreundschaft* cruises represented a brief vacation from the quotidian search. The reward for privileged workers was not so different from everyday existence in terms of *what* was consumed, but distinct in terms of the ease with which it arrived at the table.

Nostalgia for the East will fade as the proportion of the population whose lives were anchored in the decades before the fall of the Berlin Wall declines. Yet, the durability and complexity of this sentiment remain, at least for the time being, notable and the source of some controversy.[60] One does not have to be an aficionado of Proust to know that taste, smell, and recollection are intimately linked. That is why the memories of seemingly ordinary food provoke longing and a sense of a lost paradise. Some of the sentiment for the taste of the Eastern German past arose as a response to the unaffected disdain of Westerners for the flimsy and backward material culture of the East, symbolized most clearly by the infamous Trabant car (*Trabi*). Ostalgie is, in some respects, then, a backlash (*Trotzreaktion*), an expression of resentment at the easy assumption of superiority by the *Wessis*.[61] Yet, some of this contempt also reflects a disillusion with a West German image of the East before 1989, when the GDR seemed appealingly old-fashioned, a living reminder of outdated style, a kind of *Ostalgie avant la lettre*.[62] Stefan Wolle's evocation of the fragrance of plum cake alluded to earlier came in the context of a list of West German impressions of the East during the heyday of the GDR: a place where steam locomotives still chugged, the smell of household coal fires mingled with that plum cake, where telephones rang shrilly and antiquated trolleys rocked on their rails; where televisions without remote control required getting up to change channels.[63]

With regard to food, *Ostalgie* is as much about the enjoyment of food with friends and family, or in certain emotionally comfortable settings, as about the actual tastes themselves—which, if sampled years later, would likely seem bland, artificial, or uninteresting. Such experiences are available to those from other countries as well, as anyone who grew up in the United States, delighted with treats like Danish butter cookies or Bonbel cheese, can attest—but it is particularly strong in eastern Germany. This is not surprising, given the circumstances of the cultural divide brought about by the abrupt end of the Cold War and its spiritually ambiguous aftermath. Exploration of East German cuisine is, therefore, something more than a fussy historical reconstruction on the order of battle reenactment, but rather an example of contested memory of a certain period and a certain regime.

Suggested Readings

Betts, Paul. "The Twilight of the Idols: East German Memory and Material Culture." *Journal of Modern History* 72 (2000): 731–65.
Bren, Paulina and Mary Neuburger, eds. *Communism Unwrapped: Consumption in Cold War Eastern Europe*. New York, 2012.
Diewald, Martin and Heike Solga. "Soziale Ungleichheiten in der DDR. Die feinen aber deutlichen Unterschiede am Vorabend der Wende." In *Kollektiv und Eigensinn. Lebensverläufe in der DDR und danach*, ed. Johannes Huinink and Karl Ulrich Mayer, 261–305. Berlin, 1995.
Ludwig, Andreas. *Tempolinsen und P2. Alltagskultur in der DDR*. Berlin, 1996.
Merkel, Ina. *Utopie und Bedürfnis. Die Geschichte der Konsumkultur in der DDR*. Cologne, 1999.
———, ed. *Wunderwirtschaft: DDR-Konsumkultur in den 60er Jahren*. Cologne, 1996.
Stengel, Tobias and Fabian Tweder. *Deutsche kulinarische Republik. Szenen, Berichte und Rezepte au dem Osten*. Frankfurt am Main, 1998.
Thaa, Winfried, Iris Häuser, Michael Schenkel, and Gerd Meyer, eds. *Gesellschaftliche Differnzierung und Legitimätsverfall des DDR-Sozialismus*. Tübingen, 1992.
Voigt, Jutta. *Der Geschmack des Ostens. Vom Essen, Trinken und Leben in der DDR*. Berlin, 2005.
Weinreb, Alice. "Matters of Taste: The Politics of Food in Divided Germany, 1945-1971." Ph.D. diss., University of Michigan, 2009.
Wolle, Stefan. *Die heile Welt der Diktatur. Alltag und Herrschaft in der DDR, 1971-1989*. Berlin, 1998.
Zatlin, Jonathan R. *The Currency of Socialism: Money and Political Culture in East Germany*. New York, 2007.

Acknowledgments

I acknowledge with gratitude the encouragement of Justinian Jampol, director of the Wende Museum in Los Angeles, for suggesting the topic of this essay. Annalena Müller of Yale University helped me greatly with the research of this chapter in Germany. I am grateful to Carola Jülling of the Deutsches Historisches Museum (Berlin), and Andreas Ludwig and Sigrid Stenzel of the Dokumentationszentrum Alltagskultur der DDR (Eisenhüttenstadt). I benefited from the generous advice of Professors Helmut Smith of Vanderbilt University and Peter Scholliers of the Vrije Universiteit Brussel. My deepest debt is to Andrew Port, whose suggestions, observations, and encouragement were indispensable and are much appreciated.

Notes

1. Jutta Voigt, *Der Geschmack des Ostens. Vom Essen, Trinken und Leben in der DDR* (Berlin, 2005), 11. On food nostalgia of the GDR, see also Thomas Heubner, *So schmeckte es in der DDR. Ein Lach- und Sachbuch vom Essen und Trinken* (Berlin, 2004).
2. Paul Betts, "The Twilight of the Idols: East German Memory and Material Culture," *Journal of Modern History* 72 (2000): 734.
3. Voigt, *Der Geschmack des Ostens*, 127.
4. Ibid., 10.
5. Heike Solga, *Auf dem Weg in eine klassenlose Gesellschaft? Klassenlagen und Mobilität zwischen Generationen in der DDR* (Berlin, 1995), 119–24.
6. Michael Schenkel and Winfried Thaa, "Die Erosion der Zielkultur am Beispiel der Fortschrittsdiskussion in einzelnen Teilöffentlichkeiten der DDR," in *Gesellschaftliche Differenzierung und Legitimitätsverfall des DDR-Sozialismus. Das Ende des anderen Wegs in der Moderne*, ed. Winfried Thaa et al. (Tübingen, 1992), 241–430.
7. On small degrees of privilege and their importance in the GDR, see Andrew I. Port, *Conflict and Stability in the German Democratic Republic* (Cambridge, 2007), 238–70. Although they do not consider food, Martin Dewald and Heike Solga emphasize petty but symbolically significant markers of social differentiation in "Soziale Ungleichheiten in der DDR. Die feinen, aber deutlichen Unterschiede am Vorabend der Wende," in *Kollectiv und Eigensinn: Lebensverläufe in der DDR und danach*, ed. Johannes Huinink et al. (Berlin, 1995), 261–305.
8. Jonathan R. Zatlin, *The Currency of Socialism: Money and Political Culture in East Germany* (Washington, D.C., 2007), 173–74, 243–50, 260–70, 277–79; Annette Kaminsky, "Ungleichheit in der SBZ/DDR am Beispiel des Konsums. Versandhandel, Intershop und Delikat," in *Soziale Ungleichheit in der DDR. Zu einem tabuisierten Strukturmerkmal der SED-Diktatur*, ed. Lothar Mertens (Berlin, 2002), 57–79, esp. 72–76.
9. Voigt, *Der Geschmack des Ostens*, 194–95.
10. On the gherkins, see Ursula Heinzelmann, "Spreewälder Gurken: Pickled Cucumbers from the Spreewald," *Gastronomica* 4, no. 3 (2004): 18–25. On coffee in the GDR and the frustrations surrounding it, see Heubner, *So schmeckte es in der GDR*, 118–26; Katherine Pence, "Grounds for Discontent? Coffee from the Black Market to the *Kaffeeklatsch* in the GDR," in *Communism Unwrapped: Consumption in Cold War Eastern Europe*, ed. Paulina Bren and Mary Neuburger (New York, 2012), 197–225; Stefan Wolle, *Die heile Welt der Diktatur. Alltag und Herrschaft in der DDR 1971-1989* (Berlin, 1998), 199–201; Tobias Stregel and Fabian Tweder, *Deutsche Kulinarische Republik. Szenen, Berichte und Rezepte aus dem Osten* (Frankfurt/Main, 1998), 26–28. It should be noted that the pickles had a venerable pre-GDR history and have been revived since unification, whereas the low-quality brand of coffee remains merely an evocative name from the past.
11. A key concept and category noted by Ina Merkel, *Utopie und Bedürfnis. Die Geschichte der Konsumkultur in der DDR* (Cologne, 1999), 372–78.
12. Martin Ahrends, "The Great Waiting, or The Freedom of the East: An Obituary for Life in Sleeping Beauty's Castle," in *When the Wall Came Down: Reactions to German Unification*, ed. Harold James and Maria Stone (New York, 1992), 158–60.
13. "Growing up in Belfast in 1950s and 60s," Patricia Craig has written, for example, "I relished the city's old 'Burke and Hare' atmosphere (noted by Sean O'Faolain if no one else), 'the damp Lagan fogs', cobbled alleyways, coalmen's carts, sedate department

stores, raucous workingmen's pubs, late-Victorian terraces, the dripping shrubberies of Malone Road or Antrim Road villas, with mahogany seats on the lavatory and maids in the kitchen—all endangered at the time and now largely disappeared, or at least vitiated." See Patricia Craig, "Introduction," in *The Ulster Anthology*, ed. Patricia Craig (Belfast, 2006), xi.

14. On East German food culture see, in addition to the works cited earlier, Patrice G. Poutrus, *Die Erfindung des Goldbroilers. Über den Zusammenhang zwischen Herrschaftssicherung und Konsumentwicklung in der DDR* (Cologne, 2002); Ute Scheffler, *Alles Soljanka, oder wie? Das ultimative DDR-Kochbuch 1949-1989* (Leipzig, 2001); Manfred Otto, *Gastronomische Entdeckungen in der DDR* (Berlin, 1984). On consumer culture in general, see Merkel, *Utopie und Bedürfnis*; Wolle, *Die heile Welt der Diktatur*, 171–221. GDR food nostalgia has a significant web presence. See the list of recipes at http://www.daskochrezept.de/geschmacksache/multi-kulti/ddr/ (accessed 4 December 2011). Among the "Top 10 DDR Rezepte der Woche" are two kinds of *soljanka*.
15. The Deutsches Historisches Museum in Berlin has a copy of a menu from "Zum Goldbroiler" in Berlin, Schönhauser Allee, ca. 1965 (Do2 2004/1296).
16. Scheffler's *Alles Soljanka, oder wie?* is arranged chronologically and shows the changes clearly. On fish and Goldbroilers, see Voigt, *Der Geschmack des Ostens*, 115–18, 123–27.
17. Scheffler, *Alles Soljanka, oder wie?*, 116.
18. *Nasi goreng* also appears on a 28 November 1985 dinner menu from the cruise ship *Arkona* (Wende Museum Collection).
19. Deutsches Historisches Museum (Berlin), Do2 2000/1764; Bonn, Haus der Geschichte der BRD, menu collection.
20. Voigt, *Der Geschmack des Ostens*, 45–46; Michael Wildt, *Am Beginn der "Konsumgesellschaft". Mangelerfahrung, Lebenshaltung, Wohlschoffnung im Westdeutschland in den fünfziger Jahren* (Hamburg, 1994), 224–30.
21. Scheffler, *Alles Soljanka, oder wie?* 48–57. The same Palast der Republik menu with the Mexican Rumpsteak referred to earlier also offered Hungarian goulash, Moscow cheese soup, and halibut "nach Ungarischer Art" (i.e., with *letscho*). See Deutsches Historisches Museum (Berlin), Do2 2000/1764.
22. Thomas Grimm, *Das Politburo Privat. Ulbricht, Mielke, Honecker & Co aus der Sicht ihrer Angestellten* (Berlin, 2004), 55. See also Ed Stuhler, *Die Honeckers Privat. Liebespaar und Kampfgemeinschaft* (Berlin, 2005), 40–41.
23. Scheffler, *Alles Soljanka, oder wie?*, 62–67; Voigt, *Der Geschmack des Ostens*, 17–18; Klaus Steffen, *Essen wie Erich. Bevor der Ofen aus war—Das Beste aus Honeckers Hofküche* (Berlin, 1996), 20–30.
24. Victor Sebestyen, *Revolution 1989: The Fall of the Soviet Empire* (New York, 2009), 129–30; Steffen, *Essen wie Erich*, 17.
25. Grimm, *Das Politbüro Privat*, 55. On Wandlitz see Reinhold Andert, *Nach dem Sturz. Gespräche mit Erick Honecker* (Leipzig, 2001), 122–36.
26. For a comparative look at state dining occasions, see Jean-Marc Albert, *Aux tables du pouvoir: Des banquets grecs à l'Élysée* (Paris, 2009).
27. BArch Berlin, DC/20/21692, menu from 18 March 1980.
28. Tony Judt, *Postwar: A History of Europe Since 1945* (New York, 2005), 496–99.
29. Rotkäppchen is now owned by the French champagne company Mumm.
30. Steffen, *Essen wie Erich*, 72.
31. Wende Museum collection (unnumbered).

32. Wende Museum collection.
33. Wende Museum collection.
34. From the menu collection of the Leipzig branch of the Haus der Geschichte der BRD, n.d. (probably 1980s).
35. Eisenhüttenstadt, Dokumentationszentrum Alltagskultur der DDR, n.d. (probably 1980s).
36. See the two Mecklenburg specialty menus and one special event celebrating the cuisine of Frankfurt an der Oder in the Palast der Republik collection in Deutsches Historisches Museum (Berlin), Do2 2000/1767, Do2 2001/1769, Do2 2000/1766.
37. Otto, *Gastronomische Entdeckungen in der DDR; Restaurants und Gaststätten der DDR*, ed. Klaus Siedler (Berlin, 1990).
38. The Wende Museum has sixty menus from the *Völkerfreundschaft* and one from the *Arkona*. At the Haus der Geschichte in Bonn, there are twelve *Völkerfreundschaft* menus, thirty-two from the *Arkona*, and twenty-four from the *Fritz Heckert*. Three *Arkona* menus are held by the Dokumentationszentrum Alltagskultur in Eisenhüttenstadt.
39. *Urlauberschiffe: Boten der Völkerfreundschaft* (Berlin, 1961) is an illustrated description of the *Völkerfreundschaft* and its early itineraries. The book also depicts the construction and maiden Baltic voyage of the *Fritz Heckert*. For a memoir of service aboard the *Völkerfreundschaft*, see Christa Anders, *Traumreisen. Als Schiffärztin auf MS "Völkerfreundschaft"* (Kückenhagen, 2008).
40. The former *Völkerfreundschaft* and the *Arkona* are still in service. The *Völkerfreundschaft* is now called the *Athena* and belongs to Classic International Cruises of Australia; the *Arkona* sails under its old name with Aida Cruises, a German company.
41. Stefan Sommer, *Lexikon des Alltags der DDR* (Berlin, 1999), 338.
42. Bonn, Haus der Geschichte der BRD, menu collection, from 30 September 1964 to 14 October 1964. Shuffleboard is mentioned on the 27 September menu.
43. Wende Museum collection.
44. Haus der Geschichte der BRD (Bonn), menus from 26–30 September 1964.
45. Wende Museum collection.
46. Haus der Geschichte der BRD (Bonn).
47. Dokumentationszentrum Alltagskultur der DDR in Eisenhüttenstadt.
48. See, e.g., Deutsches Historisches Museum (Berlin), Do2 2000/1763 (1981); Do2 2000/1 1764 (1979).
49. Friedericke Pohlmann, *Hotel der Spione. Das "Neptun" in Warnemünde* (Schwerin, 2008), 166–68. Pohlmann describes the special status of the Neptun, which was not under the normal mediocre administration of Interhotel, and was being used by security forces. The hotel was, incidentally, the setting for some of the financial intrigues of Alexander Schalck-Golodkowski. There is an undated Hotel Neptun menu in the collection of the Dokumentationszentrum in Eisenhüttenstadt. The Wende Museum has two menus from the main restaurant of the Neptun: one from the Asian restaurant (which includes *nasi goreng* and Peking duck), and one from the Cuban restaurant. The ethnic establishments offered bilingual menus in English and German.
50. Karin Falkenberg, *Der "Waffenschmied" in Suhl. Das einzige Japan-Restaurant der DDR. Ein Jahrhundert Firmengeschichte* (Würzburg, 2000).
51. Voigt, *Der Geschmack des Ostens*, 161–64, 169–73; Heubner, *So schmeckte es*, 13.
52. Voigt, *Der Geschmack des Ostens*, 136.
53. Wildt, *Am Beginn der "Konsumgesellschaft"*, 76–108.

54. There were already significant East/West contrasts, however, in the settings and subsidies for dining and food, especially in workers' canteens and schools. See Alice Weinreb, "Matters of Taste: The Politics of Food in Divided Germany," *Bulletin of the German Historical Institute* 48 (Spring 2011): 59–82.
55. Voigt, *Der Geschmack des Ostens*, 208.
56. See, e.g., Jane and Michael Stern, *Square Meals: A Cookbook* (New York, 1984); Sylvia Lovegren, *Fashionable Food: Seven Decades of Food Fads* (New York, 1995), 168–216.
57. On these developments and especially the key importance of the 1970s, see Peter Scholliers, "Novelty and Tradition: The New Landscape for Gastronomy," in *Food: The History of Taste*, ed. Paul Freedman (London and Berkeley, 2007), 333–57.
58. For the implications of this point of view, see Betts, "Twilight of the Idols," 739–41.
59. Wolle, *Der heile Welt der Diktatur*, 221.
60. See the *Ostalgie* discussion on the H-German Listserv (http://www/h-net.org/~german/discuss/other/ostalgie).
61. See Andrew Port's contribution of 26 October 2007 to the H-German *Ostalgie* discussion cited in the previous note.
62. For a classic expression of this sentiment, see the essay on the *Niche* society by Günter Gaus, *Wo Deutschland liegt. Eine Ortsbestimmung* (Munich, 1987), 115–69.
63. Wolle, *Der heile Welt der Diktatur*, 220–21.

PART III

Constraints and Conformity
Friends, Foes, and Disciplinary Practices

CHAPTER 9

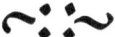

Predispositions and the Paradox of Working-Class Behavior in Nazi Germany and the German Democratic Republic

ANDREW I. PORT

Why was there not more mass protest from within the working class? Why was underground resistance to the Nazi regime not more militant or widespread? Why did that class in German society which suffered greater disenfranchisement, greater persecution and greater oppression than any other not mount at least one major challenge to the regime?... German workers ... never attempted to storm a single Gestapo office or attack Gestapo functionaries... [T]hey never translated a May Day assembly into a street battle. All of this is perfectly plausible: so why did none of it happen?
—Timothy Mason, "The Containment of the Working Class in Nazi Germany"

Thus formulated Timothy Mason with customary panache one of the most puzzling questions concerning the social history of the Third Reich.[1] It is a question made even more puzzling by the subsequent behavior of the working classes under the *second* German dictatorship. The first was a staunchly anti-Marxist regime that ruthlessly persecuted and antagonized the working class by disbanding its organizations, imprisoning its leadership, and trying to destroy its traditional social milieu. Yet, the group that the National Socialists arguably considered the greatest threat to regime stability—the group that represented the Nazis' greatest source of anxiety—failed to launch a single major challenge to their rule. The GDR was, by contrast, a self-styled "workers' and farmers' state" whose leaders lionized the working classes and claimed to rule in their name. Yet, it was that very group that posed the single greatest challenge to the regime: during the famous statewide uprising of June 1953—and then, in a much more subsidiary role, during the demonstrations that ultimately brought down the regime thirty-six years later.[2] This is a paradox that deserves explanation—especially in light of influential studies that have discreetly made workers the unsung heroes of modern German history by subtly suggesting that they were the ones ultimately responsible for the downfall of both regimes.[3]

Measuring Popular Opinion: Possibilities and Pitfalls

It is worth mentioning at the outset a number of challenges—methodological and otherwise—that make it extremely difficult to account for this apparent paradox. In the first place, it is not possible to speak of "the" working class. This was an extremely heterogeneous group, whose attitudes and experiences varied according to age, gender, region, sector, training, and political affinity, as well as familial situation and biographical background. The "working class" was, in other words, more than just stereotypically urban, industrial, and male. There were workers in the countryside, in small towns, in small factories; and not all were involved in the organized labor movement or integrated in what is generally considered the traditional working-class milieu. As Michael Schneider has pointed out, "Hardly anyone would nowadays think of describing 'the' opinion or 'the' political view of 'the' working class."[4] As a result, every (impressionistic) generalization conceals a large number of exceptions and necessarily invites a whole series of objections.

The available sources only compound these problems, for they frequently fail to include pertinent biographical information about specific individuals, or to differentiate *among* workers—or between them and other social groups. There are other serious difficulties as well. In the first place, one can find evidence under both regimes of both widespread support *and* rejection, integration *and* alienation—something that holds for entire groups as well as for single individuals, whose attitudes and behavior were often strikingly ambivalent, rendering it extremely difficult to make broad generalizations (an important point developed further later). Given the often mendacious nature of official reports and analyses, as well as the prevailing atmosphere of fear and distrust—which meant that communication and speech were not open and candid, as a rule, but rather highly inhibited—is it anyway really possible to measure and quantify intangibles such as "opinion" and "support"?

In light of this, and in the absence of reliable public opinion surveys, are there perhaps *indirect* indicators that one can use to get at such intangibles—something along the lines, for instance, of Hartmut Zwahr's innovative attempt to trace the rise of working-class solidarity in nineteenth-century Leipzig by looking at whom workers chose as godparents for their children?[5] Examining the choice of godparents will not get us very far in a highly secular society like the GDR, where outward shows of religiosity were considered suspect. But what about electoral outcomes, membership levels in official organizations, and figures regarding participation in ceremonies and other official events? These are notoriously unreliable, given the authoritarian nature of the two regimes. What, for example, do statistics about the overwhelmingly large number of young people who participated in the East German *Jugendweihe* ceremony (a secular form of youth confirmation whose "free-thinking" religious origins and working-class traditions went back to the nineteenth century) really tell us about regime support or a belief in the Socialist project, given that those who refused to participate risked a number of serious sanctions with regard to their educational and career prospects? In one Thuringian district, for example, the percentage of participants jumped from approximately 10.3 percent in 1955 to a whopping 97.4 percent by 1961. In fact, by the mid 1970s, the percentage of all East German youths who participated in the *Jugendweihe* never fell below 95 percent.[6]

Those documentary sources that do seem to shed light on popular opinion and everyday behavior (so-called *Stimmungs-, Lage-,* or *Informationsberichte*) suffer from a number of obvious limitations themselves: the randomness of what the author chose to include and exclude, for instance, the extent to which his or her own background and expectations, as well as immediate personal and professional surroundings, determined content and tenor. (This was true of official reports as well as of those submitted by members of the underground opposition.)[7] It should also be noted that the quality of the sources changed over time: the most detailed ones for the Nazi regime were produced through 1936, whereas East German ones became increasingly opaque and formulaic beginning in the late 1950s, following the end of destalinization and especially after the construction of the Berlin Wall in August 1961.[8]

Are all attempts to get at popular opinion a fool's errand, then? Those produced under both regimes give a good sense, in fact, of "what preoccupied people, what they complained about, and" (to a lesser degree) "what they were pleased with."[9] The candid descriptions of grumbling and other signs of discontent and conflict were not surprising, notwithstanding the hyperbolic tendency of these mendacious regimes to overstate their own accomplishments: officials wished to have reliable information at their disposal in order to anticipate potential sources of instability. (This was, again, also true of the underground opposition, but for patently different reasons.) As a consequence, the reports suffered from a one-sided tendency to overemphasize signs of opposition and discontent—thus leading to a distorted image of "popular opinion." In fact, as Timothy Mason once commented, "historical sources left behind by terrorist bureaucracies always document dissent better than ... consent."[10] This was true of those written by officials who saw enemy agents lurking around every corner.

as well as those of sanguine members of the opposition who could not abandon their unrealistic hopes for imminent revolution. (The more disappointed, it should be noted, bitterly emphasized instead the alleged wholesale co-option of the working classes.) Despite these pitfalls, as Ian Kershaw pointed out in his classic study of popular opinion in Bavaria, the historian benefits from the fact that both "sides," so to speak, produced reports that serve as a mutual control factor of sorts.[11] In the case of the GDR, other sources were equally revealing of popular attitudes: written complaints or petitions (*Eingaben*) to various officials, as well as the minutes of party, factory, and union meetings—all of which allow us to hear the actual and (relatively) unfiltered voices of ordinary East Germans.[12]

Opinion and Opposition under Two German Dictatorships

What do these voices tell us? And do they help us understand why it was the SED and not the Nazis who experienced a "17 June" and a "9 November"? In the first place, it is striking just how similar sources of discontent as well as forms of everyday protest were under both regimes. The same is true of the readiness with which many workers verbalized their dissatisfaction in private or semipublic spaces.[13] Most grumbling focused on everyday concerns of a material and economic nature: wage and price levels, poor working conditions, the scarcity of desired consumer goods and sufficient lodging, the absence of a "real say" in the running of one's factory, complaints about high union dues and the failure of the official unions to represent worker interests, as well as the unrelenting pressure to raise productivity and shop-floor performance. There was also much displeasure under both regimes about what were perceived to be unfair differences in income—within the working class as well as in comparison to other social groups—and in the distribution of scarce goods and social "burdens." In this regard, complaints about the "luxurious" lifestyle of supposedly more privileged groups—the *Bonzen* in Nazi Germany, the *Intelligentsia* in the GDR—were especially widespread (though especially unwarranted in the latter case). Complaints of a more purely political nature directed against the regimes as such surfaced much less frequently—not surprisingly, given that such comments were more likely to evoke a more vigorous response on the part of National Socialist and Communist security officials. But those that did usually involved calls for free elections, or, in the case of the GDR, an end to Soviet economic—and sexual—exploitation. As one East German worker—whose wife had been physically attacked three times by members of the Red Army, and who was censured for using the politically incorrect term *Russian* instead of the more acceptable *Soviets* or *friends*—wanted to know, "how could he, as a German, be a friend of the Soviets when they've taken everything away from him."[14]

Finally, frustration about the failure of the Nazis and the SED to make good on their promises—including an end to social injustice, welfare for *all*, and, during the early years of the Third Reich, continuing unemployment—were also sources of despair: ones that often gave rise, incidentally, to the instrumental use of regime propaganda. The latter was true with respect to rearmament as well. Anxiety about the possibility of another war, as well as anger about the consequent diversion of scarce resources away from consumer goods, fueled criticism of rearmament as well as pacifist sentiment both before and after 1945 (though this was, in all likelihood, less the case for those fortunate workers who had secured a job in the lucrative armaments industry). In fact, anger about rearmament played a major role in the lead-up to the uprising of June 1953.[15]

The forms of everyday opposition were also similar under both regimes, and tended to involve a general refusal to go along with the many onerous political and economic demands of the party and state. This included various forms of poor shop-floor discipline (e.g., elevated sickness rates, go-slows, and acts of minor sabotage), low turnouts at official meetings, and high levels of job turnover. Such *eigensinnig* behavior obviously involved "normal" economic struggles aimed at safeguarding or improving one's material situation and thus rarely signaled fundamental political opposition as such—even if it is difficult, of course, to separate neatly the "political" from the "socioeconomic" under these two regimes.[16] Ironically, such "anti-capitalist" behavior was widespread under "state socialism" as well, even if *das Volk* did own the means of production—which had, Marxist ideologues claimed, removed the justification for and necessity of strikes and other forms of industrial protest.

The motivation underlying such behavior was rarely clear-cut: was poor work morale a form of protest, for example, or simply a result of the excessive demands placed on German workers during the war or, after 1945, of excessive overtime resulting from severe labor shortages? There were, of course, less ambivalent, more proactive forms of protest: the spreading of rumors and jokes, refusals to contribute during state-sponsored charity drives (e.g., *Winterhilfe* during the Third Reich, so-called *Soliaufkommen* in the GDR), the casting of negative or invalid votes in public referenda or union elections, refusals to offer the Hitler greeting, clandestinely listening to foreign (including West German) media reports, the spreading of illegal pamphlets, critical graffiti, the defacing of political posters, and, last but not least, small-scale strikes. The last were, under both regimes, usually spontaneous, short-lived, defensive actions, limited to a small group of workers in reaction to a specific economic measure or unpopular policy decision.[17]

There were waves of discontent when grumbling was more pronounced, nonconformist behavior especially bold, outward signs of support even less in evidence. Security officials reported a "crisis of opinion" (*Stimmungskrise*) in 1935–36, for example, and then again twenty years later during the events that shook Poland and Hungary following Nikita Khrushchev's "secret speech" of 1956. It is also true that accents changed, e.g., complaints about continuing unemployment regularly surfaced during the early years of the Third Reich but tapered off after 1936 with the Four Year Plan and rearmament boom. At the same time, however, full employment did lead to greater insubordination.[18] In fact, a "latent feeling of disgruntlement" and "sullen noncompliance" (*mürrische Verweigerung*) were widespread under both regimes, the avowedly Marxist and anti-Marxist.[19] Most workers were apathetic, resigned, and skeptical; only a small minority was wildly enthusiastic—or involved in organized political resistance aimed at destabilizing the regime. The point is this: the striking similarity of sources of discontent and forms of everyday protest under both regimes suggest that they alone cannot account for the absence of a "June 1953" during the Third Reich.

Despite overwhelming evidence of widespread grumbling and nonconformist, "resistant" behavior, the foregoing should not suggest that all workers were uniformly opposed to or critical of the two dictatorships. Many undoubtedly rallied behind one (or even both) of these regimes, though this is difficult to quantify with any precision. So much is obvious. But there is a more nuanced point worth making, namely, that it is equally impossible to make precise claims about the sensibilities of individual workers themselves. It is not only perfectly conceivable but also highly likely that the same worker who criticized the ruling regime for one or more of the reasons discussed earlier may have also felt certain affinities for that regime. There was no doubt a broad spectrum of feelings, behavior, and practices on the part of any given individual, depending on the given circumstances or situation. As Alf Lüdtke and Detlev Peukert have reminded us, distance, resistance, and active opposition could all exist, in other words—in varying intensities, at different times, and sometimes even side by side—with various forms of support, integration, and participation.[20] Attitudes and practices are indeed "messy," and one "set" did not necessarily exclude the other. To claim otherwise would create a misleading and false dichotomy.[21]

Courting and Containing the Working Classes

All of this obviously raises important questions about the ways in which and the extent to which both regimes were able to win over and integrate the working classes. They did so in a number of ways, including, of course, the tried-and-true method of carrots and sticks. The former, which Mason has aptly referred to as "macroeconomic bribery," involved a wide range of social goodies: from subsidized vacations and other leisure activities administered by the National Socialist *Kraft durch Freude* (Strength through Joy) organization and the East German umbrella union organization (Free German Trade Union Federation, or FDGB), to a wide variety of other workplace benefits (in the tradition of German employer paternalism) and support for families.[22] Material concessions were made at specific junctures as well, most conspicuously during potentially dangerous periods of unrest and widespread discontent: the New Course of June 1953, as well as the bundle of benefits announced by the SED in December of that year, were a case in point—even if the former did fail to preempt mass unrest, as had been its intent. Memories of "June 17" fortified the willingness of the SED leadership and local officials to compromise and reach consensus in order to maintain harmony—or at least forestall serious conflict.[23] The revolutionary events of November 1918 had served as a similar reminder and monition for the National Socialists. This helped explain, for instance, why they quickly reversed a highly unpopular decision to reduce rations in 1942—or why they had hoped, more generally, to avoid fighting a protracted war that might have adversely affected living standards at home.[24] This was, after all, an important rationale for *Blitzkrieg*.

There were other, less tangible "carrots" as well, in the form of regime rhetoric and propaganda. The way in which the SED courted the working classes requires no comment. But even the National *Socialists* claimed to "care" about the working classes—and had done so ever since the party's inception. The "Socialist" wing of the party may have been sidelined by the early 1930s, but the Nazis continued once in power to employ anti-elitist rhetoric, play on traditional social resentments, sing the praises of manual labor ("Work ennobles"), and call for an end to class warfare and the creation of a harmonious "people's community" (*Volksgemeinschaft*)—all in a populist attempt to capture the hearts and minds of the *social* group it oppressed most systematically.[25]

Did these strategies work? The absence of mass unrest (apart from that of June 1953 and the fall of 1989) suggests that they largely did. But why? In many respects, the material position of the working classes did, on the whole, improve under the Nazis and the SED, though the record here is spotty. On the one hand, industrialists and factory directors became even more powerful under the National Socialists, while efforts to increase productivity intensified—and continued to do so under the postwar Socialist regime—thanks to the expansion of shift work and the introduction of industrial competitions and other strategies aimed at squeezing more and more out of the manual labor force. On the other hand, and despite attempts to freeze wages, real income began to climb beginning in 1936–37 and continued to do so even during the war, when living standards were maintained (or only declined slightly) thanks to the exploitation of those living in the occupied regions of Europe.[26] Mass unemployment finally became a thing of the past, thanks to the massive rearmament program, a development that significantly strengthened the bargaining position of the working classes.[27]

Much has been made of the possibilities for upward social mobility under both regimes, but its integrative effects have been overstated. Many of those from modest social backgrounds who benefitted from this possibility undoubtedly felt some degree of attachment or "loyalty" toward the regime—but not all: a rise in the social ranks often meant taking a position that required extensive (re)training as well as additional, burdensome responsibilities—without, necessarily, a rise in income. The stories of skilled East German workers, for example, who earned as much as or more than engineers, are well known.[28] The role that social benefits played in securing the support of the working classes has been overstated as well. They were relatively modest during the Third Reich, and availability remained limited in the GDR, especially during the Ulbricht era, when housing and childcare (not to mention staples like butter and toilet paper) continued to be in short supply.[29]

As the incessant grumbling under both regimes clearly suggests, working-class discontent about the standard of living remained widespread. That is not to deny that there was some—perhaps even a greater than heretofore—sense of social security under the Nazis and the SED. But the potentially destabilizing effects of the failure of these regimes to make good on their promises, and of the frustration that this engendered, should not be ignored or underestimated. This is a point that deserves emphasis because it provides one possible explanation for the absence of mass working-class unrest during the Third Reich: given the initially low expectations of what workers thought they might expect from a National Socialist government, the positive impression made by *any* favorable developments whatsoever must have been all the more impressive. As Ulrich Herbert has written, "the economic success of the regime, the improvement in one's own social situation [stood] in stark contrast to the predictions of the working-class movement."[30] The situation in the GDR was radically different: the expectations of what a self-styled working-class regime would deliver were not only greater but also accompanied by a greater sense of entitlement. The anger and frustration engendered by the failure of the reality to correspond to the rhetoric were therefore more pronounced. This may be the real key to understanding why a "17 June" took place *after* and not before 1945.

A number of scholars have persuasively suggested that there was a high correlation between a worker's own material situation and his or her feelings toward, and thus degree of support for (or lack of resistance against), the regime. The Nazis secured, in other words, the backing of those who secured a job. Or, to put it somewhat more crudely: "it's the economy, stupid!"[31] This type of materialist argumentation may itself be somewhat crude and reductionist, but it should not be summarily dismissed. That said, it is clearly not the end of the story, not least because *subjective* worker perceptions about their economic situation were just as, if not more, important than any "objective" economic indicators. The failure to make this distinction is, incidentally, a major shortcoming of Götz Aly's controversial study arguing that the German working class remained docile and even supportive of the regime because its members substantially benefited in a variety of material ways from its social policies.[32]

The potentially integrative aspects of regime rhetoric—as well as their potential to be destabilizing as well—have already been discussed. But what about the role played by foreign policy success and "charismatic" leadership—or racism, for that matter? These are questions that clearly apply first and foremost to the Third Reich. Hitler's successes in the international arena did enjoy positive resonance among many workers, especially his early peace overtures as well as his subsequent efforts to reestablish Germany's standing and sovereignty by reversing the more onerous aspects of Versailles. The remilitarization of the Rhineland, the outcome of the Saarland referendum, the absorption of Austria all elicited enthusiastic support. Yet, all of this was tempered by growing alarm about the possibility of a new war. (That was why the positive reaction to the rapid victory over France in 1940 was arguably a mixture of patriotism *and* relief.) In addition, much of this enthusiasm seems to have been ephemeral, quickly supplanted by more mundane concerns about the everyday. Awe for Hitler gave way to widespread anger about supply shortages a mere two weeks after the *Anschluss*, for example.[33]

As the foregoing suggests, the "Hitler Myth" apparently enjoyed purchase among many workers, though apparently to a lesser degree than it did for other social groups. The Führer was closely associated with the regime's economic and foreign policy successes, but even he did not remain immune from periodic waves of criticism. This was especially true during the latter stages of the war, following the defeat at Stalingrad and the commencement of aerial bombardment by the Allies.[34] In the end, however, the "regime held together into absolute defeat"—no doubt a result of the regime's emotional appeals to patriotic sentiment, popular anger about the Allied bombings, and paralyzing fear of the approaching Bolshevik "hordes" in the East.[35] This last point reminds us of the potentially integrative effects of the regime's racist policies. Like their compatriots, many workers apparently welcomed the discriminatory measures taken against the Jews, but rejected indiscriminate, overt acts of violence. On the whole, however, they, too, remained largely indifferent to the fate of this oppressed minority—notwithstanding, as Alf Lüdtke has argued, the supposed "appeal" that exterminating "Others" had for German workers serving on the frontlines.[36] It is possible to speculate, along similar lines, about the extent to which the racial pecking order that emerged in those factories that employed slave laborers in the 1940s promoted feelings of racial superiority and thus had a positive effect on working-class attitudes toward the regime.

There was no equivalent here for the GDR: no great foreign policy successes (international sporting events do not count!), no war to rally the masses, no charismatic leadership.[37] One can hardly imagine an East German sighing, "If

Ulbricht only knew..."—though some workers did complain "that our government certainly could not know about the supply difficulties, because if they had, they would have long ago provided assistance."[38] (This was, in all likelihood, a shrewd way in which to place low-level functionaries under pressure.) And whether the regime's anti-fascist rhetoric really hit home, given the comparisons some irate workers made between the SED and the National Socialists, the Stasi and the Gestapo, remains open to debate.[39]

Terror and Divisions, Expectations and Predispositions

This last point reminds us of the white elephant in the room, namely, the role that terror played in containing the working classes under both regimes. The fact that June 1953 took place at the high point of Stalinism, as well as the fact that the Berlin Wall fell when the Stasi was at the height of its power, suggests that repression alone cannot explain the absence of large-scale unrest in the GDR.[40] But it does not explain the absence of similar unrest under the Nazis. Could it be that the Gestapo was more brutal, more ruthless, more efficient than the Stasi?[41] Perhaps. But the more important point is that the wrath of state security forces came down most forcefully early on against the working classes, beginning with the raids that took place in working-class neighborhoods and the subsequent arrest of tens of thousands of rank-and-file members and leaders of the labor movement during the earliest months of the regime. There was no equivalent under the postwar regime, even if Social Democrats were systematically purged and arrested in the late 1940s, and even if the upheaval of June 1953 was put down with ruthless force.[42] Unlike the National Socialists, the SED never regarded or treated the working class as its primary foe. That is a significant difference, and it was what arguably made the fateful decision in June 1953 to reverse all of the unpopular policies recently adopted by the SED *except* for the one that most directly affected the working class itself—a 10 percent across-the-board hike in production quotas—so unacceptable and so explosive.[43] The irony of all this is that it was the workers' privileged ideological status itself that arguably made them more defiant and fractious in the very state that embraced them with open arms.

But that does not sufficiently account for their "containment" under the Nazis. The demoralizing defeat of 1933 made many workers feel disillusioned, resigned, powerless, and at the mercy of the new regime and its thugs—apart, that is, from the approximately one-quarter who voted for the Nazis. It also made them feel isolated: from their leaders, who now sat in jail or in exile, as well as from other social groups. To make matters worse, "the anti-Nazi working class felt that it was surrounded on all sides by positive enthusiasm for the regime and by hostility or indifference to its own economic and political interests."[44] The latter was nothing new, but the former must have been debilitating—and quite unlike the situation in the GDR, where worker grievances did not differ all that much from those voiced by other groups. Which begs the question: why did these disparate groups not come together to challenge the regime? Social resentment and jealousy—the result of many factors, including the privileged treatment of certain groups, often at the cost of others, as well as the daily struggle for scarce goods and services—prevented workers from making common cause with other social groups, and vice versa, *even though they shared many of the same grievances*. Similar factors fomented tensions among workers themselves; this was exacerbated by official production practices aimed at boosting worker output, such as the awarding of bonuses, piecework wages, Stakhanovist schemes, as well as the brigade movement, which made worker income dependent on the performance of their colleagues. In short, the East German working class was divided internally, which effectively hindered collective forms of action against the regime.[45]

Comparable social divisions existed in the Third Reich, as well as within the working class itself—and very often for similar reasons. Such divisions had already surfaced during the Weimar years between Social Democrats and Communists, for example, the skilled and unskilled, men and women; they became even more pronounced after the onset of the Great Depression. These divisions intensified during the Third Reich for a number of reasons, including the practice of wage differentiation aimed at boosting output. This divisive practice caused bad blood among workers, and continued to do so in the GDR as well. As a result, traditional forms of working-class solidarity gave way to a variety of individualistic, *sauve-qui-peut* strategies (*Lohnpolitik auf eigene Faust*).[46] This, along with state terror and the destruction of the structural conditions necessary for organized resistance (e.g., independent labor organizations), made collective challenges to the regime extremely difficult and thus highly unlikely—as they are under any political system, of course, much less in an autocratic regime that blithely employed terrorist methods against its own population. Unlikely, but not impossible, as developments in Poland in the 1980s made clear.[47]

Conclusion

It is not easy to say with any certitude why a "17 June" took place after and not before 1945. As the foregoing suggests, worker *expectations* played an extremely important role. But so, too, did their *predispositions*. The labor movement may have preached pacifism and international brotherly love, but, as the Summer of

Hate demonstrated in 1914, German workers and organized labor were, in the end, not immune to patriotic (even chauvinist) sentiment.[48] This—along with indignation and anger about the harsh terms of the Versailles Treaty, sentiments that cut across all social classes and (almost all) political allegiances— helped account for their enthusiastic approval later on of Hitler's aggressive foreign policy moves in the 1930s.

More to the point, worker behavior under each of these two regimes— whose ideologies, but not necessarily methods of control, were diametrically opposed—cannot be viewed in isolation but must be seen in relation to one another. At the risk of stating the obvious, what took place during the Third Reich had important repercussions for what followed. For example, the repertoire of everyday worker protest in the GDR included many surreptitious acts of "Schweik-like" nonconformity learned and developed long before 1945, but perfected during the Third Reich. But something else was cultivated as well under the Nazis: a visceral, racial hatred and suspicion of "the Slav."[49] German working-class culture should, in principle, have made workers in East Germany highly receptive to a workers' state. Why it did not should be a "Gretchen question" of GDR historiography. There is at least one possible explanation: years of anti-Soviet propaganda and racial indoctrination—as well as the behavior of the Red Army in 1945—meant that most Germans were predisposed to regard *any* state imposed on them by "the Russians" with suspicion and anger. In other words, in the eyes of many if not most Germans living in the East—including the working classes—the GDR was indelibly stained from the very beginning.[50]

It could be objected that the general question raised here proceeds from a false premise, namely, that German workers *should* have rebelled against these two regimes. Is this, in other words, a false *Fragestellung* similar to the one posed by generations of disillusioned Marxists who spilled a great deal of unnecessary ink trying to explain why the English working classes did not act in the normative way prescribed by Karl Marx? Besides, is a historian really equipped to answer the question of why something did *not* happen?[51] To be perfectly clear: the argument here is not that German workers necessarily tend to resist and that they should have risen up, first against the National Socialists and then against the Communists. But given the fact that hundreds of thousands did lay down their tools and take to the streets in June 1953, that they continued to complain about many of the same issues after June 1953, and, finally, that workers under the Nazis had similarly complained about many of the same issues—it is legitimate to ask why workers did not forcibly challenge authorities en masse before and then again after that date. One answer surely lies in the specific confluence of circumstances that arose in the spring of 1953, and later in the summer and fall of 1989. But, as the foregoing suggests, the answer lies as well in a messy mix of evolving expectations, predispositions, and sensibilities.

Suggested Readings

Eley, Geoff. "Labor History, Social History, *Alltagsgeschichte*: Experience, Culture, and the Politics of the Everyday—a New Direction for German Social History." *The Journal of Modern History* 61 (1989): 297–343.

Herbert, Ulrich. "Arbeiterschaft im 'Dritten Reich.' Zwischenbilanz und offene Fragen." *Geschichte und Gesellschaft* 15 (1989): 320–60.

Hübner, Peter. *Konsens, Konflikt und Kompromiß. Soziale Arbeiterinteressen und Sozialpolitik in der SBZ/DDR, 1945-1970*. Berlin, 1995.

——— and Klaus Tenfelde, eds. *Arbeiter in der SBZ-DDR*. Essen, 1999.

Kershaw, Ian. *Popular Opinion & Political Dissent in the Third Reich: Bavaria 1933-1945*. Oxford, 1983.

Kleßmann, Christoph. *Arbeiter im "Arbeiterstaat" DDR. Deutsche Traditionen, sowjetisches Modell, westdeutsches Magnetfeld (1945 bis 1971)*. Berlin, 2007.

Kopstein, Jeffrey. "Chipping Away at the State: Workers' Resistance and the Demise of East Germany." *World Politics* 48 (1996): 391–423.

Lüdtke, Alf. *Eigen-Sinn. Fabrikalltag, Arbeitererfahrungen und Politik vom Kaiserreich bis in den Faschismus*. Hamburg, 1993.

Mallmann, Klaus-Michael and Gerhard Paul. *Herrschaft und Alltag. Ein Industrierevier im Dritten Reich*. Bonn, 1991.

Mason, Tim. "The Containment of the Working Class in Nazi Germany." In *Nazism, Fascism and the Working Class*, ed. Jane Caplan, 231–73. Cambridge, 1995.

———. "The Workers' Opposition in Nazi Germany," *History Workshop Journal* 11 (1981): 120–37.

Morsch, Günter. "Streik im 'Dritten Reich.'" *Vierteljahreshefte für Zeitgeschichte* 36/4 (1988): 649–89.

Port, Andrew I. *Conflict and Stability in the German Democratic Republic*. New York, 2007.

Schneider, Michael. *Unterm Hakenkreuz. Arbeiter und Arbeiterbewegung 1933 bis 1939*. Berlin, 1999.

Acknowledgments

This chapter benefited immensely from a lively e-mail exchange that I conducted over several months with Alf Lüdtke, who kindly read and critically engaged with an earlier draft. Alf may not agree with all of my arguments, but he certainly made me fine-tune many of them.

Notes

1. Tim Mason, "The Containment of the Working Class in Nazi Germany," in *Nazism, Fascism and the Working Class*, ed. Jane Caplan (Cambridge, 1995), 234–36. According to underground Social Democratic operatives, the behavior of the working classes was "the real puzzle in Germany" during the Third Reich. See Ulrich Herbert, "Arbeiterschaft im 'Dritten Reich.' Zwischenbilanz und offene Fragen," *Geschichte und Gesellschaft* 15 (1989): 320–60 (quote on p. 320).
2. For a superb overview of recent literature on the June 1953 uprising, see Jonathan Sperber, "17 June 1953: Revisiting a German Revolution," *German History* 22 (2004):

619–43. For contrasting views about the role that East German workers played during the revolutionary events of 1989, see Linda Fuller, *Where Was the Working Class? Revolution in Eastern Germany* (Urbana, I.L., 1999); Gareth Dale, *Popular Protest in East Germany, 1949-1989* (London, 2005).
3. That is the thrust of clever studies by Tim Mason on the Nazi period and Jeff Kopstein on the GDR. In an influential book published in the 1970s, Mason argued that because of fears about worker resistance and impending worker protest, Nazi leaders—haunted by the November Revolution of 1918—decided to go to war *before* Germany was in an optimal military position to do so. By forcing Hitler's hand in 1939, workers were, by implication, ultimately responsible for Germany's defeat. Along similar lines two decades later, Kopstein argued that widespread worker intransigence had hindered East German officials from introducing salutary reforms that might have salvaged the economy. The implication here is that they were the ones who ultimately sabotaged the Socialist project—even if it took them more than forty years to do so! See Tim Mason, *Social Policy in the Third Reich: The Working Class and the "National Community,"* ed. Jane Kaplan, trans. John Broadwin (Oxford, 1993); Jeffrey Kopstein, *The Politics of Economic Decline in East Germany, 1945-1989* (Chapel Hill, N.C., 1997).
4. See Michael Schneider, *Unterm Hakenkreuz. Arbeiter und Arbeiterbewegung 1933 bis 1939* (Berlin, 1999), 684. On the traditional working-class milieu, see, e.g., Vernon Lidtke, *The Alternative Culture: Socialist Labor in Imperial Germany* (New York, 1985); Lynn Abrams, *Workers' Culture in Imperial Germany: Leisure and Recreation in the Rhineland and Westphalia* (London, 1992).
5. Hartmut Zwahr, *Zur Konstituierung des Proletariats als Klasse. Strukturuntersuchung über das Leipziger Proletatiat während der industriellen Revolution* (Munich, 1981).
6. See ThStA-Rudolstadt IV/4/10/321 and /137; Paul Betts, *Within Walls: Private Life in the German Democratic Republic* (Oxford, 2010), 72–73. Statistics about the number of Socialist, as opposed to religious, marriage ceremonies—and especially funerals, when the person in question had little to lose—might offer greater insights into the state of popular opinion. For some preliminary observations about funeral trends, see Betts, *Within Walls,* 74–77. The relevant statistics for the Thuringian town Saalfeld, which suggest a good deal of resistance to Socialist funeral ceremonies, are as follows:

Marriage Ceremonies in Saalfeld (1959–1988)

Year	Total Marriages	Socialist Ceremonies	Religious Ceremonies
1959	391	236	39
1963	436	213	53
1968	430	158	32
1969	420	7	49
1988	421	28	30

Funeral Ceremonies in Saalfeld (1965–1988)

Year	Total Deaths	Total Funerals	Socialist Ceremonies	Religious Ceremonies
1965	591	668	142	469
1970	651	786	204	457
1975	736	736	418	234
1980	787	787	332	343
1988	686	684	290	282

Source: Stadtarchiv Saalfeld 10711.

7. For a discussion of these types of issues for the Third Reich, see Ian Kershaw, *Popular Opinion & Political Dissent in the Third Reich: Bavaria 1933-1945* (Oxford, 1983), 4–10; for the GDR, see Alf Lüdtke and Peter Becker, eds., *Akten. Eingaben. Schaufenster. Die DDR und ihre Texte. Erkundungen zu Herrschaft und Alltag* (Berlin, 1997).
8. On the Nazi period, see Schneider, *Unterm Hakenkreuz*, 702; for East Germany, see Andrew I. Port, *Conflict and Stability in the German Democratic Republic* (New York, 2007), 12.
9. Christoph Kleßmann, *Arbeiter im "Arbeiterstaat" DDR. Deutsche Traditionen, sowjetisches Modell, westdeutsches Magnetfeld (1945 bis 1971)* (Berlin, 2007), 743.
10. Mason, "Containment," 252.
11. Kershaw was among the first to use systematically the so-called *Sopade* reports, which were written by Social Democrats in Nazi Germany and smuggled out to the exiled leadership. See Kershaw, *Popular Opinion*, 7–10; for the original reports, see *Deutschland-Berichte der Sopade* (Frankfurt am Main, 1980). Also see Michael Voges, "'Klassenkampf in der Betriebsgemeinschaft'. Die 'Deutschland-Berichte' der Sopade (1934–1940) als Quelle zum Widerstand der Industriearbeiter im Dritten Reich," *Archiv für Sozialgeschichte* 21 (1981): 329–88. Oppositional Social Democrats produced similar reports in the GDR for the West German *Ostbüro*, which surreptitiously kept tabs on developments in the East. These reports are available at the Archiv der sozialen Demokratie, which is housed at the Friedrich Ebert Foundation in Bonn; they are one of the main primary sources used in Kleßmann, *Arbeiter*.
12. For a systematic use of these types of minutes, see Port, *Conflict and Stability*. On East German petitions and its "culture of complaint," see Joachim Staadt, *Eingaben. Die institutionalisierte Meckerkultur in der DDR* (Berlin, 1996); Steffen Elsner, "Flankierende Stabilisierungsmechanismen diktatorischer Herrschaft. Das Eingabenswesen in der DDR," in *Repression und Wohlstandsversprechen. Zur Stabilisierung von Parteiherrschaft in der DDR und der CSSR*, ed. Christoph Boyer and Peter Skyba (Dresden, 1999), 75–86; Ina Merkel, *"Wir sind doch nicht die Meckerecke der Nation." Briefe an das Fernsehen der DDR* (Cologne, 2000); Mary Fulbrook, *The People's State: East German Society from Hitler to Honecker* (New Haven, 2005), 269–88; Jonathan Zatlin, *The Currency of Socialism: Money and Political Culture in East Germany* (New York, 2007), 286–320; Betts, *Within Walls*, 173–92.
13. For the Nazi period, the following discussion is based on Klaus-Michael Mallmann and Gerhard Paul, *Herrschaft und Alltag. Ein Industrierevier im Dritten Reich* (Bonn, 1991); Schneider, *Unterm Hakenkreuz*; Timothy Mason, "The Workers' Opposition in Nazi Germany," *History Workshop Journal* 11 (1981): 120–37; idem, "Containment"; Detlev Peukert, *Inside Nazi Germany: Conformity, Opposition, and Racism in Everyday Life*, trans. Richard Deveson (New Haven, 1987), 101–44; idem, *Der deutsche Arbeiterwiderstand gegen das Dritte Reich* (Berlin, 1990); Herbert, "Arbeiterschaft im 'Dritten Reich'"; Gunther Mai, "Die Nationalsozialistische Betriebszellenorganisation. Zum Verhältnis von Arbeiterschaft und Nationalsozialismus," *Vierteljahreshefte für Zeitgeschichte* 31/4 (1983): 573–613; idem, "'Warum steht der deutsche Arbeiter zu Hitler?' Zur Rolle der Deutschen Arbeitsfront im Herrschaftssystem des Dritten Reiches," *Geschichte und Gesellschaft* 12/2 (1986): 212–34; Günter Morsch, "Streik im 'Dritten Reich,'" *Vierteljahreshefte für Zeitgeschichte* 36/4 (1988): 649–89. For workers in the GDR, see Peter Hübner, *Konsens, Konflikt und Kompromiß. Soziale Arbeiterinteressen und Sozialpolitik in der SBZ/DDR, 1945-1970* (Berlin, 1995); Port, *Conflict and Stability*; Kleßmann, *Arbeiter im "Arbeiterstaat"*; Sandrine Kott, *Le communisme au quoti-*

dien. *Les entreprises d'Etat dans la société est-allemande* (Paris, 2001); Peter Alheit and Hanna Haack, *Die vergessene 'Autonomie' der Arbeiter. Eine Studie zum frühen Scheitern der DDR am Beispiel der Neptunwerft* (Berlin, 2004); Christoph Vietzke, *Konfrontation und Kooperation. Funktionäre und Arbeiter in Großbetrieben der DDR vor und nach dem Mauerbau* (Essen, 2008); Jeffrey Kopstein, "Chipping Away at the State: Workers' Resistance and the Demise of East Germany," *World Politics* 48 (1996): 391–423; as well as the essays in Peter Hübner and Klaus Tenfelde, eds., *Arbeiter in der SBZ-DDR* (Essen, 1999).

14. ThStA-Rudolstadt IV/7/230/1158, Protokoll der Mitgliederversammlung der SED Grundorganisation-Wema, 14 May 1952.

15. As this suggests, both world wars represented important steps in exorcising at the grassroots level whatever militarist demons had earlier plagued the German psyche. See Andrew I. Port, "Democracy and Dictatorship in the Cold War: The Two Germanies, 1949-1961," in *The Oxford Handbook of Modern German History*, ed. Helmut Smith (Oxford, 2011), 628.

16. On the concept of *Eigen-Sinn* and *eigensinnig* behavior, see the Introduction to this volume (pp. 5–6).

17. See Morsch, "Streik im 'Dritten Reich'"; Hübner, *Konsens, Konflikt und Kompromiß*, 192–205; Kleßmann, *Arbeiter im "Arbeiterstaat,"* 749–58.

18. On the waves of discontent between 1934 and 1936, and then again in 1956, see Schneider, *Unterm Hakenkreuz*, 710–17; Armin Mitter and Stefan Wolle, *Untergang auf Raten. Unbekannte Kapitel der DDR–Geschichte* (Munich, 1993), 163–295. On greater insubordination as a result of labor shortages, see Mason, *Social Policy*, 186–96; Port, *Conflict and Stability*, 178–94.

19. Quotes from Schneider, *Unterm Hakenkreuz*, 691.

20. See Alf Lüdtke, *Eigen-Sinn. Fabrikalltag, Arbeitererfahrungen und Politik vom Kaiserreich bis in den Faschismus* (Hamburg, 1993), 221–350; Peukert, *Inside Nazi Germany*, 49–66; idem, *Alltag unterm Nationalsozialismus* (Berlin, 1981), 14ff.

21. That very messiness is helpful in at least one respect: it makes the difficult question of differentiating among workers according to sector, gender, region, generation, etc. less pressing. Such differences undoubtedly existed, and are worthy of investigation, but the significance of that heterogeneity diminishes if moments of "opposition" and "integration" did indeed coexist for most, if not all, workers—*regardless* of personal background and biography.

22. Quote from Mason, "Containment," 243. On unions and tourist activities under the two regimes, see Shelley Baranowski, *Strength Through Joy: Consumerism and Mass Tourism in the Third Reich* (Cambridge, 2004); Andreas Stirn, *Traumschiffe des Sozialismus. Die Geschichte der DDR-Urlauberschiffe 1953-1990* (Berlin, 2010); (with caution) Thomas Schaufuß, *Die politische Rolle des FDGB-Feriendienstes in der DDR. Sozialtourismus im SED-Staat* (Berlin, 2011). On social benefits and the effects of such policies more generally, see Hans Günther Hockerts, ed., *Drei Wege deutscher Sozialstaatlichkeit. NS-Diktatur, Bundesrepublik und DDR im Vergleich* (Munich, 1998); Carole Sachse et al., *Angst, Belohnung, Zucht und Ordnung* (Opladen, 1982); Konrad Jarausch, "Realer Sozialismus als Fürsorgediktatur. Zur begrifflichen Einordnung der DDR," *Aus Politik und Zeitgeschichte* B20 (1998): 33–46; Beatrix Bouvier, *Die DDR—ein Sozialstaat? Sozialpolitik in der Ära Honecker* (Bonn, 2002); Gunnar Winkler, ed., *Geschichte der Sozialpolitik der DDR, 1945-1985* (Berlin, 1989).

23. The desire to reach compromise—especially on the part of officials at the grassroots level—was already widespread before the upheaval. This willingness was not, in other words, a product of June 1953—though the shock of the uprising did reinforce such conciliatory behavior. See Port, *Conflict and Stability*, 276. On the "New Course," see, e.g., Ilko-Sascha Kowalczuk, *17.6.1953. Volksaufstand in der DDR. Ursachen—Abläufe—Folgen* (Bremen, 2003).
24. See Herbert, "Arbeiterschaft," 354.
25. See, e.g., David Schoenbaum, *Hitler's Social Revolution: Class and Status in Nazi Germany, 1933-1939* (New York, 1980), 73–112; Lüdtke, *Eigen-Sinn*, 221–350; Peter Fritzsche, *Germans into Nazis* (Cambridge, M.A., 1998), 222–28.
26. See Götz Aly, *Hitlers Volksstaat. Raub, Rassenkrieg und nationaler Sozialismus* (Frankfurt am Main, 2005). This should be read in tandem with the critical review by J. Adam Tooze, "Einfach verkalkuliert," *taz*, 12 March 2005.
27. The classic, highly controversial treatment of the economic position of workers during the Nazi period is Mason, *Social Policy*. For East German workers, see Hübner, *Konsens, Konflikt und Kompromiß*; Jeffrey Kopstein, *Politics of Economic Decline*; Port, *Conflict and Stability*, 164–94.
28. See Mary Fulbrook, *The People's State: East German Society from Hitler to Honecker* (New Haven, 2005), 229–31. With respect to the question of "loyalty," see Klaus-Michael Mallmann and Gerhard Paul, 'Resistenz oder loyale Widerwilligkeit? Anmerkungen zu einem umstrittenen Begriff,' *Zeitschrift für Geschichtswissenschaft* 2 (1993): 99–116; Lutz Niethammer, Alexander von Plato, and Dorothee Wierling, *Die Volkseigene Erfahrung. Eine Archäologie des Lebens in der Industrieprovinz der DDR* (Berlin, 1991).
29. See Port, *Conflict and Stability*, 244–70.
30. Herbert, "Arbeiterschaft," 339.
31. Bill Clinton's campaign strategist James Carville coined this colorful phrase during the run-up to the 1992 U.S. presidential election. See Michael Kelly, "The Democrats—Clinton and Bush Compete to Be Champion of Change; Democrat Fights Perceptions of Bush Gain," *New York Times*, 31 October 1992.
32. See Aly, *Hitlers Volksstaat*.
33. See Schneider, *Unterm Hakenkreuz*, 729–35, 748–50.
34. See Ian Kershaw, *The "Hitler Myth": Image and Reality in the Third Reich* (Oxford, 1987), 169–225.
35. Quote from Mason, "Containment," 236.
36. See Alf Lüdtke, "The Appeal of Exterminating 'Others': German Workers and the Limits of Resistance," *Journal of Modern History* 64 (1992): 46–67. On general indifference toward the fate of the Jews, see Kershaw, *Popular Opinion*, 358–72.
37. On the role of sports in East German society, see Alan McDougall's essay in this volume, which includes references to the pertinent literature.
38. Quote from Kleßmann, *Arbeiter im "Arbeiterstaat,"* 394.
39. See, for example, Port, *Conflict and Stability*, 117. On the appeal of anti-fascism, also see the essays in this volume by Joanne Sayner and Andreas Agocs.
40. This is one of the main arguments in Port, *Conflict and Stability*.
41. On state security forces under the Third Reich and the GDR, see, e.g., Robert Gellately, *The Gestapo and German Society: Enforcing Racial Policy, 1933–1945* (Oxford, 1990); Jens Gieseke, *Die Stasi. 1945-1990* (Munich, 2011); Gary Bruce, *The Firm: The Inside Story of the Stasi* (Oxford, 2010).

42. On the early suppression of workers under the Nazis, see Heinrich August Winkler, *Der Weg in die Katastrophe. Arbeiter und Arbeiterbewegung in der Weimarer Republik 1930 bis 1933* (Berlin, 1987). On the treatment of Social Democrats in the GDR, see Beatrix Bouvier, *Ausgeschaltet. Sozialdemokraten in der sowjetischen Besatzungszone und in der DDR, 1945–1953* (Bonn, 1996); Harold Hurwitz, *Die Stalinisierung der SED. Zum Verlust von Freiräumen und sozialdemokratischer Identität in den Vorständen, 1946–1949* (Opladen, 1997).
43. See Port, *Conflict and Stability*, 78–82.
44. Mason, "Containment," 270. On working-class voting patterns under the Nazis, see Jürgen Falter, *Hitlers Wähler* (Munich, 1991), 198–230.
45. This argument is developed at length in Port, *Conflict and Stability*, esp. 195–216.
46. Herbert, "Arbeiterschaft im 'Dritten Reich,'" 324–26; Mason, "Containment," 244–52; Peukert, *Inside Nazi Germany*, 112–17.
47. See Timothy Garton Ash, *The Polish Revolution: Solidarity*, 3rd ed. (New Haven, 2002); Roman Laba, *The Roots of Solidarity: A Political Sociology of Poland's Working-Class Democratization* (Princeton, 1991).
48. For a nuanced discussion of German reactions to the outbreak of war in 1914 that downplays popular enthusiasm, see Jeffrey Verhey, *The Spirit of 1914: Militarism, Myth, and Mobilization in Germany* (New York, 2006).
49. See Wolfgang Wippermann, *Die Deutschen und der Osten. Feindbild und Traumland* (Darmstadt, 2007), as well as the essays in Gregor Thum, ed., *Traumland Osten. Deutsche Bilder vom östlichen Europa im 20. Jahrhundert* (Göttingen, 2006).
50. On East German views about the "Russians," as well as relations between the "occupiers" and "occupied," see Silke Satjukow, *Besatzer. "Die Russen" in Deutschland 1945 bis 1994* (Göttingen, 2008); idem, *Befreiung? Die Ostdeutschen und 1945* (Leipzig, 2009); Port, *Conflict and Stability*, 117–19. On the Soviet occupation more generally, see Norman Naimark, *The Russians in Germany: A History of the Soviet Zone of Occupation, 1945–1949* (Cambridge, M.A., 1995).
51. This surely commits at least one of the fallacies of question-framing identified in David Hackett Fischer, *Historians' Fallacies: Toward a Logic of Historical Thought* (New York, 1970), 3–39.

CHAPTER 10

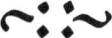

Israel as Friend and Foe
Shaping East German Society through Freund- and Feindbilder

DAVID G. TOMPKINS

The construction and reception of external friends and enemies made up an essential element of the Communist worldview. By providing models to be emulated and rejected, party officials and sympathizers utilized these *Freund-* and *Feindbilder* to shape the new Socialist society, as well as to claim legitimacy for their aims. These images saturated the public space, and their presentation and manipulation were a constant of life under socialism, as the parties sought to mobilize and dominate their populations. But ordinary citizens were not merely passive objects of this propaganda, for they brought their preexisting ideas, as well as opinions formed by exposure to Western media, to this struggle over attitudes, outlooks, and worldviews.

This essay focuses on East Germany, and more specifically on the case of Israel as an example of a country whose representation in the GDR evolved considerably: from that of a left-leaning state filled with kibbutzim to a rapacious imperialist ally dominated by its bourgeoisie. The transformation of this image in the East German context from the late 1940s through the late 1960s is a particularly compelling one, since the two countries shared a number of similarities as relatively small countries, both undergoing (re)construction with an anti-fascist ideology and on the front lines of conflicts against much larger enemies. The transformation over time of Israel's image from friend to foe challenged fundamental aspects of Communist self-understanding, as it called into question the usual Manichaean worldview of positive and negative camps. This evolving representation of an Israel moving away from the Soviet bloc thus destabilized the basic notion that socialism would be ultimately victorious, for it weakened the core idea of the correctness of the Communist path. This, along with the fact that a formerly sympathetic country was not only increasingly tied to the "imperialist" powers, but had also come to dominate militarily Soviet-bloc allies—the Arab countries of the region—all posed a further threat to the idea promoted by East German leaders of a powerful, monolithic Communist community. Since Israel fell into the imagined space just below more prominent and consistent friends and enemies such as the USSR and United States, the shaping and reception of its image was an important site for working out just what it meant to be Communist in the Communist bloc. And finally, German anti-Semitism offered a rich but dangerous set of symbols that officials had to grapple with in an attempt to influence the worldviews of East German citizens through the representation of Israel.[1]

With a focus on the image of Israel in East Germany from the late 1940s through the late 1960s, this essay will examine one prominent example of Socialist discourse about external friends and enemies, analyze the attempt to influence society through the construction of this symbol, and explore responses by the East German populace. SED officials were relatively successful in this effort, despite unexpected stumbles and surprising forms of resistance. The essay examines three periods: the Stalinist years around 1950, the decade from the mid 1950s to the mid 1960s, and, finally, the 1967 Six-Day War and its aftermath. During the early postwar years, Israel received positive notice in eastern Germany and throughout the Soviet bloc, enjoying an image as a progressive country working against the forces of "imperialism" and "reaction," to employ the terminology of the day. Around 1950, this image began to darken, as the Soviet Union and its allies focused on a supposed Zionist threat. But the GDR found additional reasons to resent Israel as well. Increasingly, Israel was linked to the imperialist powers, and its image assumed a patina of aggression and exploitation. This portrayal slowly intensified in the later 1950s and into the 1960s, as the Soviet bloc, drawing ever closer to Israel's Arab neighbors, increasingly emphasized a dichotomy between "progressive" and "imperialist" forces in the region. A negative image of Israel climaxed with the Six-Day War, when nearly all Socialist countries officially broke diplomatic relations with Israel—effectively turning the country into a full-fledged enemy in East German discourse.

Israel as Potential Ally

Following the leadership of the Soviet Union, the Communists in eastern Germany supported the UN resolution on the creation of Israel in late 1947, as well as the birth of the state in May 1948. Soviet leaders were willing to overlook their traditionally Leninist rejection of Zionism in order to support a blow to the regional colonial power Great Britain, and thus favored the creation of Israel for broader strategic reasons.[2] Indeed, the USSR and Czechoslovakia were the first two countries to recognize Israel formally, with the other Soviet-bloc states not far behind—though not, of course, the Soviet Zone of Occupation, which did not become an independent state until the fall of 1949. More specifically, the leading role of leftist parties in Israel gave the Soviet bloc hope that the fledgling country would become an ally in this strategically important part of the world. Eastern German press reports on developments in the Middle East were positive toward Israel, emphasizing the Israeli working class's right to a national state. A wave of support emanating from political officials and elites swept over the population through the press.

The Socialist Unity Party (SED) expressed clear enthusiasm for the new state of Israel around the time of its founding. Its press agency released an announcement in May 1948 that celebrated the Jewish struggle against "USA imperialists" and the "fascist elements" of the Arab Legion.[3] Politburo member Paul Merker was a particularly vocal Israel supporter who, in party circles as well as in the broader press of the late 1940s, depicted the foundation of Israel in a positive light and stressed the anti-fascist and anti-imperialist affinities between the East German Communists and Jews building a state in Palestine.[4] In a typical article in *Neues Deutschland*, the leading daily newspaper of the party, he wrote, "The Jewish population [in Palestine] deserves the sympathies and energetic help of all progressive forces. Especially the democratic forces in Germany have the duty to express their sympathies and cooperation."[5] He also wrote the introduction to an informational brochure from June 1948 that also included positive words about Israel from Wilhelm Pieck, soon to become president of the GDR. Merker's contribution supported Israel's existence as part of a worldwide "progressive struggle" and depicted the heroic Jewish working class as fighting bravely against American and British imperialism and their Arab allies.[6] Newspaper articles in *Neues Deutschland* consistently praised the Israeli fight for national independence, and the weekly *Weltbühne* featured a number of longer articles that portrayed Israel as a small but brave, progressive entity struggling against a huge sea of right-wing forces.[7] The struggle over Palestine was described in clearly ideological terms in this range of publications, with Israel as the politically sympathetic actor fighting both global imperialism and local reactionary forces. In a powerful symbolic statement, the Israeli flag began to fly on official holidays from the buildings of the Jewish community.[8]

The image presented to the eastern German public in the late 1940s was of Israel as a young and heroic country that was a potential member of the Socialist camp and indeed, in certain ways, even a model to be emulated. Like East Germans and Communists throughout the world, the Jews of Palestine (and later the state of Israel) were engaged in combat with the forces of reaction at home and those of imperialism more generally. The picture of workers building a better future for themselves in a difficult situation provided a pedagogical example for East Germans in their own struggle to build socialism in a world of powerful imperialist interests allegedly striving to stunt those efforts.

Growing Tensions

Already in the late 1940s, this positive representation of Israel began to be undermined by events internal and external to East Germany. At home, Communist leaders throughout the Soviet bloc became worried about the attraction of Israel as a potential source of divided loyalties for Jews living in their own countries. The founding of Israel prompted expressions of support from Soviet and Soviet-bloc Jews, most famously in the spontaneous demonstration of enthusiasm for Israel's first ambassador to the Soviet Union, Golda Meyerson (later Meir) in Moscow in the fall of 1948. Many Jews did, in fact, seek to emigrate to the new country, prompting fears about the loss of manpower and expertise at a time of reconstruction.[9] A further damper on Soviet-bloc favor came in 1950, when Israel supported the United States over the conflict on the Korean peninsula. Growing national movements in the Arab countries also offered Communist states an attractive opening for influence in the region—and thus presupposed a turn away from Israel. As a further stumbling block in the specific East German context, Israel presented demands for reparations to authorities in the two Germanys in 1951, and the SED resisted these calls. As part of a more general turn against enemies throughout the Soviet bloc in the context of the escalating Cold War conflict, attention shifted to Jews, Zionism, and Israel, which were increasingly seen as part of an international network seeking to undermine communism. Increasing anti-Semitism throughout the bloc, both politically motivated and related to traditional prejudices, culminated in the Rudolf Slánský trial in Czechoslovakia in late 1952 and the so-called Doctors' Plot in the Soviet Union in early 1953, both of which significantly affected the official presentation of Israel in the GDR.

In the early 1950s, the issue of German reparations to Israel became a focal point of attention, and the SED decided it would not pay them, ostensibly because it was already supporting victims of fascism—including Jews—at home; furthermore, it did not recognize Israel's right to speak for Jews more generally. In this context, the linking of Israel to capitalist, imperialist powers functioned as a further justification for refusal. Also, SED leaders asserted repeatedly and loudly their anti-fascist policies and actions to uproot Nazis and Nazism from (East) German soil. The press condemned the 1952 agreement between the Federal Republic and Israel, whereby the former agreed to pay "reparations" to the latter, as a treaty between "West German and Israeli *Großkapitalisten*" that would only benefit Israeli war industries and U.S. imperialists—a link that would be ceaselessly asserted in the years to come.[10]

This increasingly negative picture of Israel culminated in the publicity surrounding the 1952 trial of Rudolf Slánský and his alleged coconspirators in neighboring Czechoslovakia. The East German daily press repeatedly linked Israel and Zionism with "American imperialism" and the capitalist threat. An extended article in a party journal and a related 103-page pamphlet alleged that "the Zionist movement has nothing in common with the goals of true humanitarianism. It is controlled, directed, and commanded by American imperialism, and serves only its interests and those of Jewish capitalists."[11] Israel was termed a "vassal state" of the Americans, who were advancing their menacing goals through it. Very aware that their anti-Israel position could be perceived as anti-Semitic, East German officials then and later consistently sought to deny this interpretation by claiming to focus on class and not race, i.e., that their negative view of Israel was based on the state's capitalist and imperialist affinities.[12] Nonetheless, anti-Semitic tropes about Jews and Zionists as perfidious, sneakily dangerous, and exploitative abounded at the time and later, as we shall see, all in an attempt to tarnish the image of Israel.[13]

Vitriol aimed at Israel died down somewhat after Josef Stalin's death, which marked the abrupt end of speculation about a so-called Doctors' Plot supposedly involving malevolent Jewish doctors intent on killing the Soviet dictator. This, along with the subsequent political thaw introduced by Stalin's successors, helped reduce some of the overheated rhetoric about threats to socialism. A renewed focus on Israel in the public space picked up once again during the Suez Canal crisis in the fall of 1956, when Israel joined the British and French in taking military action against Egypt, thereby definitively aligning itself with the other Cold War camp. East German press articles and official government statements portrayed Israel in a negative light, even if often as a semi-unwitting tool of the imperialist powers of Britain and France, as well as of "international monopoly capitalism" more generally.[14] The SED leadership maintained that the Federal Republic's support for Israel through reparations allowed the latter to undertake such aggressive actions, thus strengthening the notion that West German payments meant imperialist oppression and were consequently a threat to world peace.[15]

All across the country, officials worked to communicate the party line on Israel, and sought to assess and guide the population's reaction to unfolding events. The linkage of Israel to the imperialist powers fit well into a larger narrative at this time of crisis in the Soviet bloc: the Hungarian Revolution had taken place concurrently, and the SED was seeking to blame the West for attempting to undermine communism. Officials claimed a strong and negative reaction to Western and Israeli intervention in Suez across the GDR: from workers, the intelligentsia, and young people, as well as from Rostock in the north to the small town of Meiningen in the south, and to cities and factories in between.[16] Some workers echoed the line that the Israelis were like the reactionary capitalists, fomenting trouble in Hungary. Others even claimed that they had, at first, thought the Hungarians were genuinely unhappy, but the events in Suez convinced them that the imperialists were indeed behind everything.[17] The portrayal of Israel as an imperialist power attempting to undermine left-leaning Egypt served as a timely pedagogical tool for teaching about supposedly similar Western designs on Hungary.

But SED officials were unable to control the discourse around Israel completely, and, in fact, a number of East Germans expressed openly anti-Semitic opinions. According to one worker, for instance, it was a "Jewish bandit-state (*Räuberstaat*)."[18] More extreme anti-Semitic views and actions surfaced as well. This included the wish, expressed in several factories, that Adolf Hitler should have killed more Jews so that they could not have attacked Egypt; the claim that the fascists were correct in alleging that "Jews always incited new wars"; or the fact that some people in the northern town of Wismar had used the Israeli attack as an occasion to agitate against Jews.[19] In later years (see below), official discourse drew parallels between Israel and Nazi Germany, building on the potential already existing in the population—such as that of one Magdeburger, who compared Israel's actions in Egypt to Hitler's attacks.[20] The Nazi past was also not far from the minds of the minority of East Germans who expressed negative views of Egypt's leader Gamal Abdel Nasser, who was sometimes compared to Hitler—or criticized for having former Nazis as advisers.[21] And while officials encouraged citizens to draw acceptable parallels, they sought to suppress undesirable ones—as in the case of several individuals who felt that if Nasser deserved Suez, then the East Germans had every right to regain the eastern territories ceded to Poland after World War II.[22] In the aftermath of Suez, informal interviews and the monitoring of individual opinions painted a picture of a population that broadly shared a critical view of Israel as an aggressor state in league with imperialist powers.[23] By this time, the SED could claim some success at creating a negative image of Israel—and at using it to influence the worldviews of the East German population in a manner largely consistent with the party's aims of promoting and preserving the Socialist project and resisting imperialist encroachments.

The views of Victor Klemperer, a philologist of Jewish descent who had converted to Protestantism and survived the Third Reich by virtue of being in a "mixed marriage" (as well as some lucky escapes), are worth noting for their similarity to the party's negative representation of Israel. He had long been critical of Zionism, and, in the mid 1950s, he condemned Israel and its actions toward the Arabs. In 1955, he wrote in his diary that Israel was "[o]n the warpath against Egypt and Arabia, with tanks and jet fighters. Cock fighting. The Israelis have American masters and American blades in their claws."[24] And in 1957, he asserted that the Israelis were "worse than the Nazis" and would wind up "in the penultimate circle of hell."[25]

Focus returned to the region with the trial of Adolf Eichmann in 1961. In its aftermath, a well-publicized book appeared on the proceedings, written by Friedrich Karl Kaul, the East German representative there. While the book and the contemporary reporting focused on linking Eichmann to leading West Germans and condemning the Federal Republic as fascist, the fifth chapter provided a highly critical interpretation of Israel's prehistory. It claimed that Zionism was a creation of the Jewish bourgeoisie aimed at deflecting the aspirations of the Jewish working class, and drew links between Zionism and imperialism.[26] The source for this chapter was a book that had a revealing history in the GDR: Konstantin Iwanow and Zinovii Scheinis's *The State of Israel: Position and Politics*, published in 1959 in the Soviet Union. The book was updated and translated into German, and published in the GDR in 1960. After half of its 6,000 copies had been delivered to libraries and bookstores, leading SED functionary and Politburo member Albert Norden—whose father had been a rabbi—decided in the spring of 1961 to recall them seemingly because it was overly critical of Israel and due to protests by the Communist Party of Israel.[27] That some of its essential and contentious arguments were included in Kaul's book two years later demonstrates how the representation of Israel was becoming overwhelmingly negative.

One significant reason for the emergence of a more sharply critical image of Israel was the development of links between the Arab world and the Soviet bloc in the 1950s and 1960s. This relationship was particularly important for the GDR as it tried to gain international recognition in the face of the Hallstein Doctrine, the West German policy establishing that it would not maintain diplomatic relations with any state recognizing the GDR; the numerous Arab states were consequently a sought-after prize for East German leaders,[28] and efforts to draw closer to the Arab world increased at this time. This led, for example, to a flattering 1959 exhibition in Berlin on the Arab independence movement, which condemned Israel as an imperialist base in the Middle East.[29] East German leader Walter Ulbricht's high-profile trip to Cairo in late February 1965 brought more opportunities to refine the negative image of Israel: during this visit, he publicly called it an "advanced position of the imperialists," and emphasized purportedly dangerous links between West Germany and Israel.[30] Ulbricht even went so far as to state that Israel was founded by the imperialist powers to hinder the progress of the Arab states, a rabidly anti-Israel statement that went beyond the Soviet bloc's official ideological line and that even drew a sharp protest from the Israeli Communist Party.[31]

SED ideologues concurrently produced material for party members and for broader discussion that elaborated on the view of Israel as aggressive in nature and in league with imperialism; it was claimed, at the same time, that its workers were exploited by greedy capitalists.[32] The lesson of the situation was made more immediately relevant as Israel was compared to West Berlin: both were portrayed as outposts of capitalism and imperialism that good Communists were obliged to struggle against.[33] A cascade of articles in *Neues Deutschland* reinforced a negative image of Israel in league with the enemies of the GDR and the Communist world. A particularly notable point in this campaign was a painting in a Dresden exhibition of Arab artists that featured Jesus on the cross with a naked prostitute holding the Israeli flag.[34]

From the mid 1950s through the mid 1960s, SED officials continued to spread a negative image of Israel—one against which East Germans were encouraged to define themselves. This effort peaked with the publication of an official collection of documents from the preceding years that was aimed at crystallizing this image. In essence, these claimed that East Germans were members of the Socialist world, working against the capitalist exploitation and aggressive imperialism manifested in Israel and its supporters Great Britain, France, the United States, and West Germany.[35] Still, recent German history presented considerable problems to using Israel in this way, for such criticism could potentially foster anti-Semitic views that might muddle the GDR's proclaimed anti-fascist identity. All of these issues came further into relief with the momentous events of late spring 1967.

Israel as Enemy: The Six-Day War in June 1967

The Six-Day War provided the tipping point for the consolidation and dissemination of "*Feindbild* Israel." Deepening the already highly negative image of Israel in light of the conflict, SED officials now portrayed Israel as a rapacious vassal state in league with the ever more imperialist Americans, who themselves were allegedly becoming increasingly involved in Vietnam, as well as with the Federal Republic, the GDR's rival next door, in a thickening web of worldwide aggression. SED officials employed this representation of a hawkish Israel to offer an example against which supposedly peace-loving, justice-minded East Germans should define themselves, as well as to try to rationalize the failures of the Soviet bloc and its defeated allies in the region.

From the first days of the conflict, a wide-ranging media offensive spread this more fully negative representation of Israel. In fact, the Politburo itself provided guidelines to press, radio, and television outlets aimed at magnifying the party line.[36] Party officials worked assiduously to communicate a consistent portrayal across the media landscape that would "condemn the aggressor and expose his barbaric goals of conquest, inhuman methods, and the fanatic support from Bonn."[37] Walter Ulbricht himself gave a major, highly publicized speech on the subject in mid June, and the party published a booklet featuring a related article, as well as information on the history of the conflict that once again portrayed Israel as aggressive and imperialist.[38] Perhaps the most disturbing example was a poem published in a Magdeburg newspaper that depicted Israel teaching its children to rob and steal, and nailing a figure of peace onto a cross.[39]

Party officials orchestrated a wide-ranging campaign in daily newspapers all across the country aimed at labeling Israel as an aggressor in league with imperialist forces.[40] Articles in *Neues Deutschland* were particularly harsh at this time, emphasizing the idea of Israel as a savage actor that conducted barbarous acts on the battlefield.[41] Politburo member Albert Norden called for the press to make explicit comparisons to Nazi atrocities, including one with Germany's surprise attack against the Soviet Union in 1941.[42] One of the cruder examples came from a factory newspaper that showed a cartoon of Defense Minister Moshe Dayan grasping for Gaza and Jerusalem—while an approving Hitler looked on.[43] Articles continually reinforced the trope of Israel as an imperialist power working to contain the progressive development of its Arab neighbors and, more generally, serving the interests of the United States and West Germany. Both countries had allegedly "pumped" capital and weapons into Israel in a long-planned effort to create both an "imperialist beachhead" and a "spearhead of NATO," an oft-invoked image. These imperialist powers also intentionally supported bourgeois, chauvinist circles in Israel who feared the working class, and who, more generally, dominated the Israeli economy.[44] Some articles described statements from mass organizations that condemned Israeli aggression and its imperialist aims, while other reports claimed that East Germans were united in their disapproval of Israel.[45] One of the more powerful and attention-grabbing pieces was the "Declaration of GDR Citizens of Jewish Background," which was organized by Norden and attacked Israel in uncompromising language.[46]

A recurring column in *Neues Deutschland* answered reader questions in a similar manner, and was considered so effective that party officials directed regional newspapers to adopt this same strategy of "public education."[47] These letters not only offered the opportunity to show ordinary East Germans what their fellow citizens thought of the conflict, but also provided a forum to drive home the message about Israel's aggressive nature while emphasizing its alleged links to imperialism during the present conflict as well as since its founding.[48] One response explained that Israel's kibbutzim were not Socialist, but rather a relic of earlier days that were currently exploited by the bourgeoisie and that served as a cover for capitalist exploitation.[49] Hubert Windisch from Gera wanted to know how the Israelis had achieved their military victories, and was told that a surprise attack was a dangerous, insidious move typical of imperialist states—and that one must always be prepared to deal with the "perfidiousness of imperialist aggressors."[50]

Windisch's letter—assuming that he was the actual author—revealed an undercurrent of anxiety among ordinary East Germans, as well as their leaders. How had "their" side lost the conflict so spectacularly, and what did that mean for the Soviet bloc and socialism more broadly? A number of citizens expressed fears that the GDR was also vulnerable, or that the Socialist camp was weak.[51] A particular representation of Israel served an important purpose here, as it had in the fall of 1956 during the Suez crisis: to provide a narrative that asserted the ultimate strength of the Communist world and that stressed the need for solidarity. Israel could only win because of its devious, criminal tactics and the unfair and disproportionate support of its aggressive imperialist allies, especially the United States and West Germany.[52]

To counter these fears and communicate its portrayal of Israel more fully, SED officials sought to reach out to party members and the broader population through more direct means such as public meetings. Authorities in Berlin prepared extensive materials for these occasions that emphasized Israeli aggression as part of a larger imperialist plot for regional domination.[53] University officials and the Free German Youth (FDJ) organized protest actions and expressions of solidarity with the Arab countries among young people; in Dresden alone, 10,000 students took to the streets.[54] The national trade union (FDGB) undertook an extensive program to educate workers about the conflict. In factories throughout the country, officials organized educational meetings and solidarity "actions" that sought to brand Israel as an aggressor in league with American and West German imperialism. Speakers were prepared with extensive materials to drive home the representation of Israel as a major hindrance to "peace, democracy, and progress."[55] In a direct reference to the situation of East Germans themselves, citizens were again encouraged to view opposition to Israel as somehow equivalent to the resistance against Western "aggression" in Berlin in August 1961. These meetings also produced collections of donations for the Arab countries, as well as thousands of resolutions and telegrams that condemned Israel for its "brutal fascist methods" and *Soldateska*, a term evoking an undisciplined, marauding army.[56]

Officials claimed an outpouring of support for the GDR, and for the Soviet bloc more generally, because they had backed the anti-imperialist side in the conflict.[57] They pointed to the cascade of protest resolutions from around the country with slogans like "Down with Israeli aggression!" and noted the words of individual workers who condemned Israel—such as Kurt Stüwe, head designer at the Karl-Marx-Werk in Babelsberg: "the criminal acts of war of the Israelis ... bring forth deep indignation and disgust."[58] If official reports are taken at face value, citizens in East Berlin seemed to have been particularly convinced of links between Israel and American imperialism, perhaps a result of their exposed position on the front line of the Cold War. Party officials reported "great outrage and a broad wave of protest" that included meetings and events in workplaces of all kinds that "unanimously condemned the aggression."[59] The SED claimed that even more workers had embraced the party line following Ulbricht's virulently anti-Israel speech on June 15, and "condemned Israel's aggression as an imperialist war of conquest…" In fact, they were now reportedly prepared to work even harder to support the GDR in light of the conflict.[60]

Officials were occasionally unable to secure unanimous votes for protest resolutions.[61] For example, only half of thirty-five workers signed a protest resolution at a ball-bearing factory in Zella-Mehlis, the VEB Thüringer Kugellagerfabrik—and three even left the hall during the discussion.[62] Two-thirds of the foremen did not support a protest resolution at VEB Werkzeugfabrik, a tool factory in Königsee, and only seven out of sixty-two workers in the union group at the VEB Grubenlampe in Zwickau voted to support a resolution condemning Israel. Officials at this mine lamp factory organized a second discussion and worked to convince staff members to sign, but five people still voted against it and a large group continued to abstain.[63]

Such dissent, at least in such an open and public form, was rare—or, at least, rarely reported. But other dissenting voices appeared in less formal settings, with a significant minority of East Germans expressing their support for Israel. Some sympathizers asserted that Israel was a victim of Arab aggression, though party officials worked hard to convince them otherwise.[64] Others felt that East Germany should support Israel in light of Nazi atrocities during World War II.[65] Additional expressions of solidarity with Israelis were framed in light of Jewish suffering more generally, or with reference to a Jewish right to a homeland. According to others, Jews were, after suffering so many years of oppression, fighting a just war for their very existence and needed adequate land and resources.[66] These views seem to have been in the minority, but their regular appearance in reports shows that the official image of Israel encountered some opposition.

One source of support for Israel came from practicing Christians, though party officials claimed that the overwhelming majority supported the SED's position.[67] Some Christian citizens seemed to base their opinions on the Bible, claiming the Israelis deserved that land or were its true heirs.[68] A professor of theology in Berlin believed East Germans should support Israel because of German actions in World War II, and asserted, furthermore, that the Israelis had "built themselves roads, [and] work[ed] for social progress."[69] The organist at the Paulus Church in Halle hung a sign in his apartment window saying "Practice solidarity with Israel," and prayers were said for Israel at a church in Ribnitz during a youth service.[70]

Another deviation from the party's official representation of Israel took the form of anti-Semitic statements, not unlike what had happened a decade earlier. Several factory workers opined that more Jews should have been gassed by the Nazis.[71] Others claimed that Hitler had been correct: Jews were bad and also responsible for the two world wars.[72] According to several people in

Schwerin, "we can expect nothing good from world Jewry."[73] One individual living in the countryside claimed that the Israeli aggression meant that too many Jews had been "left over" (*übrig geblieben*) after World War II.[74] As it had earlier, the SED consistently claimed that its criticism of Israel—a capitalist and imperialist state—was not anti-Semitic, but rather a question of class (*Klassenfrage*) and not race (*Rassenfrage*).[75] Officials also sought to make this distinction in an attempt to undercut sympathy for Israel among those citizens who felt that East Germany needed to atone for Nazi crimes.[76]

In the aftermath of the Six-Day War, SED officials took a survey of attitudes about the conflict based on a societal cross-section drawn from six factories in Leipzig and Dresden. The respondents were roughly half workers, a third were in managerial positions, and the rest were members of the "intelligentsia." They retained anonymity, and the questions lacked an overt bias. Clear majorities agreed with the party-sponsored image of Israel, but significant minorities held alternate views. Roughly 56 percent thought Israel had been the aggressor, but nearly a third blamed both sides, and about one in ten expressed sympathy for Israel. Surprisingly, only two-thirds of the respondents agreed with the SED's representation of Israel as an imperialist state, while about 15 percent said that was not the case and another 15 percent that they did not know.[77] After over a decade of exposure to a negative image of Israel, and after a summer of frequent and lengthy public propaganda about Israel's supposed perfidy, it would appear that most but not all citizens of the GDR saw Israel as a country not to be admired and emulated.

Conclusion

Such surveys and the related internal reports explored here offer valuable insights into both the ambitions of party officials and the attitudes of ordinary citizens. Historians have begun to analyze and carefully utilize such reports to gain a deeper understanding of the worldviews of East Germans.[78] The attempt to gauge public opinion in a dictatorship using such sources is of course problematic, for respondents were likely guarded in their responses, given the repressive nature of the regime.[79] But the fact that such surveys and reports—with opinions that diverged significantly from what party officials would have hoped—existed, combined with careful attention to context, make these sources a useful window into popular attitudes in the East German dictatorship.

The negative image of Israel spread in 1967 continued to be propagated over the next two decades with unabated intensity. Despite the Arab surprise attack that started the so-called Yom Kippur War of 1973, Israel was once again labeled the aggressor. And during the 1982 invasion of Lebanon, the East

German press made frequent and exaggerated comparisons between Israeli and Nazi "crimes."[80] This *Feindbild*, which had coalesced over the 1950s and 1960s in a manner both planned and in response to real events, continued to be an effective tool for educating East Germans about the imperialist foe nearly to the end of the GDR.

In the two decades after World War II, the image of Israel in East Germany was transformed from that of a friend to that of a bitter enemy of the Communist world. Party officials and educated elites worked to formulate these portrayals of Israel: initially sympathetic, as a progressive country fighting reactionary forces, but increasingly, after 1950, as aggressive, exploitative, and linked to capitalist and imperialist powers like the United States and West Germany. The broader population then encountered these manifold images in public settings and the media in various forms. By offering both positive and negative examples, the evolving image and symbolic picture of Israel served a pedagogical function meant to mobilize society for the building of socialism and shore up the legitimacy of the SED at home. In addition, it helped the party explain its interpretation of the world—and the place of East Germans in it—in the context of the long Cold War struggle between communism and capitalism. This constructed representation of Israel occupied a significant space in the self-conception of both ordinary citizens and their leaders, and suggests another way in which the former gradually "became" East Germans over the four decades of the GDR's history.

Suggested Readings

Aust, Marin and Daniel Schoenpflug, eds. *Vom Gegner lernen. Feindschaften und Kulturtransfers im Europa des 19. und 20. Jahrhunderts*. Frankfurt, 2007.

Bachmann, Wiebke. *Die UdSSR und der Nahe Osten. Zionismus, ägyptischer Antikolonialismus und sowjetische Außenpolitik bis 1956*. Munich, 2011.

Haury, Thomas. *Antisemitismus von links. Kommunistische Ideologie, Nationalismus und Antizionismus in der frühen DDR*. Hamburg, 2002.

Herf, Jeffrey. *Divided Memory: The Nazi Past in the Two Germanys*. Cambridge, M.A., 1997.

Jahr, Christoph, Uwe Mai, and Kathrin Roller, eds. *Feindbilder in der deutschen Geschichte. Studien zur Vorurteilsgeschichte im 19. und 20. Jahrhundert*. Berlin, 1994.

Port, Andrew I. *Conflict and Stability in the German Democratic Republic*. New York, 2007.

Niven, William. *Facing the Nazi Past: United Germany and the Legacy of the Third Reich*. New York, 2002

Satjukow, Silke, and Rainer Gries, eds. *Sozialistische Helden. Eine Kulturgeschichte von Propagandafiguren in Osteuropa und der DDR*. Berlin, 2002.

Satjukow, Silke, and Rainer Gries. *Unsere Feinde: Konstruktionen des Anderen im Sozialismus*. Leipzig, 2004.

Timm, Angelika. *Hammer, Zirkel, Davidstern. Das gestörte Verhältnis der DDR zu Zionismus und Staat Israel*. Bonn, 1997.

Notes

1. For more on how the GDR dealt with the legacy of Nazism, see William Niven, *Facing the Nazi Past: United Germany and the Legacy of the Third Reich* (New York, 2002); Jeffrey Herf, *Divided Memory: The Nazi Past in the Two Germanys* (Cambridge, M.A., 1997).
2. For more on Lenin and Stalin's rejection of Zionism as reactionary, bourgeois, and nationalist, see especially Thomas Haury, *Antisemitismus von links. Kommunistische Ideologie, Nationalismus und Antizionismus in der frühen DDR* (Hamburg, 2002), 210–52. On the Bolshevik struggles with the Zionists and Bundists, see Zvi Gitelman, *Jewish Nationality and Soviet Politics: The Jewish Sections of the CPSU* (Princeton, 1972).
3. Helmut Eschwege, *Fremd unter meinesgleichen. Errinerungen eines Dresdner Juden* (Berlin, 1991), 64.
4. Herf, *Divided Memory*, 98–99. He would later pay for this support with imprisonment and expulsion from the party. See Herf, *Divided Memory*, 106–61.
5. *Neues Deutschland*, 24 February 1948, quoted in Angelika Timm, *Hammer, Zirkel, Davidstern. Das gestörte Verhältnis der DDR zu Zionismus und Staat Israel* (Bonn, 1997), 84.
6. Eschwege, *Fremd*, 63.
7. Haury, *Antisemitismus*, 325–26; Timm, *Hammer*, 86–87.
8. Eschwege, *Fremd*, 65.
9. Wiebke Bachmann, *Die UdSSR und der Nahe Osten. Zionismus, ägyptischer Antikolonialismus und sowjetische Außenpolitik bis 1956* (Munich, 2011), 134; Karin Hartewig, "Jüdische Kommunisten in der DDR und ihr Verhältnis zu Israel," in *Jenseits der Legenden. Araber, Juden, Deutsche*, ed. Wolfgang Schwanitz (Berlin, 1994), 130.
10. "Wiedergutmachung—für wen?," *Neues Deutschland*, 25 November 1952, cited in Timm, *Hammer*, 132.
11. "Lehren aus dem Prozeß gegen das Verschwörerzentrum Slansky," in *Einheit* 8/3 (1953): 203–16. See also Timm, *Hammer*, 116.
12. On how the GDR claimed to separate anti-Semitism from its anti-Zionist stance, see Peter Dittmar, "DDR und Israel (I): Ambivalenz einer Nicht-Beziehung," in *Deutschland Archiv* 10/7 (July 1977), 739–40.
13. The literature on anti-Semitism and the GDR is extensive. Two of the most important recent works are Haury, *Antisemitismus*, and, in English, Herf, *Divided Memory*.
14. Timm, *Hammer*, 144.
15. Dittmar, "DDR und Israel (I)," 750–51.
16. Stiftung-Archiv der Parteien und Massenorganisationen der DDR im Bundesarchiv (SAPMO-BArch), DY-27, 6518, Stimmungsbericht, Cottbus, 14 November 1956, and Bericht, Meiningen, 10 November 1956; DY-30, IV 2/5/582, Fernschreiben (FS) 220, Rostock, 1 November 1956; DY-30, IV 2/5/694, FS 127, Cottbus, 2 November 1956, and Informationsbericht Nr. 19/56, Cottbus, 1 December 1956; DY-30, IV 2/5/732, FS 32, Magdeburg, 30 October 1956, and FS 34, Magdeburg, 31 October 1956.
17. SAPMO-BArch, DY-30, IV 2/5/732, FS 32, Magdeburg, 30 October 1956 and FS 2, Magdeburg, 2 November 1956.
18. SAPMO-BArch, DY-30 IV 2/5/732, FS 34, Magdeburg, 31 October 1956.
19. SAPMO-BArch, DY-30 IV 2/5/732, FS 1, Magdeburg, 1 November 1956; DY-30 IV 2/5/694, FS 127, Cottbus, 2 November 1956, 202; DY-30 IV 2/5/582, Stimmungsbericht, 12 November 1956.

20. SAPMO-BArch, DY-30, IV 2/5/732, FS 3, Magdeburg, 1 November 1956.
21. SAPMO-BArch, DY-27, 6518, Stimmungsbericht, Cottbus, 14 November 1956; DY-6, 4721, "Informationsbericht für die Zeit vom 15.10 bis 31.10.1956," Neustrelitz; DY-30, IV 2/5/732, "Bericht über die Stimmung der Bevölkerung," Magdeburg, 13 November 1956.
22. SAPMO-BArch, DY-30, IV 2/5/582, Stimmungsberichte from Rostock.
23. SAPMO-BArch, DY-27, 6518, Stimmungsbericht, 14 November 1956; Bericht, Meiningen, 10 November 1956. See also SAPMO-BArch, DY-30, IV 2/5/582, DY-30, IV 2/5/694, and DY-30, IV 2/5/732.
24. See the entry from 3 September 1955 in Victor Klemperer, *The Lesser Evil: The Diaries of Victor Klemperer, 1945-1959* (London, 2003), 455.
25. See the entry from 23 November 1957 in ibid., 501.
26. Friedrich Karl Kaul, *Der Fall Eichmann* (Berlin, 1963).
27. SAPMO-BArch, DY-30, 19236; see also Timm, 161–62 and 421 n.59; Eschwege, 194. Timm notes that the book was nonetheless held by libraries and could be checked out.
28. See also Herf, 190–200. GDR leaders especially tried to gain the official recognition of the Arab states after their angry reaction to the establishment of official West German–Israeli relations in May 1965, though recognition was not achieved until 1969 or later. See also William Glenn Gray, *Germany's Cold War: The Global Campaign to Isolate East Germany, 1940-1969* (Chapel Hill, 2003).
29. Wolfgang Schwanitz, "Judenargwohn? Zum Israel-Bild in SED-Akten über arabische Länder (1948-1968)" in *Orient* 35/4 (1994): 646.
30. *Neues Deutschland*, 24 February 1965, cited in Peter Dittmar, "DDR und Israel (II): Ambivalenz einer Nicht-Beziehung," in *Deutschland Archiv* 10/8 (August 1977): 848–49.
31. SAPMO-BArch, DY-30, IV A 2/20/829, 70. In fact, the party split shortly thereafter over the harsh criticism by the Soviet bloc about Israel's nature and policies. A largely Jewish faction led by Moshe Sneh and Shmuel Mikunis broke with a mostly Arab faction led by Meir Vilner and Tawfik Toubi; the latter supported the Soviet bloc and its policies and took a highly critical view of Israel. For more on this and on the relations between the KPI and the SED, see Dittmar, "DDR und Israel (II)," 856–58.
32. SAPMO-BArch, DY-30, A 2/9.02/17, Informationsdienst, nr. 88, April 1965.
33. SAPMO-BArch, DY-30, IV A 2/15/306, Halbmonatsmeldungen Nr. 4/65, 12.3.65 and Nr. 5/65, 19 March 1965; DY-30, IV A 2/9.02/45, Argument der Woche, 15 March 1965.
34. Eschwege, *Fremd*, 106–7.
35. SAPMO-BArch, DY-30, IV A 2/9.02/55, "Dokumente zur Haltung der DDR gegenüber der aggressiven Politik des Staats Israel," 15 January 1967.
36. SAPMO-BArch, DY-30, J IV 2/2A/1228, Protokoll der Sitzung des Politbüros, 7 June 1967; DY-30, J IV 2/2A/1230, Protokoll der Sitzung des Politbüros, 13 June 1967.
37. SAPMO-BArch, DY-30, IV A 2/9.02/55, various telegrams (quote from FS-Telegramm), 15 June 1967.
38. Walter Ulbricht, *Antwort auf aktuelle Fragen* (Berlin, 1967).
39. Konrad Weiß, "'Du hast den Frieden frech ans Kreuz geschlagen...' Israelfeindschaft und Antisemitismus in der DDR," in *Deutschland und Israel. Solidarität in der Bewährung,* ed. Ralph Giordano (Gerlingen, 1993), 78–79.

40. SAPMO-BArch, DY-30, IV A 2/20/832, Fernschreiben-Telegramm, 7 June 1967 (plus other telegrams sent during the following days).
41. Dittmar, "DDR und Israel (II)," 850.
42. SAPMO-BArch, NL 4182, 1339, letter from Albert Norden to Werner Lamberz, 9 June 1967.
43. "*Das hat's bei uns nicht gegeben!*" *Antisemitismus in der DDR. Das Buch zur Ausstellung der Amadeu Antonio Stiftung* (Amadeu Antonio Stiftung, 2010), n.p.
44. "Dokumentation: Israel—Vorposten des internationalen Monopolkapitals" and "...dominieren die USA-Gruppen," *Neues Deutschland*, 15 June 1967, in SAPMO-BArch, DY-34, 7973.
45. SAPMO-BArch, DY-34, 7973.
46. Albert Norden organized the letter and signatures; a number of prominent citizens of Jewish background refused to sign. See Karin Hartwig, "Jüdische Kommunisten," 134–35.
47. SAPMO-BArch, DY-30, IV A 2/9.02/55, FS-Telegramm, 11 June 1967.
48. Peter Lorf, "Lange vorbereitet," *Neues Deutschland*, 12 June 1967, and Lothar Killmer, "Speerspitze gegen den Nahen Osten," *Neues Deutschland*, 10 June 1967, in SAPMO-BArch, DY-34, 7973.
49. Lothar Killmer, "Tarnkappe der Konzerne. Was steckt hinter Israels 'Sozialismus'?" *Neues Deutschland*, 11 June 1967, in SAPMO-BArch, DY-34, 7973.
50. Lothar Killmer, "Woraus erklären sich die militärischen Erfolge…?," *Neues Deutschland*, 15 June 1967, in SAPMO-BArch, DY-34, 7973.
51. SAPMO-BArch, DY-30, IV A/9.02/44, "Information über Berichte, Argumente und Probleme der Bevölkerung," 13 June 1967; DY-30, IV A 2/5/22, "4. Kurzinformation über die Stimmung der Bevölkerung zur Aggression Israels gegen die VAR und andere arabischen Staaten," 13 June 1967.
52. SAPMO-BArch, DY-30, IV A 2/5/22, "3. Kurzinformation über die Stimmung der Bevölkerung zur Aggression Israels gegen die VAR und andere arabischen Staaten," 7 June 1967.
53. SAPMO-BArch, DY-30, IV A 2/20/832, "Material for Aufklärung über die Hintergründe, Absichten und Ziele der imperialistischen Aggression," 7 June 1967.
54. SAPMO-BArch, DY-06, 4543, "Information über Meinungen zur imperialistischen Aggression Israels gegen die arabischen Staaten," 13 June 1967.
55. SAPMO-BArch, DY-34, 7973, "Referentenmaterial für das Auftreten in Gewerkschaftsversammlungen zur imperialistischen Aggression in Nahen Osten," 16 June 1967.
56. SAPMO-BArch, DY-30, J IV 2/2A/1228, Protokolle der Sitzung des Politbüros, 7 June 1967; DY-34, 7973, telegrams, "Referentenmaterial," and numerous "Informationen"; DY-30, IV A 2/5/22, "Information der BL [Bezirksleitung] Berlin über erste Stimmungen und Meinungen zur Aggression Israels gegen die VAR," 6 June 1967, and "3. Kurzinformation über die Stimmung der Bevölkerung zur Aggression Israels gegen die VAR," 7 June 1967; also see the telegrams in SAPMO-BArch, DY-30, 7973.
57. SAPMO-BArch, DY-6, 1028, "Sonderinformation über die Reaktion der Werktätigen zur Aggression Israels gegen die arabischen Staaten," 8 June 1967; "2. Sonderinformation über Stimmung und Meinungen zur Aggression Israels gegen die arabischen Staaten," 12 June 1967; SAPMO-BArch, DY-6, 4543, "Information über Meinungen zur imperialistischen Aggression Israels," 13 June 1967; also see the reports in SAPMO-BArch, DY-30, IV A 2/5/22 and IV A 2/9.02/44.

58. SAPMO-BArch, DY-6, 1028, "2. Sonderinformation über Stimmung und Meinungen zur Aggression Israels gegen die arabischen Staaten," 12 June 1967; SAPMO-BArch, DY-30, IV A 2/5/22, "1. Kurzinformation über die Stimmung der Bevölkerung zur Aggression Israels...," 5 June 1967.
59. SAPMO-BArch, DY-30, IV A 2/5/22, "Information der BL Berlin über erste Stimmungen und Meinungen zur Aggression Israels gegen die VAR," 6 June 1967.
60. SAPMO-BArch, DY-6, 1028, "Information über die Reaktion der Werktätigen auf die imperialistische Aggression der israelischen Regierung gegen die arabischen Staaten," 22 June 1967.
61. SAPMO-BArch, DY-30, IV A 2/5/22, "Information an die Mitglieder und Kandidaten des Politbüros," 14 June 1967; "Information der BL Berlin über erste Stimmungen und Meinungen zur Aggression Israels gegen die VAR," 6 June, 1967; DY-6, "Sonderinformation über Stimmung und Meinungen zur Aggression Israels gegen die arabischen Staaten," 12 June 1967.
62. SAPMO-BArch, DY-6, 1028, "Stimmungen und Meinungen zur Vorbereitung der Volkswahlen," 26 June 1967.
63. SAPMO-BArch, DY-30, IV A 2/5/22, "Information an die Mitglieder und Kandidaten des Politbüros," 14 June 1967.
64. SAPMO-BArch, DY-6, 1028, "Stimmung und Meinungen zur Vorbereitung der Volkswahlen," 26 June 1967.
65. SAPMO-BArch, DY-30, IV A 2/5/22, "Information der BL Berlin über erste Stimmungen und Meinungen zur Aggression Israels gegen die VAR," 6 June 1967; SAPMO-BArch, IV A 2/15/308 "Information zur Aggression des Staates Israel," 10 June 1967.
66. SAPMO-BArch, DY-30, IV A 2/15/308, Abteilung Organisation, Gruppe Parteiinformation, 7 June 67; SAPMO-BArch, DY-30, IV A 2/5/22, "Information der BL Berlin über erste Stimmungen und Meinungen zur Aggression Israels gegen die VAR," 6 June 1967; "2. Kurzinformation über die Stimmung der Bevölkerung zur Aggression Israels gegen die VAR," 6 June 1967; "3. Kurzinformation über die Stimmung der Bevölkerung zur Aggression Israels gegen die VAR," 7 June 1967; SAPMO-BArch, DY-6, 1028, "Sonderinformation über die Reaktion der Werktätigen zur Aggression Israels gegen die arabischen Staaten," 8 June 1967; "2. Sonderinformation über Stimmung und Meinungen zur Aggression Israels gegen die arabischen Staaten," 12 June 1967.
67. For more on the relationship between the Protestant church and Jews and Israel, see Irena Ostmeyer, *Zwischen Schuld und Sühne. Evangelische Kirche und Juden in der SBZ und DDR, 1945-1990* (Berlin, 2002).
68. SAPMO-BArch, DY-30, IV A 2/9.02/44, "Information über Berichte, Argumente und Probleme in der Bevölkerung," 13 June 1967; "Information über aktuelle Fragen, Argumente und Probleme der Bevölkerung," 22 June 1967; SAPMO-BArch, IV A 2/15/038, "2. Bericht über die Meinungsbildung zur israelischen Aggression gegen die arabischen Staaten," 8 June 1967; SAPMO-BArch, DY-6, 4543, "Information über Meinungen zur imperialistischen Aggression Israels gegen die arabischen Staaten," 13 June 1967.
69. SAPMO-BArch, DY-30, IV A 2/15/38, "Zweiter Bericht über die Meinungsbildung zur israelischen Aggression gegen die arabische Staaten," 8 June 1967.
70. SAPMO-BArch, DY-30, 2/5/22, "3. Kurzinformation über die Stimmung der Bevölkerung zur Aggression gegen die VAR und anderer arabischen Staaten," 7 June 1967, and "4. Kurzinformation über die Stimmung der Bevölkerung zur Aggression gegen die VAR und anderer arabischen Staaten," 13 June 1967.

71. SAPMO-BArch, DY-34, 7973, "Information;" SAPMO-BArch, DY-30, IV A 2/5/22, "Dritte Kurzinformation über die Stimmung der Bevölkerung zur Aggression Israels gegen die VAR."
72. SAPMO-BArch, DY-30 IV A 2/15/308, "2. Information zur Aggression des Staates Israel," 10 June 1967.
73. SAPMO-BArch, DY-30, IV A 2/15/38, "Zweiter Bericht über die Meinungsbildung zur israelischen Aggression gegen die arabische Staaten," 8 June 1967.
74. SAPMO-BArch, DY-30, IV A 2/5/22, "Information der BL Berlin über erste Stimmungen und Meinungen zur Aggression Israels gegen die VAR," 6 June 1967.
75. This formulation appears frequently. See, e.g., SAPMO-BArch, DY-34, 7973, Aktenvermerk, 14 June 1967; "Referentenmatierial für das Auftreten in Gewerkschaftsversammlungen zur imperialistischen Agression im Nahen Osten," 16 June 1967.
76. SAPMO-BArch, DY-30, IV A 2/9.02/44, "Information über Berichte, Argumente und Probleme der Bevölkerung," 13 June 1967.
77. SAPMO-BArch, DY-30, 5202.
78. Jens Gieseke, "Bevölkerungsstimmungen in der geschlossenen Gesellschaft. MfS-Berichte an die DDR-Führung in den 1960er- und 1970er-Jahren," in *Zeithistorische Forschungen/Studies in Contemporary History*, Online-Ausgabe, 5/2 (2008) (URL: http://www.zeithistorische-forschungen.de/16126041-Gieseke-2-2008) (accessed 29 June 2011); Andrew I. Port, *Conflict and Stability in the German Democratic Republic* (New York, 2007); see also Heinz Niemann, *Meinungsforschungforschung in der DDR. Die geheimen Berichte des Instituts für Meinungsforschung an das Politbüro der SED* (Cologne, 1993).
79. For a thoughtful overview of a similar issue with respect to the Nazi period, see Ian Kershaw, *Popular Opinion and Political Dissent in the Third Reich. Bavaria 1933-1945* (Oxford, 2005 [1983]), 5–10.
80. Timm, *Hammer*, 236–42 and 280–85.

CHAPTER 11

Humiliation as a Weapon within the Party
Fictional and Personal Accounts

PHIL LEASK

In its attempt to transform those living in the German Democratic Republic (GDR) into "East Germans," the Socialist Unity Party (SED) used a combination of force and more subtle means of persuasion. Though many aspects of this have already been extensively researched, the party's use of humiliation as a weapon to punish people directly, as well as to instill fear and ensure compliance, has so far been largely overlooked. Analyzing fictional and personal accounts, this essay considers the party's humiliation of its own members, not the everyday humiliation of ordinary people or the vast program of humiliation undertaken by the Ministry for State Security (MfS, or Stasi).[1] Victims of humiliation in the SED reacted with bewilderment, outrage, and a strong sense of injustice, but tended to blame individual functionaries or the remnants of Stalinism—not the party itself—for their plight. Only rarely was there a hint that the practice of humiliation might have been a result of the party's Leninist origins; even critical party members did not normally make this connection. They instead constructed in their minds the concept of an ideal party faithful to the utopian vision of Vladimir Ilich Lenin and refused to consider that the Leninist structures and practices of the actual party, themselves, might have made it impossible for that vision ever to be achieved.

Fiction, Personal Accounts, and "History"

Despite the pressure to conform to Socialist realism, the novels discussed in this essay portray in an imagined, carefully constructed form some of the many possible ways of living in the GDR. Literary historians stress that party requirements as well as censorship and self-censorship led to the production of books largely supportive of efforts to build socialism.[2] They argue that it is possible to understand aspects of the society from textual analysis and that this can make a contribution to the writing of GDR history.[3] To consider the way in which the texts present humiliation requires some sensitivity to political, historical, social, and generational contexts.[4] It also requires consideration of the narrative voice and the method of narration in order to identify the narrator's attitude toward the events or characters depicted.

Using a variety of examples from different time periods, certain patterns of humiliation emerge, which can then be compared with the patterns detected in personal accounts. Unless intended for publication, the latter did not necessarily have to adhere strictly to party requirements, but were still likely to be influenced by dominant attitudes toward literary form and content. Yet, as is the case with all such documents, they were not objective accounts. They included letters whose authors seem to have done little to structure or shape them, as well as ones apparently designed to achieve a particular result, and, finally, memoirs written in order to make sense of events retrospectively, to right wrongs, or to "set the record straight." Patterns can nevertheless be identified here as well. What is most striking is that fictional incidents of humiliation by the party not only closely resembled the similar stories related in personal accounts, but also extended and amplified them through their heightened capacity for interiority and metaphor, their different narrative techniques, and their determination to explore concerns that were considered taboo. This gave a broader significance to what was being recounted about humiliation.

A Brief Theory of Humiliation

In common usage, humiliation appears to mean much the same as embarrassment or shame or ignominy, while "being humbled" is also treated as akin to being humiliated. This reflects uncertainty over the nature of humiliation. For Gabriele Taylor and William Ian Miller, humiliation is an "emotion of self-assessment." Diane Trumbull refers to it as the "trauma of disrespect," while Evelin Lindner considers it the "nuclear bomb of the emotions," but also an act, a feeling, and a process.[5] What these and other definitions have in common is that they see power—and the connection between the use of power and the emotions that result from it—as central to humiliation.[6] It can help, therefore, to consider humiliation not as an emotion in itself, but rather as a specific exercise of power with predictable emotional consequences. This exercise of power causes a perceptible, often extreme change for the worse in the position of the victim and in the victim's feelings about himself and his relationship to the world.

Humiliation consistently involves a number of elements: the stripping of status in the eyes of others, rejection or exclusion, unpredictability or apparent arbitrariness, and a personal sense of injustice for which there is no remedy. In the texts considered in this essay, all of these elements of humiliation are present, even where German terms equivalent to humiliation (e.g., Demütigung or Beschämung) are not used.[7]

All of the elements of humiliation are connected. Arbitrary behavior in itself is not necessarily humiliation; for example, a law might be only sporadically, arbitrarily, or unpredictably enforced, but when it is enforced, those who are its "victims" are simply unlucky. They are not humiliated since they were always aware that power might be used legitimately against them. Humiliation takes place when arbitrary behavior involves a breach of law or of accepted norms, so that behavior—which was until then known to be acceptable—is suddenly redefined as unacceptable. Since the victim is powerless to save himself from what is being done and since no appeal or remedy is available, he feels a deep sense of injustice. Barrington Moore has suggested that this sense of injustice is probably universal, since "every human society does have a conception of unjust punishment and a specific way of deciding why the punishment is unjust"—such as when the punishment "violates a rule or norm accepted by those subject to the authority that inflicts the punishment."[8]

Except in minor cases, humiliation cannot be simply shrugged off. It is frequently experienced as traumatic, and its consequences can be extreme and long-lasting, perhaps even permanent. Humiliation commonly engenders in the victim rage, a longing for revenge, a desperate desire to belong once again, and a sense of impotence, sometimes leading to obsessive behavior, depression, and an inability to function as before. Humiliation is different from shame. Each involves the loss of status: shame for a wrong that has been committed, humiliation for a wrong done to oneself.[9] They are often connected, however, particularly when someone feels shame for having participated in humiliating someone else, or for having failed to intervene when humiliation was taking place. At the heart of these feelings is the perception that power has been used unjustly.

The Problem of Justice and Power

The humiliation of party members by the party was something of a paradox, since a commitment not to humiliate either those who had been defeated or one's political enemies was one of the GDR's founding principles.[10] For example, in a short story by Friedrich Wolf, "Siebzehn Brote" (Seventeen Pieces of Bread), the narrator, a German Communist in a Red Army propaganda unit near Stalingrad, makes it clear to his Soviet friends that the humiliation of his fellow Germans must be avoided. In accordance with the new morality of a future German workers' and farmers' state, and explicitly in the name of Lenin, fairness and dignity—not arbitrary punishment or the desire for revenge resulting from the earlier humiliation of the Red Army—must prevail. Only in this way can the cycle of humiliation, revenge, and further humiliation be broken.[11]

The challenge faced by the SED was to ensure respectful treatment of its political enemies while, at the same time, carrying out a revolution that lacked the support of much of the population. Article 6 of the 1949 East German Constitution reflected the tension between these two aims: while stating that "all citizens have equal rights before the law," it then defined a wide range of activities as criminal, such as incitement to boycott democratic institutions and organizations, as well as "all other activities directed against equal rights."[12] This gave officials great scope for arbitrarily redefining as contrary to the Constitution what would, in the West, have usually been considered ordinary democratic or social activities. In turn, this led to the imposition of humiliating punishments, including exclusion from participation in society. Those convicted under Article 6, which theoretically protected their democratic rights, lost the right to jobs in the public service, to hold higher positions in economic and cultural activities, to vote, or to stand for election.[13] The 1968 Constitution was even more explicit in its guarantees of rights and the respect for individual dignity that should have made humiliation by the party or state impossible.[14] But Article 1 also ensured a class-based approach to the conception and management of society, entrenched the power of the party over the state, and therefore excluded from the party and from full participation in society all who wished to see a different approach.[15]

The SED's understanding of the nature of power—and thus of justice—was class-based at its core. The purpose of the party, following Lenin's precepts, was to gain control of state power in the form of a dictatorship of the proletariat.[16] What Mike Dennis has called the "undoubted primacy of politics over law" followed logically from this position. Erich Mielke, the head of the Stasi, declared in 1979, "Power is the most important position from which to fulfill the historical mission of the working class, to establish Communist society ... Socialist law is an important instrument of exercising, enhancing and consolidating power."[17] There is a clear gap here between Marxist-Leninist ideology and John Rawls's theory of "justice as fairness." What Rawls called his "guiding idea" was that the principles of justice for a society arise from an imagined original agreement. These are the principles "that free and rational persons concerned to further their own interests would accept in an initial position of equality as defining the fundamental terms of their association.... This way of regarding the principles of justice I shall call justice as fairness."[18] In justice as fairness, no one knows the position or views or interests of the other members of society, so that the principles of justice "are chosen behind a veil of ignorance."[19] Rawls believed that this was the basis for bringing about the fairest possible and most equal distribution of goods (in the widest sense of the term) in a society. As Michael Sandel notes, "Rawls argues that distributive justice is not about rewarding virtue or moral desert. Instead, it's about meeting the legitimate expectations that arise once the rules of the game are in place."[20]

The "rules of the game" in the GDR were determined by the SED, but they implied a social contract arising out of the party's anti-fascist myth: in return for accepting party rule in an anti-capitalist society, the people would be washed clean of their Nazi-era sins and granted the benefits of living in a society based on equal dignity, equal responsibility, and equal opportunity.[21] For this to be effective, the people needed to have confidence in the new system of Socialist justice.

Sensing Injustice: Examples from the Texts

Fictional and personal representations of the GDR suggested that, on the one hand, ordinary people believed—without expressing it in such terms—that there was a commitment from both the party and the people to a Rawlsian view of justice as fairness and to the rules of the game following from it, and that, on the other hand, they saw these rules being arbitrarily broken by the SED. In line with Barrington Moore's theory, they apparently felt that their sense of what justice should mean in the specific circumstances of the GDR had universal applicability. When Peter Urack in Stefan Heym's *Collin* (1979)—a novel dealing with feelings of shame about complicity in the humiliation of party members during the show trials of the late 1950s—declares to his Stasi father that "coercion is coercion, injustice is injustice, then as now, in the West as here,"[22] he echoes what was also expressed in many East German memoirs and letters about the use of humiliation: the sense not only that people have suffered as a result of actions taken by the regime, but also that the power that had caused this suffering and stripped them of their status in their community or society had been used arbitrarily—in conflict with accepted norms and in a way that was both irresistible and unjust. The elder Urack, the senior Stasi officer in *Collin*, uses Marxist dialectics to define justice as that which maintains the power needed to build socialism: "Let's be clear: injustice is not simply injustice. It all depends on who's doing what and to what end."[23] He explicitly justifies the use of illegal acts by the state and regrets the subsequent rehabilitation of his political enemies: "It wasn't wrong that we wrongly arrested, charged, and convicted people. How could something be wrong that was done for the dictatorship of the proletariat?"[24]

In Monika Maron's *Flugasche* (Flying Ashes), a 1981 novel about the journalist Josefa Nadler's attempts to get East German authorities to close down a dangerously polluting power station, the protagonist's obsession with injustice is rooted in the humiliation of her grandparents under the Nazis.[25] Her obsession turns to rage as her struggle against injustice is blocked by those concerned with abstract concepts and a constantly postponed better future rather than with their stated commitment to justice and equal dignity in the present. She sees herself as the victim of injustice with no possibility of redress, and her sense of impotence leads her to a position of extreme mental instability. Excluded from the party, she can return to some sense of normality only by abandoning her fight and accepting defeat and a lower position in society, a classic trajectory for someone who has been humiliated. Christoph Hein's *Horns Ende* (The End of Horn), published in 1985, is the story of a long duel between the local party representative, Kruschkatz, and a politically disgraced historian, Horn, who finally kills himself rather than endure a second humiliation. As if commenting on Josefa Nadler's position, Kruschkatz, the party realist, asserts that there is no remedy available to Horn other than to accept what was done to him, declaring that justice requires the greater good of society, even if the innocent suffer: "After all, even the law isn't perfect. The most terrible sacrifice that the march of history demands is the death of the innocent. That is the toll in lives that progress costs."[26] Humiliation, Hein's narrator suggests throughout the novel, can involve literal death, but also a kind of death-in-life. Besides occasional direct and brutal interventions, a series of small and large acts, leading to apparently minor disappointments and frustrations, amount to a constant, deliberate, and humiliating thwarting of the full development of the personality, as well as to the undermining of a sense of individual worth and of the possibility of justice.

Of these three novels, all from the supposedly more liberal period under Erich Honecker in the 1970s and 1980s, two (*Collin* and *Flugasche*) were not published in the GDR. They portray concern among committed Socialists that the party was not abiding by its stated principles and that it was willing to use humiliation as one of its ways of holding on to power. The party reacted to this concern with great hostility and by committing acts of humiliation itself, including the stripping of Wolf Biermann's GDR citizenship in 1976 and the persecution of those who subsequently objected to this. *Horns Ende* and *Flugasche* suggest indirectly that humiliation in the GDR followed logically from the experience of humiliation as an exercise of power during the Nazi period, and that, as people "became" East Germans, there was historical continuity from the Nazi era to Walter Ulbricht and then Honecker—though they do not suggest, of course, that humiliation in the GDR was remotely on the scale of that of the Nazi period. Highly popular novels from the Ulbricht period, ostensibly supportive of the Socialist project, were also striking, as we shall see, for the number of examples of humiliation of SED members by the party itself.

Humiliation and Injustice in the "Bitterfeld" Novels

At the first so-called Bitterfeld Conference in 1959, held in a chemical complex in the Saxon-Anhalt town of Bitterfeld, the SED attempted to encourage writing by industrial and agricultural workers, as well as to impose further requirements on professional writers. The latter were expected to write about the work of building socialism, to be among the workers and write about their experiences, and to demonstrate, in line with the principles of Socialist realism, their commitment to the party and its aims.

In several of the "Bitterfeld" novels published in the 1960s, the main characters observe humiliation or are themselves the victims of it, while others live in fear of humiliation. Erik Neutsch's *Spur der Steine* (Traces in Stone), a novel set in an expanding chemical works, depicts the eventual conversion to the party of the charismatic but anarchistic construction worker, Hannes Balla, largely through the work of the dedicated party secretary, Werner Horrath. Less conventional is the depiction of Horrath himself, who becomes preoccupied with the party's tendency to act unjustly. Horrath is initially attacked for ignoring the sacred economic Plan in order to raise productivity instead. The party's view is that this was beneficial but contrary to the rules, and gives him a formal reprimand (*Rüge*).[27] This in itself should not have been felt as a form of humiliation, since Horrath accepts the party's rules. The ferocity of the attack and his own underlying sense of justice nevertheless make him feel that he has been humiliated.[28] Later he is savagely criticized at a party meeting for his excessive patience with Balla, leaving him in a state of impotent fury at the apparent injustice. The whispered words of another party member highlight both the ordinariness of the party's use of humiliation, as well as the fear that it engenders: "Don't take it to heart—that was really nothing. Last time the mayor was down on his knees, howling his head off..."[29] It is Horrath's adulterous relationship with the young engineer, Kati Klee, that causes his eventual downfall. Accepting that the party has the right to quiz its members about their moral standards, he effectively lies to the party by not admitting he is the father of Klee's child and by ensuring that the party's hostility is directed toward her, not him. Feeling great shame for this, he later sees that it was wrong for the party to judge the relationship between them since love is not a collective matter and cannot be a moral failing.[30] He has nonetheless lied to the party and, when this is revealed, he is stripped of his position by the pitiless Heinz Bleibtreu, his eventual successor, who asserts the party line on justice and correct behavior: "Every moral weakness, my friend, ... serves as a target for the class enemy.... Clean and honest living are indispensible for the hardened cohorts of the revolution."[31] Horrath becomes an ordinary building worker, but is punished again after interfering in the name of justice to countermand Bleibtreu's destructive instructions. His ejection from the site by Bleibtreu offers a clear example of the type of excessive, unreasonable punishment designed to reduce Horrath and other "offenders" to the status of an outcast—an act of humiliation carried out, of course, by someone imbued with an unshakeable, unquestioning loyalty to the party.[32]

Initiation, Humiliation, and Hierarchy

An important way of inculcating loyalty to the party was through the ritualized process of initiating party members, particularly those likely to become leading functionaries. This was significant because initiation rituals frequently have a clear and dangerous purpose: to transmit both the capacity and the desire to humiliate. The person who appears to be accepted after the initiation is, in fact, a "lesser" member in the established hierarchy and power structure, and is prone to sense that the power of those above him might be arbitrarily used against him. His membership depends on having been humiliated, on the fear of further humiliation, and on being prepared to prove himself by humiliating those who come after him.[33] This is likely to establish a sense of mutual support or solidarity, as in an army or in a Marxist-Leninist party, where the initiate is welcomed into a brotherhood of the excluded or self-excluded, who see themselves as different from, not part of, "ordinary" society, and as living by different rules.

In the 1920s, 1930s, and 1940s, Communists from outside the Soviet Union were trained to be active revolutionaries under conditions of illegality and extreme danger. Their commitment to the party and its aims was required to be absolute; personal interests and relationships were seen to be secondary at best—and dangerous at worst. Though this approach was made even more rigorous under Josef Stalin, it grew out of the experience of the Bolsheviks under Lenin: above all their need to survive prior to the revolution, and then to win the civil war and ensure the survival of the new Soviet Union. This emotional and physical commitment to the party, as well as the willingness to accept torture and brutality as facts of life, are graphically spelled out in Willi Bredel's *Die Prüfung* (The Test) of 1934, Anna Seghers's *Das siebte Kreuz* (The Seventh Cross, 1946), and Bodo Uhse's 1954 novel *Die Patrioten* (The Patriots).[34]

Wolfgang Leonhard's memoir *Die Revolution entlässt ihre Kinder* (Child of the Revolution) is part of an ongoing argument that the author, a former high-level party functionary who fled the GDR for his own safety, attempts to have with his comrades back in the GDR.[35] His aim is to denounce Stalinism and praise Yugoslavia's alternative approach to socialism. This inevitably affects his interpretation of events, but the memoir is still useful because Leonhard does not identify the party's use of humiliation as such as problematic. Describing his time at the Comintern school in a remote location in the Soviet Union in

1942 and 1943, Leonhard shows how the party initiated its future functionaries in a way that both humiliated and rewarded them so that they were ready to repeat this exercise of power themselves over those beneath them in the carefully established party hierarchy. The process involved eliminating a sense of personal closeness, trust, and integrity; inculcating a willingness to act ruthlessly against perceived enemies, including friends and family; and developing a commitment to follow the party line absolutely and to change one's views immediately and unquestioningly whenever the party demanded it.[36]

The initiation was required to be a painful process involving criticism and self-criticism, a Leninist technique widely used by Communist parties to subjugate their members.[37] Leonard describes his first, unexpected "self-criticism" as a brutal experience in which he was relentlessly attacked without knowing why, in the manner of the Inquisition. His response was to deny the horror of the humiliation and reduce the pain of it by identifying, in part, with the values and views of the humiliator, leading him to feel guilt and shame for what he had seen as entirely innocent actions or comments during his time up to then at the Comintern school.[38] He sensed that he had become permanently changed by the process of "self-criticism" and that his integrity had been compromised: "How could we be honest when every innocent word, 'objectively considered', was taken to be a hostile remark?"[39] A similar act of power was used against each of his fellow students; they became no longer cheerful and enthusiastic, but instead earnest, wary of one another, and watchful of every word.

The initiation of party members is central to Stefan Heym's *Die Architekten* (The Architects), a novel published in 2000 but written during the early 1960s about the personal and political consequences of the compromises that exiled German Communists had made in the Soviet Union in the 1930s and 1940s. Arnold Sundstrom, a top GDR architect, is a loyal Communist who reshapes his behavior at any time according to the wishes of the party. Over the years, Sundstrom has carefully and methodically initiated Julia, the daughter of a German Communist who had been a victim of Stalin (thanks, in part, to Sundstrom), to believe implicitly in the party and in Stalin. The process of political initiation also involved child abuse and sexual abuse, something that Julia eventually recognizes as humiliating. In fact, Sundstrom has groomed Julia not just for the party but also for himself, so that the compliant "daughter" becomes the obedient wife, for whom the process of initiation has to continue: "training a young person to think correctly was a never-ending task."[40]

In Maron's *Flugasche*, Josefa Nadler is persecuted by her boss Siegfried Strutzer, whose unswerving commitment to the party line, as well as his willingness to humiliate, follow directly from his humiliation as a boy in a boarding school, where he was subjected to initiation rituals and sexual abuse. When asked why he did not run away, Strutzer makes it clear that he enjoys the power that humiliating initiation rituals provide him with: "He had felt it to be okay,

Strutzer had replied. His sense of justice was not disturbed by it. Later, when he had become one of the bigger students, he, too, had put shoe polish on the genitals of the smaller ones."[41] Josefa sees the connection between this and the way in which the party initiates its members: "Strutzer had studied. Strutzer had been at the party school. Strutzer had never again shown an interest in a girl whom someone higher than he had his eye on. He could distinguish with certainty who was higher and who was lower. At the *Illustrated Weekly*, Strutzer belonged to the higher ones."[42] Because the party hierarchy is clearly established, Josefa, a more junior member, will always be treated as such by Strutzer.

Humiliation and Inner-party Discipline

Once loyalty to the party was established through the initiation, education, and training of individual members, internal disciplinary practices ensured it was maintained. One of these was "democratic centralism," a process attributed to Lenin, whereby decisions made at the top filtered down through the ranks of the party and required everyone to implement every decision.[43] In principle, those occupying the highest echelons were accountable to and periodically elected by delegates from lower levels, and their decisions were supposed to take into account the wishes of those below.[44] In East German novels and personal accounts, democratic centralism is usually portrayed as a process in which the decisions are made at the top and passed down—without taking into account the opinion of lower functionaries or the rank-and-file and without providing adequate explanation. A sense of vulnerability is, as a result, ever present among lower party officials. They fear that they will be blamed and humiliated for not doing what they should be doing, but also for doing something they were instructed to do—but that is suddenly no longer official party policy.

In Erwin Strittmatter's *Ole Bienkopp*, a 1963 Bitterfeld novel about the early years of the agricultural cooperatives, the protagonist for whom the novel is named is humiliated by his class enemies, as well as by his class allies, while other important characters also suffer from, or are complicit in, acts of humiliation.[45] For instance, the local party secretary, Jan Bullert, is a victim of his failure to understand the subtleties of democratic centralism. After participating in the exclusion of Ole from the party for having formed a cooperative in contravention of party policy, Bullert attends the party Conference with a mandate to criticize such initiatives. He enthusiastically tells Herbert Wunschgetreu, the SED District Secretary, about his planned speech—only to encounter the unpredictability of those above him: "Wunschgetreu gave a slight smile: the world moves on; what was wrong yesterday can be right tomorrow."[46] Hearing the conference speakers eagerly embrace the concept of the agricultural cooperative he was primed to condemn, Bullert rushes out in confusion, realizing that he was about to be utterly humiliated.[47] Wunschgetreu subsequently praises Bienkopp and distances himself from the earlier decision to expel him. He proceeds to punish Bullert for the speech he had prepared, and humiliates him by removing him from his party post. Elsewhere in the novel, Wunschgetreu and the lower party functionary Willi Kraushaar are portrayed as anxious and almost paralyzed by the need to satisfy the unpredictable wishes of those above them in the party hierarchy.[48] For Wunschgetreu, this is associated with shame for his part in the humiliation and early death of one of the party's heroic figures, who was called to task for having supposedly criticized the Soviet Union.[49]

Party discipline required members to abide absolutely by the Party Statute, or rule book, which made them fear humiliation for having infringed the rules—even inadvertently. One technique party officials used to ensure discipline was to write ostentatiously in a black notebook when a party member was doing or saying something. This instilled a fear of humiliation and possible sanctions, and frequently paralyzed the individual concerned, who did not know what he or she was doing that might be wrong. Wunschgetreu and the new local party secretary Frieda Simson both realize this. For Simson the black notebook is a symbol and a source of her power, and she is happy to use it for her own benefit. Wunschgetreu, for his part, comes to see it as representing a particularly malevolent way of exerting power within the party—one that makes him doubt whether the party is indeed "always right" and that causes further shame about the part he plays in humiliating fellow members.[50]

Irreconcilable Contradictions: The "Ideal" versus the "Real" Party

Even when SED members, such as the fictional Horrath, Nadler, and Wunschgetreu, started to suspect that the party might not always be right and that humiliation might be lying in wait for them should they make mistakes, the texts considered here suggest that most remained loyal. Since the fear of humiliation is, above all, the fear of rejection and exclusion, of a life-changing event that is not of one's own choosing and cannot be reversed, particularly dedicated members dreaded most the ultimate sanction: the exclusion from, and thus loss of connection to, the party. When members could no longer deny the party's faults and shortcomings, they tended to idealize aspects of the SED and sought to realize this idealized version—while not entirely rejecting the actual version of the party. The imagined "ideal" party was the source and protector of the utopian vision originally formulated by Marx and Engels and then brought within reach by Lenin. The real party, with its links to the Soviet Communist Party, was the gatekeeper to Lenin and to the practical realization of that vision. While the real party could exist without the ideal party, the reverse was not true. This was what made it so hard for those who believed in the vision to reject the party root and branch—and what made the fear of exclusion so powerful. Discussing the biographies of veteran Communists and the "fundamental dynamic" between these members and the party leadership, Catherine Epstein concludes that the KPD/SED "ruthlessly exploited its most committed followers, who in turn willingly sacrificed their personal interests for the supposed good of the party."[51]

Joachim Goellner, who was born in 1926, provides an example of a minor SED functionary with an unshakeable belief in the ideal party. His autobiography, which revolves around three acts of humiliation, clearly reveals his sense of injustice at being rejected by the party.[52] Writing in the late 1990s, he displays continuing enthusiasm for Marxism-Leninism, hatred for "Stalinism," and rage at his treatment by the SED. The account is highly subjective, of course, and retrospectively applies his later view of Stalin to earlier events. Nevertheless, since he was not always aware of what was being done to him and its implications, his autobiography provides a powerful case study of the uses and consequences of humiliation, from the earliest to the last days of the GDR. Appended to the memoir are copies of correspondence with people in power, which demonstrate the devastating psychological impact of what he endured.

Goellner "converted" during his time in a Soviet prisoner of war camp, joined the SED upon his return to Germany, and worked in the shipbuilding industry in Rostock. By 1953 he was the party functionary responsible for cultural activities in the shipyards, but had become increasingly anti-Stalinist.[53] His first humiliation arose not from political differences, but from what the party called morally unacceptable behavior: in 1961 he divorced his wife and married a much younger woman, who was pregnant. The party organization, keen to demonstrate its commitment to Ulbricht's Ten Commandments of Socialist Morality, gave him a severe reprimand (*strenge Rüge*), stripped him of his position in the SED, and sent him to perform hard physical work in primitive conditions on the shop floor, which temporarily crippled his right arm. Though Goellner tried to believe that he had not been treated badly, he reveals his anger at his humiliation when complaining that he had been "'hurled back down' into the proletariat." He describes his working conditions as "slavery within 'modern' socialism" while criticizing hypocrisy within the party, since "higher state and party functionaries often got their secretaries pregnant."[54]

Dorothee Wierling notes that for party members from the generation of the "1929ers" (which included Goellner), the SED functioned well into the 1960s as the primary "disciplinary institution of setting the rules, sanctioning all transgressions, and granting or denying forgiveness and community."[55] Andrew Port's study of adultery in the early years of the GDR confirms the gap between theory and practice that so outraged Goellner. The party embraced a strong line on "moral infractions," and its members had to account for their behavior at special meetings of the SED factory committee: often assuming an air of moral superiority, the interrogators posed surprisingly lurid and intrusive questions, delving into the most personal areas of the man's private life. Such queries were generally accompanied by a lecture admonishing the profligate for not "finding his way" to the party for support, and, more seriously, for damaging the reputation of the SED in the eyes of the masses.[56]

Punishments involved what would, in other circumstances, be seen as humiliation: "official party sanction, the cancellation of political or professional training, removal from positions of responsibility, and, in the case of white-collar workers, delegation to the shop floor were all customary."[57] Apparently paradoxically, it was the attitude of the party member himself that determined whether such treatment amounted to humiliation. In cases where the member's commitment to the party included an unconditional acceptance of the party's right to define the way he should lead his private life and according to which moral standards, the breaching of those standards and a sense of letting down the party was a source of shame. Where there was no such acceptance, the party was seen as interfering inadmissibly in one's private affairs, and any punishment was felt as humiliation. The same applied in cases where the punishment was felt to be disproportionate, or where higher SED officials supposedly acted similarly without being punished.

Goellner's second humiliation in 1976 was more clearly political in nature. Again in a party post but "increasingly conscious of the contradiction between Marxist-Leninist theory and GDR practice," he was critical of a theatrical production by someone higher up in the party who interpreted the criticism as a contravention of the requirements of party discipline and democratic centralism.[58] After being dismissed, he slipped into apathy and depression, but—despite feeling a strong sense of injustice—retained his faith in the ideals of socialism: "I don't call the socialism of Marx and Lenin into question, rather the way it is being implemented, which, by now, is turning against the old masters themselves."[59]

In 1979, back in his old job in the shipyards, he became more dissatisfied and embittered, and started drinking heavily. After leaving his wife (who attempted suicide), he got another party job in Rostock, with a "Stalinist" boss.[60] Over the years, the cumulative effects of his humiliation and his responses to humiliation (anger, depression, loss of empathy for others, alcohol dependency) resulted in serious mental problems and led to another episode of humiliation, one that he provoked himself. At a function in Berlin, he tried to force his way through a security cordon to talk to the party leaders, claiming to be their equal and therefore to be entitled to mix with them. After being summoned to appear before the party, he was then excluded from it. Goellner knew that his behavior was self-destructive, but sensed that it was because of the way he had been treated over the years.⁶¹ He continued to suffer from depression and apathy. Family tragedies then ensued: his favorite son tried to cross into Poland to reach the West German Embassy to flee to the Federal Republic, but was arrested, imprisoned, and then expelled to the West.

Goellner, sensing that his son was deeply depressed, made many unsuccessful requests to be allowed to visit him. After his son committed suicide in 1987, Goellner became seriously mentally ill himself. Several documents and letters archived along with his account give a clear idea of his condition. In a "Statement to the Stasi," he admitted that he tried twice to commit suicide, in December 1987 and July 1988.⁶² Consumed by impotent rage, a common consequence of humiliation, he was desperate to turn things back to the way they ought to have been, wanting everything to have been different, wanting his son not to have killed himself, wanting the authorities to have allowed him to visit his son, wanting the GDR not to have treated people the way it did. Pushing for change in the GDR, he wrote letters constantly: to Erich Honecker; the editor of *Neues Deutschland*; Hans-Joachim Vogel, the leader of the SPD faction in the West German Bundestag; the SED Central Committee; as well as the editor of *Sputnik* in Moscow—a Soviet magazine banned in November 1988 in the GDR because of its critical articles inspired by Mikhail Gorbachev's reform policies.

After the *Wende*, Goellner, still a believer in Marxism-Leninism, raged against both the new society and the old. He was particularly angry at the thought that those who had persecuted him in the past were again in positions of power and supposedly still persecuting him.⁶³ With his faith in the "ideal" party intact, however, he declared that socialism was the blueprint for society that most persuasively offered the prospect of a dignified life for all people in all parts of the world, now and in the future.⁶⁴

Joachim Goellner's account provides a striking example of the humiliation of someone representative of a typical subgroup in the party: the postwar "convert" (like the fictional Wunschgetreu) who became a minor party functionary with absolute loyalty to and an unshakeable belief in the "ideal" party. As a prisoner of war, Goellner claimed to have learned from direct experience with the Soviet people the importance of not seeking revenge or humiliating one's defeated enemies. This made his subsequent humiliation by the party to which he had devoted himself all the more poignant. Goellner was the victim of arbitrary and vindictive action that conflicted with the norms and values to which he believed he and the party were committed. His frustration over his rejection by the party carried with it a deep sense of injustice and an awareness that he could do nothing to counter the way in which power was being used against him. Indeed, his naive attempt to speak to party leaders underscored the extent to which the actions of the party had undermined his own mental stability. The postwar convert nevertheless remained loyal to the end—to the "ideal" party, however, not to the incarnation of the party that had repeatedly humiliated him.

A Prophecy of Doom: *Ole Bienkopp*'s Critique of Lenin

Like fictional supporters of the "ideal" as opposed to the "real" party (Josefa Nadler in *Flugasche*, Horrath and Klee in *Spur der Steine*, the persecuted Havelka in *Collin*), Goellner blamed the Stalinization of the party for its failure to live up to its ideals. A rare alternative critique is presented in Strittmatter's *Ole Bienkopp*. In this case, the way in which examples of the party's humiliation of its own members are presented (e.g., with comments by the narrator) amounts to an attack on key structures and core beliefs that go back to Lenin. In other words, the narrator's critique implies that the Leninist party as such might be fatally flawed since it contains elements that are irremediably destructive and self-destructive. These include the inevitable misuse of power arising from democratic centralism, the humiliating demand for self-criticism, and the use of humiliation more generally as a central feature of party discipline. But the narrator also implies that the path to socialism remains the only morally proper way forward for society, and that socialism can only be achieved through the party. Once again, the inherent contradiction is apparently resolved by a belief in the ideal party—which pursues Lenin's vision while rejecting some of the more questionable methods Lenin introduced. Several characters convey this idea, most notably Anton Dürr: tireless, incorruptible, utopian, and passionately committed to achieving the ends he supports without using means that make their achievement impossible. Anton is a substitute Lenin figure for the party in the village, able to do no wrong and always a point of reference for what is right, even after his death. Ole Bienkopp becomes his equally idealistic but more fallible successor. Significantly, the representatives of the ideal party *both* die. Anton is killed by an external enemy; Ole, the utopian humiliatingly defined twice as an internal enemy, dies because of actions by Frieda Simson, the representative of the "real" party.

The voice of the narrator is significant here, commenting sometimes ironically, sometimes intrusively, sometimes portentously, but also positively about the chaotic and mismanaged efforts to build socialism. The narrator reaches out to embrace the readers with a comforting voice that not only retains a clear sense of a grander vision, but also expresses sorrow at the way in which the party's representatives disconnect themselves and the SED from the full, generous, pleasurable life that the party should be promoting. As "comrades," the narrator suggests, the readers will share the position of superiority he has adopted over the characters and his commitment to the ideals that guide the best of them. The narrator also assumes that the readers are, like him, believers in the ideal party, declaring that this imposes a responsibility to ensure that rigid functionaries are not the ones who ultimately control the SED. But he gives no hint of how to resolve the contradiction between the ideal vision and the current strategy for achieving it: the remorseless use of power based on Leninist principles, most particularly "democratic centralism" and the "dictatorship of the proletariat."

It can be inferred from *Ole Bienkopp* that the party's need to humiliate its perceived internal enemies arises from its fear that what is being argued by even the SED's most benign critics represents a serious challenge to the very existence of the Leninist party.[65] This is a pessimistic prophecy: the party cannot achieve what it is, in principle, aiming to achieve, and cannot, by its very nature, be reformed.[66] Members who retain their utopian Socialist vision and believe that only the party can achieve it will be dispensed with by the party while it still has the power to do so, or will be seen as irrelevant to further political struggles once the Leninist principles are eventually discarded. This prophecy was ultimately validated by a number of events: the undermining of Communist control in the Soviet Union following Gorbachev's abandonment of key Leninist tenets in the late 1980s; the SED's refusal to follow Gorbachev because it understood that, shorn of its Leninist character, the party would collapse; the call from prominent GDR intellectuals in 1989 for continuing efforts to build the ideal party's version of socialism; and, finally, the disappearance of the political structures and support that, they believed, might have made this possible.[67]

Conclusion

The texts considered here suggest that the party consciously used humiliation as a weapon against its own members to secure their loyalty and to ensure that party loyalty took precedence over other values in their lives, such as loyalty to family and friends, or their commitment to dignity, respect, and fairness. The texts also suggest that party members retained a sense of justice, which conflicted with the party leadership's view that whatever was necessary to maintain the dictatorship of the proletariat was, by definition, just. The unpredictable, apparently arbitrary behavior of the leadership sometimes paralyzed SED functionaries, for whom the fear of humiliation was a fear of rejection and exclusion by the party. When action was taken against them for their supposed errors, they felt this was unjust, but were powerless to resist—and were subsequently consumed by impotent rage at their humiliation. The response to this—a belief in an "ideal" party, i.e., a more perfect form of the "real existing" party—did not help them to look closely at their beliefs or at the basis of the party's actions, i.e., the Leninist principles and practices that were designed to ensure the party could seize and hold power, but that did not set out a practical route for achieving the supposedly more humane ideals of Karl Marx and Friedrich Engels. The supporters of the ideal party wanted to bring about the socialization of the means of production through the support and cooperation of ordinary people—not through the "real" party's dictatorship of the proletariat. They preferred discussion to administrative measures that prevented or punished the expression of alternative views. Instead of democratic centralism, they wanted real democracy within the party that guaranteed the rights of all members—with loyalty being a two-way street.[68] They nevertheless continued to see the SED as the only instrument to achieve their ideals, and had no strategy to resolve the contradiction between their desires and the reality of the party's everyday practices. Even attempting to devise such an alternative would have prompted serious questions about whether the party's use of power had become an end in itself. Apart from any painful personal and social consequences, this left potential opponents of the leadership intellectually and politically incapacitated. Humiliation was thus an effective weapon, but one that ruled out both the option of internal party renewal *and* the possibility of state power being used to find a different path to socialism.

Suggested Readings

Emmerich, Wolfgang. *Kleine Literaturgeschichte der DDR*. Leipzig, 1996.
Engelmann, Roger and Clemens Vollnhals, eds. *Justiz im Dienst der Parteiherrschaft. Rechtspraxis und Staatssicherheit in der DDR*. Berlin, 1999.
Glaeser, Andreas, *Political Epistemics. The Secret Police, the Opposition, and the End of East German Socialism*. Chicago, 2011.
Just, Gustav. *Zeuge in eigener Sache. Die fünfziger Jahre in der DDR*. Frankfurt am Main, 1990.
Leonhard, Wolfgang. *Die Revolution entlässt ihre Kinder*. Cologne, 1962.
Loest, Erich. *Durch die Erde ein Riß. Ein Lebenslauf*. Leipzig, 1981.
Lokatis, Siegfried. *Der Rote Faden. Kommunistische Parteigeschichte und Zensur unter Walter Ulbricht*. Cologne, 2003.
Margalit, Avishai. *The Decent Society*. Trans. Naomi Goldblum. Cambridge, M.A., 1996.
Moore, Barrington, Jr. *Injustice: The Social Bases of Obedience and Revolt*. London, 1978.
Rawls, John. *A Theory of Justice*. London, 1973.
Rorty, Richard. *Contingency, Irony and Solidarity*. Cambridge, 1989.
Sandel, Michael J. *Justice: What's the Right Thing to Do?* London, 2009.
Taylor, Gabriele. *Pride, Shame and Guilt. Emotions of Self-assessment*. Oxford, 1985.
Weber, Hermann, *Die DDR 1945-1990*, 3rd ed. Munich, 2000.

Notes

1. For an extended discussion of these accounts, see Phil Leask, *Power, the Party and the People: The Significance of Humiliation in Representations of the German Democratic Republic* (Ph.D. thesis, University College London, 2012).

2. See, e.g., Simone Barck, Martina Langermann, and Siegfried Lokatis, eds., *"Jedes Buch ein Abenteuer."* Zensur-System und literarische Öffentlichkeit in der DDR bis Ende der sechziger Jahre (Berlin, 1998); Siegfried Lokatis, *Der Rote Faden. Kommunistische Parteigeschichte und Zensur unter Walter Ulbricht* (Cologne, 2003); for a satirical view, see Volker Braun, *Hinze-Kunze-Roman* (Frankfurt am Main, 1988), 147–50.
3. Peter Uwe Hohendahl and Patricia Herminghouse, eds., *Literatur und Literaturtheorie in der DDR* (Frankfurt am Main, 1976), 8–9; Wolfgang Emmerich, *Kleine Literaturgeschichte der DDR* (Leipzig, 1996), 17–20.
4. Catherine Epstein, *The Last Revolutionaries: German Communists and Their Century* (Cambridge, M.A., 2003), 212. Mary Fulbrook and Dorothee Wierling point to the significance of the "1929ers." Many of the party members considered in this essay belonged to that generation. They saw the SED as a new protector, but always had to prove their loyalty. See Dorothee Wierling, "How Do the 1929ers and the 1949ers Differ?" in *Power and Society in the GDR, 1961-1979. The "Normalisation of Rule"?* ed. Mary Fulbrook (New York and Oxford, 2009), 207–8; Mary Fulbrook, *Dissonant Lives: Generations and Violence through the German Dictatorships* (Oxford, 2011).
5. Gabriele Taylor, *Pride, Shame and Guilt: Emotions of Self-assessment* (Oxford, 1985), 1; William Ian Miller, *Humiliation, and other Essays on Honor, Social Discomfort, and Violence* (Ithaca, N.Y., and London, 1993), x; Diane W. Trumbull, "Humiliation: The Trauma of Disrespect," *Journal of the American Academy of Psychoanalysis and Dynamic Psychiatry* 36/4 (2008): 643–60; Evelin Lindner, *Making Enemies: Humiliation and International Conflict* (Westport, C.T. and London, 2006), xiii, 19.
6. See, e.g., Richard Rorty, *Contingency, Irony and Solidarity* (Cambridge, 1989), 89–92.
7. It was often a whole set of actions that added up to humiliation. Christoph Hein was an exception in often using the word *Demütigung*. See his novels *Der fremde Freund* (Berlin and Weimar, 1982), 14; *Horns Ende* (Berlin and Weimar, 1985), 66; *Der Tangospieler* (Frankfurt am Main, 1989), 131, 203. Even here, key events revealed to be acts of humiliation are not explicitly described as such.
8. Barrington Moore, Jr., *Injustice: The Social Bases of Obedience and Revolt* (London, 1978), 31.
9. See Linda M. Hartling and Tracy Luchetta, "Humiliation: Assessing the Impact of Derision, Degradation and Debasement," *The Journal of Primary Prevention* 19/4 (1996): 262–63; Virginia Held, "Terrorism and War," *The Journal of Ethics* 8/1 (2004): 75.
10. This is a theme in classic texts such as Anna Seghers, *Das Siebte Kreuz* (Amsterdam, 1946); Willi Bredel, *Die Prüfung* (Berlin and Weimar, 1981).
11. Friedrich Wolf, "Siebzehn Brote," in *Erzähler der DDR*, vol. 1 (Berlin and Weimar, 1985), 9–15.
12. Hermann Weber, *Dokumente zur Geschichte der Deutschen Demokratischen Republik 1945-1985* (Munich, 1986), 158.
13. Ibid.
14. See, e.g., Articles 19 and 20 in ibid., 300.
15. Ibid., 299.
16. See the entry "marxistisch-leninistische Partei" in Kollektiv von Mitarbeitern des Dietz Verlages, ed., *Kleines politisches Wörterbuch* (Berlin, 1973), 515–18.
17. Mike Dennis, *The Stasi: Myth and Reality* (Harlow, 2003), 61.
18. John Rawls, *A Theory of Justice* (London; Oxford; New York, 1973), 11.
19. Ibid., 12.
20. Michael J. Sandel, *Justice: What's the Right Thing to Do?* (London, 2009), 161.

21. Alan L. Nothnagle, *Building Mythology and Youth Propaganda in the German Democratic Republic, 1945-1989* (Ann Arbor, 1999), 101–2; Antonia Grunenberg, *Antifaschismus—Ein deutscher Mythos* (Reinbek, 1993), 132.
22. Stefan Heym, *Collin* (Munich, 1979), 97.
23. Ibid., 98.
24. Ibid., 234.
25. Monika Maron, *Flugasche* (Frankfurt am Main, 1981).
26. Hein, *Horns Ende*, 73.
27. Erik Neutsch, *Spur der Steine* (Halle, 1966), 165.
28. Ibid., 173–74.
29. Ibid., 230.
30. Ibid., 530.
31. Ibid., 872.
32. Ibid., 903.
33. See the discussion of these processes and their long-term consequences in Pierre Clastres, *La Société contre l'État. Recherches d'Anthropologie Politique* (Paris, 1974), 156–58; Avishai Margalit, *The Decent Society*, trans. Naomi Goldblum (Cambridge, M.A., and London, 1996), 195–96; Leask, "Power, the Party, and the People," 43–44, 203–9.
34. Bodo Uhse, *Die Patrioten* (Berlin, 1955).
35. Wolfgang Leonhard, *Die Revolution entlässt ihre Kinder* (Cologne and Berlin, 1962).
36. Leonhard, *Revolution*, 199; also see the self-examination of the old Bolshevik Rubashov in Arthur Koestler, *Darkness at Noon* (London, 1980) and the interviews in Lutz Niethammer, Alexander von Plato, and Dorothee Wierling, *Die volkseigne Erfahrung. Eine Archäologie des Lebens in der Industrieprovinz der DDR* (Berlin, 1991), e.g., 585–86.
37. Weber, *Dokumente*, 189; *Kleines Politisches Wörterbuch*, 773.
38. Leonhard, *Revolution*, 226–29.
39. Ibid., 229.
40. Stefan Heym, *Die Architekten* (Munich, 2000), 79.
41. Maron, *Flugasche*, 118.
42. Ibid., 119.
43. Institute of Marxism-Leninism, Central Committee of the CPSU, "Preface," in V.I. Lenin, *Selected Works*, vol. 1 (Moscow, 1970), 16; *Kleines politisches Wörterbuch*, 149.
44. *Kleines politisches Wörterbuch*, 148–50.
45. Erwin Strittmatter, *Ole Bienkopp* (Berlin and Weimar, 1965).
46. Ibid., 231.
47. Ibid.
48. See, e.g., Ibid., 320, 330–32, 342–43.
49. Ibid., 328–29.
50. Ibid., 329–30.
51. Epstein, 212.
52. Joachim Goellner, *Autobiographie*. "Die wundersame Reise des Odysseus des XX. Jahrhunderts." For the original typed manuscript, with personal photos and documents, see Kempowski Biografienarchiv Berlin 6860/1.
53. Ibid., 76.
54. Ibid., 91, 93.
55. Wierling, 207.
56. Andrew I. Port, "Love, Lust, and Lies under Communism: Family Values and Adulterous Liaisons in Early East Germany," *Central European History* 44 (2011): 484.

57. Port, "Love, Lust, and Lies," 485.
58. Goellner, 107.
59. Ibid.
60. Ibid., 113.
61. Ibid., 116.
62. Kempowski Biografienarchiv 6860/2, Joachim Goellner, *Dokumente*, "Stellungnahme an Stasi," 29 August 1988.
63. Kempowski Biografienarchiv 6860/1, Goellner to Judge Lange (Amtsgericht Rostock), 8 July 2003.
64. Kempowski Biografienarchiv 6860/1, Goellner, 165.
65. Among the many critical responses to *Ole Bienkopp*, only one suggested that the novel pointed to a contradiction between original Marxist ideals and the actions of the party in practice: Inge v. Wangeheim, *Die Geschichte und unsere Geschichten* (Halle, 1966), 77, quoted in Reinhard Hillich, "Aufforderung zum Mitdenken. Erwin Strittmatters Roman 'Ole Bienkopp,'" in *Werke und Wirkungen. DDR-Literatur in der Diskussion*, ed. Inge Münz-Koenen (Leipzig, 1987), 100.
66. Sigrid Meuschel makes this argument in *Legitimation und Parteiherrschaft in der DDR* (Frankfurt am Main, 1992).
67. The political critique contained in *Ole Bienkopp* is not undermined, as such, by Strittmatter's membership in an SS police regiment during World War II—something he did not reveal during his lifetime. See Sven Felix Kellerhoff, "War auch Erwin Strittmatter in der SS?" *Welt Online Kultur*, 9 June 2008; Annett Gröschner, "Dann nahmen wir das Dorf und brannten es nieder," *Welt Online Kultur*, 14 August 2012.
68. Epstein, 223–27.

CHAPTER 12

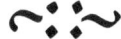

Playing the Game
Football and Everyday Life in the Honecker Era

ALAN MCDOUGALL

In April 1989 the leader of the football section at Traktor Hochstedt, a sports club in a village halfway between Erfurt and Weimar, sent a petition to the district council (*Bezirksrat*) about the "very bad conditions" at the club's ground. Officials had campaigned unsuccessfully for more than a decade for a clubhouse with changing-room facilities. The only building currently available was a community hall 500 meters from the pitch. It had no sanitary facilities beyond an outside toilet and was also used by the table tennis and chess sections, as well as by various mass organizations and the fire brigade. When the hall was double-booked on the day of a league game against Molsdorf, the Hochstedt team was forced to retreat to the section leader's garage to get changed. "In my opinion," he asserted, "that is not right after 40 years of the GDR."[1]

Complaints about inadequate sports facilities were commonplace during the last decade of the Honecker era, part of an upsurge in petitions (*Eingaben*) to the authorities on all manner of consumer issues that reached the astonishing annual figure of more than one million in the late 1980s.[2] Amid political stagnation and economic decline, and in a period when the GDR's international standing was closely tied to the phenomenal success of its Olympic teams, the lack of running water or indoor toilets at a small football ground in rural Thuringia was not a priority for Communist leaders. But such problems mattered greatly to the many GDR citizens who organized and played recreational sports. They are also of considerable value to social historians of the GDR, as a window onto the contradictions between rhetoric and reality under consumer socialism and the festering socioeconomic grievances that left the ruling SED (Socialist Unity Party) with so few supporters in the autumn of 1989. Recent work on mass sports provision in the GDR's twilight years emphasizes the dismal reality of neglect and deterioration behind the SED's loudly trumpeted claim to offer sports for all.[3]

Such scholarship forms part of a growing body of work on what the SED termed "free time and recreational sport" (*Freizeit- und Erholungssport*).[4] Studies of football as a mass participatory activity, though, are conspicuous by their absence. Much has been written about the persistent international shortcomings of East German football and the triumphs and tribulations of the domestic league (*Oberliga*), accounts of which tend either to focus on secret police (Stasi) infiltration of the game or to present individual club histories that are understandably limited in range and ambition.[5] Considerable work has also been undertaken on fan culture, with an emphasis on the problems caused by trouble-making supporters in thrall to the "English disease" of hooliganism during the 1970s and 1980s.[6]

The following study turns attention away from *Oberliga* stars and unruly supporters to the problems faced by ordinary citizens in playing football under Communist rule. It first outlines football's central role in mass sports provision in the GDR—its popularity, the resentment sometimes caused by its prominence, and state-driven initiatives to promote the game. An examination of recreational football in the Ulbricht era then follows, showing that complaints about poor facilities were not inventions of the 1970s and 1980s. Making particular use of sports-related petitions to the authorities, the main section of this essay examines the financial and material difficulties that compromised football at the grassroots level during the final two decades of the regime.

The key arguments advanced here highlight football's significance as a marker of the complex relationship between state and society in Honecker's East Germany. The game provided a means by which citizens could safeguard or develop a sense of their "own interests" (*Eigen-Sinn*), interests that did not necessarily accord with, or were largely detached from, SED goals.[7] This space was opened up by what might be termed the self-imposed limits of the SED dictatorship, i.e., its apparent, at first sight surprising, willingness to grant relatively free rein to certain spheres of cultural and social life. In a "honeycomb state" where the organizational apparatus was so vast and multilayered that the line between regime and society was often unclear, Communist power was "societalized" (that is to say, delegated to citizens as active carriers of the system) more often than it was uniformly imposed from on high.[8] This was particularly apparent in mass sports, which relied strongly on volunteer activism. Innovation and improvisation, rather than enforced central planning, were the norm here.[9]

Situated in an ambiguous public/private sphere that was neither radically dissenting nor regime-endorsing, football was a hugely popular liminal activity, at once dependent on the centralized state and curiously detached from it. Football's "betwixt and between" existence allowed practitioners to "be themselves" in ways that were not possible in the more institutionalized and regulated areas of a small, relatively stable society such as the GDR.[10] Players' lives were ultimately governed by a constrained autonomy that suggests that a full understanding of the GDR's social history cannot be upheld by either top-down theories of totalitarianism or the idea of inner emigration associated with Günter Gaus's "niche society."[11] Playing the game meant probing and negotiating the uncertain boundaries between *Eigen-Sinn* and authority. The results illustrated football's often unintended ability to act as a thorn in the side of dictatorial governments.

"King Football": The Game as *Massensport* (Mass Sport) in the GDR

Football's uniqueness in the GDR, as in many other countries, stemmed from its vast appeal as both a spectator and participatory sport. In many of the country's largest sports associations (*Sportvereinigungen*, or SVs), such as the army club Vorwärts and the railway industry club Lokomotive, the game was consistently the most popular sport in terms of registered players, sections, coaches, and referees.[12] In 1990, on the eve of its dissolution, the East German Football Association (DFV), numbered 5,534 clubs, 30,200 teams, and 424,587 members.[13] In other words, roughly one in every forty GDR citizens was a footballer. This estimate excludes the many others who played informally, such as the steelworkers in the town of Thale, who organized matches beyond the DFV's purview, and the fans of Union Berlin, who founded a league in 1981 without official support or sanction, playing wherever pitches were available.[14]

Football's deep roots in East German society can be traced to the factors that made it the world's foremost sporting activity in the twentieth century. "A simple and elegant game, unhampered by complex rules,"[15] football was easy to organize and relatively cheap to play. Basic facilities were widely available. In a survey of young people's sporting habits in 1987, the Central Institute for Youth Research (ZIJ) in Leipzig found that football pitches (including those without permanently installed goals) were more readily reachable within twenty minutes than any other type of sports facility in the republic.[16] Many smaller communities lacked indoor swimming pools or tennis courts, but most of them had football grounds of one type or another. Football's ubiquity was reinforced by its established status as a spectator sport. Even in the dog days of the 1980s, average attendance at *Oberliga* games was between 10,000 and 12,000. Big televised matches, such as Dynamo Dresden's clash with West German giant Bayern München in the European Cup in 1973, could attract almost 60 percent of the total viewing audience.[17] Contrary to stereotypes of the armchair fan, there was substantial crossover between those who watched and those who played the game.[18]

The predominance of football in the GDR's sporting discourse was not always to the SED's liking. Commenting in 1963 on trade union neglect of mass sports, the party leadership in the town of Guben noted that "often the entire sporting activity [within a factory] consists only of football."[19] A textile factory that employed 1,750 women in the East Berlin district of Lichtenberg was criticized in 1956 for allotting the majority of its sporting budget to the "trump card" of football, more specifically the factory-sponsored men's team, which played in the second district division and had only three factory workers among its members.[20] A winning side displayed local patriotism, and brought glory to the individual factory or institution that supported it. But the focus on football could retard or exclude the development of other sports, thereby undercutting the SED's plans to create a healthy, motivated, and collective-minded workforce through regular exercise.

Following the Soviet model, the GDR's sporting structures were centered on the workplace. Factories funded their own sports club (*Betriebssportgemeinschaft*, or BSG), within which football frequently made up the largest section. The Free German Trade Union Federation (FDGB) sponsored a cup competition that, like the Football Association Challenge Cup in England, was open to "people's" (i.e., amateur) teams, as well as to the cream of GDR football. Nearly 6,000 teams entered the 1967–68 tournament.[21] Individual sports clubs, such as SV Stahl (representing the steelworkers), ran fiercely contested nationwide competitions for recreational players.[22] Youth football, an area in which the GDR excelled internationally, also received strong backing. The football *Spartakiad* in the largely rural county (*Kreis*) of Seelow in 1975, for example, contained matches in five age groups. Teams such as Traktor Letschin and Traktor Gusow, finalists in the tournament for 15- and 16-year-olds, paid an entry fee of one mark and only had to bring along a team sheet, identification cards, and a "useable" football in order to compete.[23]

On paper, the provision of structures and facilities enabling East Germans to play football looked impressive. In its five-year plan for the 1961–65 period, the football authorities in Erfurt promised "no sports festival without football," announced cup competitions for Free German Youth (FDJ) and Young Pioneer teams, and encouraged a higher profile for the so-called Golden Tractor tournament in the countryside.[24] In reality, such ambitious plans were only as strong as the network of unpaid administrators, coaches, and referees available to carry them out. Football's large volunteer corps often made up for shortfalls in state support. It also spread the game to constituencies largely beyond the SED's influence and interest. This was most clearly apparent in the growth of women's football during the 1970s and 1980s, an expansion that was almost entirely driven by grassroots initiatives.[25]

Recreational Football in the Ulbricht Years

Though not a football fan, Walter Ulbricht liked to portray himself as a "friend of German athletes." Publications emphasized his sporting roots in Leipzig, where he joined a workers' gymnastics club at the age of fourteen.[26] In 1959 he publicly demonstrated his commitment to mass sports by pushing his stolid frame around a volleyball court in East Berlin at an event organized to launch an SED campaign to encourage "everyone everywhere" to "play sport once a week" (*Jedermann an jedem Ort, einmal in der Woche Sport*).[27]

In her study of Communist attempts to mobilize support via sports in the 1950s, Molly Wilkinson Johnson argues that SED commitment to mass sports was stronger then than at later dates, when Olympic glory, and concomitant generous funding of performance sports, were given priority.[28] Yet, many of the problems faced by sports functionaries in the 1970s and 1980s—decrepit or misappropriated facilities, equipment shortages, and neglect of mass sports in favor of the elites—had bedeviled their predecessors too. Following the June 1953 uprising, for example, athletes from SV Chemie complained about the high price and irregular availability of equipment (most notably tennis balls and football boots), the preferential treatment accorded to army and police football teams, and the use of sports grounds for nonsporting purposes.[29]

There are also similarities across the decades in how these ongoing problems were resolved. In the 1950s, as in the 1980s, a self-help culture ensured that things got done when the state lacked the resources or commitment to build or expand sports facilities. Footballers, gymnasts, hockey players, and skiers all devoted volunteer hours to rebuilding war-ravaged sports grounds and clubhouses in the GDR's early years, as the authorities encouraged recreational athletes to fashion their own goalposts and volleyball nets.[30] Voluntarism served both the needs of the state, saving money and offering uplifting propaganda examples, and its citizens, providing much-needed facilities and a bond forged through shared goals.[31] It also dovetailed with the self-identity of the *Aufbau* (construction) or Hitler Youth generation, i.e., those who had lived through Nazism and World War II and subsequently found pragmatic common ground with the Communist leadership in raising the GDR from the rubble. The "reconstruction myth" was based on hard work and a broad sense of political conformity.[32] In the sporting arena, it also encouraged grassroots initiatives that were a source of considerable local pride. Individual histories of ex-GDR sports clubs often emphasize the modest, community-based origins of postwar facilities and activities: the first usable grass pitch at Eintracht Mahlsdorf's ground on the outskirts of Berlin, laid with the help of a local farmer and his two horses, for example—or the "Sisyphus work" undertaken by volunteers at what later became the sports club (*Sportgemeinschaft*, or SG) Rotation Leipzig 1950 to send the men's football team to a tournament in Bautzen despite transport and petrol shortages.[33]

Footballers, like other sportspersons, eventually expected something in return for their hard work and were unafraid to voice displeasure when perceived needs were not met. Letters dispatched to the Central Committee (ZK) sports department between August 1959 and January 1960 complained about the neglect of rural sports clubs, the limited availability of facilities such as swimming pools, and the lack of state funding for BSGs.[34] With rationing now ended and the GDR supposedly set fair on the path to socialism, there was a growing tendency to call the state to account, particularly regarding the upkeep of facilities.

An instructive case from the world of football involved BSG Lokomotive Weißenfels. In February 1963 officials from the club's football section wrote to the Halle district council to protest about ongoing problems with their ground. Four years earlier it had been plowed up during the season for the installation of a sewage system; making it playable again required 1,800 hours of labor on the part of BSG members. In 1960 the club was promised a new sports ground, but—despite press publication of the financial plan for this undertaking—"it remained only a promise." At the urging of football section leaders, the move to a new facility was finally granted in 1962. But the old pitch on which the club continued to play in the meantime was dug up again, without consulting the BSG leadership, in order to drain off excess water. League fixtures were disrupted. The players once more stepped in, clearing building materials and mounds of earth from the playing surface, so that matches involving four Lok Weißenfels teams could resume.[35]

The communication from Lok Weißenfels contained many of the features that would later characterize petitions about mass sports during the Honecker era. The authors emphasized the self-help ethos that the SED lauded: not only the volunteer sacrifices that made the ground playable, but also the grassroots pressure that finally forced through the start of construction on a new facility in late 1962. Unresponsive or politically unreliable officials populated the narrative. The first county councilor with whom the club dealt absconded to West Germany. His successor showed "no interest" in Lok's problems and allowed the factory that owned the land where the original facility was located to ignore agreements to respect playing schedules during construction. Local rivalry played a role as well. Lok Weißenfels's anger was fed by the fact that a newly founded neighboring BSG, Traktor Bürgwerben, was given 10,000 marks in 1960 for a sports ground "that is still not finished today"—a largesse, it was implied, which the more established club would have put to better use.[36]

Supplying mass sports facilities was problematic long before Honecker came to power in 1971. It is thus difficult to confirm Jonathan Grix's argument that the provision of such services declined "from the late 70s onwards."[37] There were certainly more complaints by then. But this most likely reflected increased citizen awareness of the power of petitions (a law included in the 1974 constitution required all letters of complaint to be answered within four weeks),[38] as well as a growing intolerance of second-rate facilities, rather than a clearly quantifiable decline. What might have been acceptable in the "reconstruction" era of the 1950s was no longer good enough in the supposedly more prosperous and stable period of "real existing socialism." Perceptions of the state's shortcomings changed, rather than the shortcomings themselves. Petitioners adopted a "rhetoric of decline" that reflected a growing skepticism about the SED's ability to create a more egalitarian society.[39] Their correspondence with the state became more confrontational, more sarcastic, and more assertive, foreshadowing the revival of civil society and popular disrespect for authority that characterized the protests of 1989.[40]

Football and Everyday Life in the Honecker Era

The transition years between Ulbricht and Honecker were marked by the SED's increased commitment to both elite and mass sports. In 1969 the Politburo created a hierarchical system of resource distribution that gave medal-rich Olympic sports such as athletics and swimming the lion's share of state funding, while the likes of tennis, basketball, and ice hockey fell by the wayside. Football was included in the favored Sport I category, but only grudgingly, thanks to its popularity rather than its efficacy, ranking as low as sixteenth on the list of priorities.[41] The new policy bore fruit at the 1972 Munich Olympics, where the GDR finished third in the medal table behind the Soviet Union and the United States and just ahead of West Germany.[42] With the introduction a year later of a comprehensive system for finding and training young talent, the bedrock of the East German "sports miracle" was in place.[43]

At the same time, the SED expanded its commitment to recreational sports. The five-day workweek was introduced in the GDR in 1967. That same year an ambitious mass sports program was announced at a sports science congress in Leipzig, and the party leadership increased the recommended exercise dosage for citizens from once to "several times" a week.[44] Starting in the early 1970s, the East German sports federation (*Deutscher Turn- und Sportbund*, or DTSB) created joint sports programs with the FDGB and the FDJ that organized successful mass sports festivals, as well as events such as the "table tennis tournament for thousands" and the jogging campaign *Eile mit Meile* ("make haste with miles").[45]

It was clear which was the more important of these two branches of Socialist sports. Olympic athletes were the GDR's most successful export, giving the regime an international prestige that it enjoyed in few other areas. In comparison, the organization of local bowling or football leagues was a minor concern, to be left as before to volunteers working in their spare time. What changed, though, were people's expectations. As Dan Wilton argues, the apparent "opening up" to a wider range of popular interests in sport and music during this period increased hope among citizens that "more personalised and localised concerns... should and could be resolved."⁴⁶ The regime thus became hostage to ambitions that, in the field of mass sports, it often lacked the time and money to fulfill. Popular disappointment about broken promises was almost inevitably the result. Though hard to quantify on a national level, the number of sports-related petitions appeared to increase steadily during the 1970s. The police sports club SV Dynamo, for example, received a total of 14 petitions in 1968, 60 in 1974, and 118 in 1977.⁴⁷ A "culture of complaint" entrenched itself more firmly among sports practitioners and fans.⁴⁸ It reflected a growing impatience with the SED regime on the part of citizens no longer sustained by the more optimistic, or less expectant, spirit of the construction generation—a holding to account that could be seen in numerous areas of everyday life in this period, from housing shortages to the availability of drinkable coffee or Mediterranean oranges.⁴⁹

Football featured prominently in sporting petitions. From the late 1970s onward, the dominant topic was public anger at the favoritism shown toward the Stasi club, Berliner FC Dynamo (BFC), which won the league title for ten consecutive seasons between 1979 and 1988 amid widespread accusations of corruption that earned it the sobriquet *Schiebemeister* (crooked champions). Following the controversial 1985 cup final between BFC and bitter rival Dynamo Dresden, the DFV and its newspaper *Die Neue Fußball-Woche* ("The New Football Week") received roughly 700 letters of complaint about alleged officiating bias toward the team from Berlin. Public outcry was so strong that the football association, after studying video footage of the game, banned the referee from all international and *Oberliga* matches for a year.⁵⁰

Fans complained more frequently, and were complained about more frequently, than players. Other recurrent themes include the forced transfer of players from small clubs to larger ones; the miserable performances of the national team in World Cup and European Championship qualifying matches; ticket distribution problems (particularly for strictly policed matches against West European teams); and public order disturbances caused by young, irreverent, and often drunk *Schlachtenbummler* (away fans) in and around grounds across the GDR. But football-related petitions were also submitted by East Germans who played or coached the game themselves. They detailed spats between local rivals over ground sharing or player poaching, or protested against the DFV's imposition of disciplinary measures. Angry football section representatives at BSG Fortschritt Heubach, a small community in the southwestern district of Suhl, portrayed sanctions imposed upon the club—after a referee had been forced to abandon a Heubach game in March 1986—as part of a plot to ensure that local competitor Heßberg was promoted from the second county division instead.⁵¹ Other petitioners were more constructive. In 1983 a thrift-minded referee from Halle wrote to Honecker suggesting the use of waste material rather than valuable resources such as chalk or construction lime to mark out football pitches.⁵²

Much has been written about the centrality of petitions, in the absence of conventional democratic markers, as a means of registering complaints about life under East German socialism—and about the problems that historians face in analyzing such stylized forms of discourse with the state.[53] Based around conflict and conflict resolution, petitions showcased "disturbances in everyday life" rather than everyday life itself.[54] They did not discuss, for example, the fact that football facilities in many parts of East Germany were often adequate and sometimes very good. When the journalist Doug Gilbert visited a factory sports club near Leipzig in the mid 1970s, he noted the "beautiful layout" of football pitches in constant use by the club's largest section, which had ten teams in operation.[55] People of all ages were usually within close reach of a place where they could go to kick a ball around cheaply.

If petitions only focused on the problematic sides of everyday existence, the language in which they were written did not necessarily reflect, or fully reflect, popular attitudes toward the GDR. Petitioners became adept at "speaking Socialist."[56] The rhetorical tricks deployed by citizens who wrote to the popular consumer rights television program *PRISMA* about problems with housing, work, holidays, and foodstuffs were likewise adopted by petitioners writing about mass sports: an introduction outlining the writer's commitment to socialism, followed by a specific and detailed complaint. This complaint was sometimes accompanied by a threat or by a choice quotation from a high-ranking individual (Honecker, for example) or public document (the GDR Constitution) that highlighted discrepancies between what the party said and actually did.[57] To obtain a helpful response, petitioners portrayed themselves in ways that were likely to gain or maintain the sympathy of the authorities. Most of the complainants about BFC in the 1980s described themselves as loyal citizens, even as their criticisms of the refereeing situation became increasingly outspoken—an outspokenness that was starkly apparent in petitions on other subjects at this time. Sports petitioners were part of a wider community of correspondents with the state. After all, they were also *PRISMA* watchers, Trabant drivers, coffee drinkers, and apartment seekers.

Taking into account the caveats, the millions of letters of complaint penned by citizens remain a highly valuable source for historians. They offer detailed insights into the private lives of East Germans and highlight the "patterns of individualization" that often undermined the collectivist goals of the GDR.[58] Whatever constraints shaped the dialogue between the state and its citizens, both sides generally took the petition process seriously. Nor were these constraints necessarily a barrier to blunt, often insightful critiques of Communist rule. Petitions illustrated what people wanted from the regime and what they wanted for themselves—expectations that changed over time in mass sport and other areas. As indices of the relationship between *Eigen-Sinn* and authority, they are critical to understanding how East Germans questioned the legitimacy of the SED dictatorship.

Though the GDR faced some difficulties in supplying the population with boots and balls, systemic equipment shortages were less problematic for recreational footballers than for tennis players, skiers, or runners. "I hadn't gathered," one petitioner from Brandenburg dryly wrote in 1983, "that the *Eile mit Meile* movement was in fact a jog through the city's shops!"[59] Football section leaders used petitions to complain about facilities rather than footwear. With many indoor pools across the republic in serious disrepair by the late 1970s and the 1980s, and priority access at functioning venues accorded to performance athletes, recreational swimmers did much the same. When Friday-night swims at Dynamo's swimming pool at the Sportforum facility in East Berlin were discontinued in 1979, the city's SED leader, Konrad Naumann, received an indignant petition signed in the name of "many friends of swimming." There were not enough pools in the rest of Berlin, it argued, for Dynamo to exclude the public in this arbitrary manner.[60] Football was not in such dire straits as swimming, but infrastructural problems in the two sports were part of the same discussion, one in which citizens queried the gap between Communist rhetoric and reality, and highlighted the gulf that separated performance athletes—the sporting equivalent of the party *Bonzen* (bigwigs)—from their recreational peers.

Three petitions sent to officials between 1978 and 1989 help illuminate this discussion of football facilities in the Honecker era. The first was written in August 1978 by the football section leadership at Dynamo Forst to Erich Mielke, the head of the Stasi; the second consists of a pair of letters dispatched by the football section leadership at BSG Tiefbau Berlin to the head of the ZK sports department, Rudi Hellmann, in November 1981 and October 1982; the third is the aforementioned petition from the football section leadership at BSG Traktor Hochstedt to the Erfurt district council in April 1989.

The three petitions raised similar issues. As we have already seen, failure to build the long-promised clubhouse and changing rooms at Traktor Hochstedt had obliged players to share a community hall 500 meters from the football ground with everyone from the fire brigade to the chess club—and on one occasion to change for a match in the coach's garage for want of other available space.[61] Petitioners from Dynamo Forst complained that there was only one pitch for seven football teams at the club's ground. Changing facilities were limited, the heating system unreliable, and the access road in such a poor state that children were barred from using it in rainy weather. The section lacked money for footballs, gear, and regular transport to away games.[62] The chief concern at BSG Tiefbau was the lack of electricity at the club's ground in Gosen on the eastern fringes of Berlin. As a result, players (including, it was emphasized, children) were forced to change in a primitive hut, wash with cold water, and hold team talks by candlelight.[63]

The tone of these communications was one of polite exasperation, displaying a sense of entitlement to greater support from a regime that repeatedly expressed the importance of sports. The act of writing was itself presented as a final plea for help that had been too long in coming. In the most extreme case, the 1981 petition from BSG Tiefbau Berlin claimed that the club had been trying to get an electricity supply for its ground since 1958.[64] Blame for delays and broken promises was widely dispersed: the leadership of SG Dynamo Forst and its parent organization Dynamo Cottbus in the example of the Forst football section, and the state electricity suppliers, the sponsoring factory, and the local party leadership in Tiefbau Berlin's case.[65] Mass sport in East Germany encouraged among its practitioners a mixture of independence from the (often inattentive) state and ultimate reliance upon its munificence, creating the environment of constrained autonomy that governed footballers' experiences under communism.

The dual nature of citizens' relationship to the state was reflected in the stylistic approach of the petitioners, who professed loyalty and distance in almost the same breath. A sense of local pride was framed within a wider narrative of their section's contribution to socialism. Functionaries at Traktor Hochstedt, for example, highlighted the successes under trying conditions of its schoolboy, youth, and men's teams, and requested help "in the interests of [GDR] football in general and especially for football in Hochstedt."[66] Using a rhetorical device common to petitioners on many subjects, football leaders at Dynamo Forst—after emphasizing their contribution to SV Dynamo's development—implied that the SED regime was failing to uphold Socialist ideals. Facilities there, they claimed, were "no advertisement" for a Dynamo sports club, before adding the politically loaded reminder that the team's home had formerly been a "workers' sports ground."[67]

A sense of optimism giving way to disillusionment was particularly marked at BSG Tiefbau Berlin. In its first petition to Hellmann in November 1981, the football leadership noted that, despite terrible conditions at the club's ground, "enthusiasm for sport had previously won out. But today's young people have no more patience for that."[68] A second petition in October 1982, prompted by the fact that nothing had changed in the intervening period, expressed a brusquer sense of anger and disappointment: "We cannot and will not just accept that we are being left alone with our difficulties, in a stadium in which our sports club with its 160 members is threatened with dissolution for the reasons mentioned in our correspondence of 17 November 1981. Is nobody then interested in our continued existence? Can you in that case so hugely disappoint the sportspersons and functionaries who for years and decades have voluntarily given themselves to the development of sport?" The petitioners then drew attention to the "crass contradiction" between what was offered to ordinary East Germans and what was offered to the elites: "We might rightly rejoice in the great successes of our leading sportspersons. But doesn't mass sport, the work done in factory sports clubs and sections, play a decisive role in these successes that are the envy of so many countries throughout the world?"[69]

There are echoes here of not only standard party and trade union laments about the undervaluing of recreational sporting activities (especially prevalent in the 1950s), but also of complaints directed by Soviet officials during the 1930s at the Spartak sports society, which was accused of neglecting mass sports to support top athletes, including players in the club's popular football team.[70] The feelings of Tiefbau officials were shared by disgruntled citizens in other sports, such as the aspiring marathon runner from Rathenow who found that training shoes were only available to elite athletes—or the recreational swimmers in Dresden who were barred from using a local pool because they had apparently made it too dirty for the high-performance swimmers there.[71] A parallel can also be drawn between growing resentment of SED elitism in the provision and maintenance of sports facilities, and the populist strand that underpinned supporters' anger about the declining fortunes of BSG football teams such as Chemie Leipzig and Sachsenring Zwickau in the same period.[72] Both suggested that citizens sometimes internalized, or at least knew how to use, the egalitarian ideals of socialism better than the Socialist regime itself. The end result, though, was disengagement among mass sport functionaries, a turning inward to resolve problems that the SED could not resolve in order to satisfy local sporting needs.[73] Failing facilities pointed to the larger failings of the Socialist project. It is difficult not to see something of significance in the incredulous comments about primitive sporting conditions made by petitioners at Tiefbau Berlin ("and this in the year 1981!") and at Traktor Hochstedt ("that is not right after 40 years of the GDR").[74]

The responses to the petitions from Forst, Gosen, and Hochstedt confirmed that skepticism about party promises was not misplaced. They also shed light on the often dysfunctional character of Communist rule. Bureaucratic inertia was particularly hard for Tiefbau Berlin to overcome, as the club's second petition from October 1982 made clear. Despite protracted discussions involving the district DTSB and SED leaderships, top officials at the club's sponsoring factory, and the putative energy suppliers (the Berlin energy combine), negotiations to ensure an electricity supply to the ground in Gosen were still not finalized eleven months after the BSG's initial petition.[75] It was a similar story of delays and buck-passing at Traktor Hochstedt. The Erfurt district council emphasized in June 1989 the need for the "strongest principles of thrift" in any clubhouse construction proposals, essentially redirecting the BSG's request for help to the same village and county authorities who had provided so little support during the previous decade—a hugely frustrating process that was commonly replicated in citizens' attempts to seek redress of the most contentious of all petition issues, the housing situation.[76] Dynamo Forst's petition was given shortest shrift. The Dynamo Cottbus leadership declared that an extension to the changing-room facilities at Forst's ground was "unnecessary," while expansion of the training area into a second full-sized pitch would have to be undertaken by club volunteers. Problems were attributed primarily to recent difficulties in finding a groundskeeper, though Forst footballers were also rebuked for not doing enough toward the upkeep of their ground. No further monies were to be made available for equipment or gear. Dynamo Forst's football section, the district organization asserted, already received generous financial support.[77]

The responses highlighted the financial constraints that governed mass sports provision during the last decade of the Honecker era. The best that officials in Erfurt could offer Traktor Hochstedt was possible inclusion in the district's 1990 financial plan. But any clubhouse project, it was emphasized, would have to be subsidized with manual labor on the part of BSG members.[78] Not much had changed since the early 1950s in this regard, when functionaries in Leipzig, Plauen, and elsewhere promoted mass voluntary work actions on stadia as a means of saving money.[79] Low-cost sport in East Germany was predicated on this ingrained volunteer ethos. As Doug Gilbert noted in the late 1970s, "GDR mass sports clubs have a very good record of taking care of themselves."[80] It was what kept Tiefbau Berlin's football section going, despite the lack of a regular electricity supply since the late 1950s. It was what allowed Traktor Hochstedt's youth team to stand undefeated at the top of the county league table in the 1988–89 season. It was what prevented the heating system at Dynamo Forst's ground from freezing during the winter of 1977–78.[81]

In all three cases, mass sport functionaries were left to their own devices until such time as they felt compelled to call on the state for help. Even at Dynamo Forst, which was part of a sports organization that was run on tighter lines than ordinary BSGs, micromanagement was not the order of the day—as suggested by the lack of urgency in permanently filling the position of club groundskeeper and by the unwillingness to support an upgrade to the access road that was churned up by farm vehicles ("we cannot have any influence on changing this state of affairs").[82] We see again the limited presence of the SED dictatorship in mass sports, a hands-off attitude that was particularly feasible in football, with its large volunteer body of referees, coaches, and administrators. This approach worked if basic levels of state support, or at least perceptions of such support, were maintained.

During the 1980s, though, the unspoken social contract between East German citizens and the regime began to break down, less because facilities were any worse than in the 1950s (they were generally better) than because football, swimming, and tennis section leaders were less willing to accept subpar conditions, especially given the resources that were being pumped into the GDR's Olympic program. The state's commitment to mass sport now came back to haunt it, creating—or at least fueling—a sense of resentment among the people whom it short-changed. In their second petition to Rudi Hellmann in late 1982, football leaders at Tiefbau Berlin bitterly remarked that "we seem to lack all credibility in the eyes of our sportsmen, as we cannot give them concrete information about when or even if we are going to get a supply of electricity." If all areas of society, they concluded, were run in "such a complicated and irresponsible" manner, "where would we be then!"[83] The petitioners were closer to the truth than they knew. The SED's grip on power was less secure and all-encompassing than it seemed. The regime's inability to either effect or control change, in mass sports as in other areas from housing to travel, was swiftly and dramatically exposed in the autumn of 1989.

Conclusion

In December 1989 New Forum, one of the political organizations that emerged as the SED dictatorship began to collapse, noted that "sport in the GDR—an enormous feather in the cap of both the Party and the government—is not rooted in the people."[84] This was a damning indictment for a regime that portrayed mass sports as a key component in forging a healthy Socialist society. In reality, as the petitions of the Honecker era reveal, the central organs of state power had limited influence on, and interest in, everyday sporting activities. The volunteers who did the legwork in football and other sports were part of the state structure, but they were not necessarily regime loyalists. An unintended consequence of the SED's desire for a comprehensively ruled society was to open up the ever-expanding state apparatus to elements whose support for socialism was conditional. The condition, in the case of mass sports, was that the voluntarist culture that kept football and other sections thriving would be supplemented when necessary with state funding for essential items such as buildings and equipment. By the 1980s, the SED could not keep up its end of the bargain, as the GDR's planned economy—hobbled by a plummeting currency, ubiquitous shortages, corruption, bottlenecks, and low worker morale—went into steep decline.[85] There was not enough money to maintain existing sports structures, let alone build new ones.[86] This had been true of the 1950s, too; the big shift in the intervening thirty years was a growing impatience with restrictions and deficiencies that, if SED propaganda were to be believed, should have long since been eradicated.

The history of the GDR was not static. Nor were the responses of its citizens to the problems that they negotiated in their everyday lives. The sporting self-help strategies developed during the first decade of Socialist reconstruction survived into the final decade of the GDR's existence, but in a manner that reflected growing popular detachment from Socialist goals. It is instructive to note that numerous BSGs in the 1980s turned away from traditional, Communist-approved offerings and embraced instead politically suspect "trend sports" such as karate, aerobics, skateboarding, and windsurfing.[87]

"Tell me how you play and I'll tell you who you are," wrote the Uruguayan novelist and football fanatic Eduardo Galeano.[88] What can "playing the game" ultimately tell us about East Germany and East Germans during the Honecker era? Football did not bring down communism. But the testy dialogue between the authorities and recreational players in petitions from the late 1970s and the 1980s sheds light on both the material shortcomings of socialism and East Germans' increasingly lucid intolerance of such shortcomings. The state of the game—not only the underfunded facilities, but also other unresolved problems such as hooliganism and BFC's deeply unpopular preeminence—thus constituted an important part of the crumbling backdrop for the momentous events of the summer and fall of 1989. Football also highlights salient themes about the nature of the relationship between state and society in the GDR: the limits of the totalitarian paradigm in explaining and understanding social and cultural activities; the fuzzy boundaries between rulers and ruled that were particularly prevalent in leisure time pursuits; and, finally, the importance of a flexible and robust *Eigen-Sinn* in shaping and defending recreational interests. Football, rather like the church or popular music, occupied a liminal space between the public and the private, where ways of being were not determined solely, or even primarily, by the dictates of the state.

"Playing the game" meant, of course, quite literally just that for many thousands of ordinary East Germans: the playing of football matches at all levels and among all age groups throughout the Socialist republic—even on shoddy pitches, using balls without plastic covering, and wearing imported Adidas boots. Whereas fans and elite players were often subject to extensive state surveillance—and thus to a more constrained form of the constrained autonomy that characterized football in the GDR—lower-level footballers, with rare exceptions, led a less encumbered existence. For them football was a social bond, a fun and low-cost form of exercise and competition, and a source of local pride. Post-*Wende* accounts of numerous clubs illustrate that, even when facilities were far from ideal in the GDR, the game survived. BSG Berliner Werkzeugmaschinenfabrik (machine tools factory) Marzahn, today FC Nordost Berlin, kept a football section going, despite losing its home ground to the construction of new concrete-block (*Plattenbau*) apartments in Marzahn during the early 1980s. BSG Rotation Leipzig 1950 (today SG Rotation Leipzig 1950) did likewise after the DTSB evicted the club from its home ground in 1979 and turned the latter into a site for an elite sports school.[89] In defending and following individual or local interests through a combination of engagement with, and detachment from, Communist power, footballers safeguarded a sporting *Eigen-Sinn* that, in many cases, outlasted the country in which they lived and played. In the end, the people's game was far more resilient than the people's state.

Suggested Readings

Betts, Paul. *Within Walls: Private Life in the German Democratic Republic*. Oxford, 2010.
Braun, Jutta. "The People's Sport? Popular Sport and Fans in the Later Years of the German Democratic Republic." *German History* 27/3 (2009): 414–28.
——— and René Wiese. "DDR-Fußball und gesamtdeutsche Identität im Kalten Krieg." *Historische Sozialforschung* 30/4 (2005): 191–210.
Dennis, Mike. "Behind the Wall: East German Football between State and Society." *GFL-Journal* 2 (2007): 46–74.
Gilbert, Doug. *The Miracle Machine*. New York, 1980.
Grix, Jonathan. "The Decline of Mass Sport Provision in the German Democratic Republic." *The International Journey of the History of Sport* 25/4 (2008): 406–20.
Hinsching, Jochen, ed. *Alltagssport in der DDR*. Aachen, 1998.
Horn, Michael and Gottfried Weise. *Das große Lexikon des DDR-Fußballs*. Berlin, 2004.
Johnson, Molly Wilkinson. *Training Socialist Citizens: Sports and the State in East Germany*. Leiden, 2008.
Klaedtke, Uta. *Betriebssport in der DDR. Phänomene des Alltagssports*. Hamburg, 2007.
Kluge, Volker. *Das Sportbuch DDR*. Berlin, 2004.
Leske, Hanns. *Erich Mielke, die Stasi und das runde Leder. Der Einfluß der SED und des Ministeriums für Staatssicherheit auf dem Fußballsport in der DDR*. Göttingen, 2004.
Merkel, Ina, ed. *"Wir sind doch nicht die Mecker-Ecke der Nation." Briefe an das DDR-Fernsehen*. Cologne, 1998.
Willmann, Frank, ed. *Fußball-Land DDR. Anstoß, Abpfiff, Aus*. Berlin, 2004.
Wilton, Dan. "The 'Societalisation' of the State: Sport for the Masses and Popular Music in the GDR." In *Power and Society in the GDR, 1961-1979: The 'Normalisation of Rule'?* ed. Mary Fulbrook, 102–29. Oxford, 2009.

Notes

1. Thüringisches Hauptstaatsarchiv Weimar (ThHStAW), Bezirkstag und Rat des Bezirkes Erfurt Altregistratur Nr. 46939/1, petition from the football section at BSG Traktor Hochstedt to Erfurt district council, 21 April 1989.
2. Paul Betts, *Within Walls: Private Life in the German Democratic Republic* (Oxford, 2010), 189.
3. Jutta Braun, "The People's Sport? Popular Sport and Fans in the Later Years of the German Democratic Republic," *German History* 27/3 (2009): 414–28; Jonathan Grix, "The Decline of Mass Sport Provision in the German Democratic Republic," *The International Journey of the History of Sport* 25/4 (March 2008): 406–20.
4. See, e.g., Uta Klaedtke, *Betriebssport in der DDR. Phänomene des Alltagssports* (Hamburg, 2007); Jochen Hinsching, ed., *Alltagssport in der DDR* (Aachen, 1998); Molly Wilkinson Johnson, *Training Socialist Citizens: Sports and the State in East Germany* (Leiden and Boston, 2008); Dan Wilton, "The 'Societalisation' of the State: Sport for the Masses and Popular Music in the GDR," in *Power and Society in the GDR, 1961-*

1979: *The 'Normalisation of Rule'?*, ed. Mary Fulbrook (Oxford and New York, 2009), 102–29.
5. For an overview of existing literature, see Mike Dennis, "Behind the Wall: East German Football Between State and Society," *GFL-Journal* 2/2007: 46–74. On the *Stasi and football*, see Hanns Leske, *Erich Mielke, die Stasi und das runde Leder. Der Einfluß der SED und des Ministeriums für Staatssicherheit auf dem Fußballsport in der DDR* (Göttingen, 2004). An insightful club history is Jens Fuge's account of underdogs Chemie Leipzig, *Leutzscher Legende. Von Britannia 1899 zum FC Sachsen* (Leipzig, 1992).
6. See, e.g., Mike Dennis, "Soccer Hooliganism in the German Democratic Republic," in *German Football: History, Culture, Society*, eds. Alan Tomlinson and Christopher Young (London, 2006), 52–72; Frank Willmann, ed., *Stadionpartisanen. Fans und Hooligans in der DDR* (Berlin, 2007).
7. On the concept of *Eigen-Sinn*, see, e.g., Alf Lüdtke, *Eigensinn. Fabrikalltag, Arbeitererfahrungen und Politik vom Kaiserreich bis in den Faschismus* (Hamburg, 1993); Thomas Lindenberger, ed., *Herrschaft und Eigen-Sinn in der Diktatur. Studien zur Gesellschaftsgeschichte der DDR* (Cologne, 1999).
8. Mary Fulbrook, *The People's State: East German Society from Hitler to Honecker* (New Haven, 2005), 235–36, 247–48; Wilton, "The 'Societalisation' of the State," 102–5.
9. Jochen Hinsching, "Der Bereich 'Freizeit- und Erholungssport' im 'ausdifferenzierten' Sport der DDR," in *Alltagssport in der DDR*, 16.
10. On the concept of liminality see Victor Turner, *The Forest of Symbols: Aspects of Ndembu Ritual* (Ithaca, N.Y., 1967), 93–111. On the liminal (or in-between) character of football crowds in the Soviet Union, see Robert Edelman, *Spartak Moscow: A History of the People's Team in the Workers' State* (Ithaca, N.Y., 2009), 99.
11. Corey Ross, *The East German Dictatorship: Problems and Perspectives in the Interpretation of the GDR* (London, 2002), 19–25, 32–36; Dan Wilton, "Regime Versus People? Public Opinion and the Development of Sport and Popular Music in the GDR, 1961-1989" (Ph.D. diss., University College London, 2005), 120–22.
12. Stiftung Archiv der Parteien und Massenorganisationen der DDR im Bundesarchiv (SAPMO-BArch), DY 12/2440, Organisationsstatistik des Deutschen Turn- und Sportbunds: Armeesportvereinigung "Vorwärts," 31 December 1972; SAPMO-BArch, DY 12/2416, Mitgliederstatistik des Deutschen Turn- und Sportbunds: SV Lokomotive, 30 September 1960.
13. Archivgut des Deutschen Fußballverbandes der DDR (DFV), Konzeption des DFV der DDR zur Vorbereitung der Beratung der beiden Präsidien DFV-DFB am 19.05.1990 in Berlin (West), 7 May 1990; DDR-Bezirksverbände, n.d.
14. Uwe Karte, "An der Basis," in Frank Willmann, ed., *Fußball-Land DDR. Anstoß, Abpfiff, Aus* (Berlin, 2004), 171; http://www.eisern-union.de/union-liga/index.htm.
15. Eric Hobsbawm, *Age of Extremes: The Short Twentieth Century 1914-1991* (London, 1994), 198.
16. SAPMO-BArch, DC 4/716, Körperkultur und Sport—fester Bestandteil der sozialistischen Lebensweise der Jugend der DDR (Untersuchung "Jugend und Massensport 1987"), December 1987 (Tables 55 and 56).
17. Michael Horn and Gottfried Weise, *Das große Lexikon des DDR-Fußballs* (Berlin, 2004), 420; Dennis, "Behind the Wall," 57–58.
18. SAPMO-BArch, DC 4/721, Neuere Ergebnisse zum Verhältnis Jugendlicher zum Fußball (Fanverhalten)—Expertise des ZIJ zur Untersuchung "Sport '87," March 1988.

19. Brandenburgisches Landeshauptarchiv (BLHA), Rep 930 Nr. 911, Einschätzung der Erfüllung des Beschlusses der Bezirksleitung vom 15.2.1962 "Die Aufgaben bei der Entwicklung von Körperkultur und Sport bis 1965 im Bezirk Cottbus," sowie des gegenwärtigen Standes der Wahlen im DTSB, 22 March 1963.
20. SAPMO-BArch, DY 34/3879, Den Massensport weiterentwickeln!, 21 August 1956.
21. SAPMO-BArch, DY 34/17719, Einschätzung der Pokalwettbewerbe, n.d. (1968).
22. On the SV Stahl football tournament (1955–57), see SAPMO-BArch, DY 46/2411.
23. BLHA, Rep 731 Nr. 977, 11. Kreis-, Kinder- und Jugendspartakiade 1975 im Fußball der Nachwuchsmannschaften, 4 June 1975. Named after the Roman gladiator Spartacus, the *Spartakiade* were contested in various disciplines at the county, district, and national levels to promote competitive sports among young East Germans.
24. ThHStAW, Bezirkstag und Rat des Bezirkes Erfurt KK 24, Perspektivplan für 1961-1965, n.d.
25. See, e.g., Gertrud Pfister, "The Challenges of Women's Football in East and West Germany: A Comparative Study," *Soccer and Society* Vol. 4, No. 2/3 (April/June 2003): 128–48; Carina Sophia Linne, *Freigespielt. Frauenfußball im geteilten Deutschland* (Berlin, 2011).
26. Johnson, *Training Socialist Citizens*, 46.
27. Volker Kluge, *Das Sportbuch DDR* (Berlin, 2004), 178–79.
28. Johnson, *Training Socialist Citizens*, 203.
29. SAPMO-BArch, DY 34/3665, Auswertung der durchgeführten Instrukteureinsätze und Berichte aufgrund der Vorkommnisse am 16. und 17.6.1953, 6 July 1953.
30. Johnson, *Training Socialist Citizens*, 125–33.
31. Ibid., 113–24.
32. Dorothee Wierling, "The Hitler Youth Generation in the GDR: Insecurities, Ambitions and Dilemmas," in *Dictatorship As Experience: Towards a Socio-Cultural History of the GDR*, ed. Konrad Jarausch (Oxford and New York, 1999), 312–17.
33. http://www.bsv-eintracht-mahlsdorf.de/Verein/verein3.htm; Rolf Beyer, *Rotation Leipzig 1950: 50 Jahre* (Leipzig, 2000), 7–8.
34. SAPMO-BArch, DY 30/IV 2/18/1, Analyse der Post aus der Bevölkerung seit Anfang August 1959, 6 January 1960.
35. Landeshauptarchiv Sachsen-Anhalt, Abteilung Merseburg (LHASA, MER), RdB Halle, Nr. 9418, petition from the football section at BSG Lokomotive Weißenfels to Halle district council, 13 February 1963. There is no reply to the petition in the file.
36. Ibid.
37. Grix, "The Decline of Mass Sport Provision," 409.
38. Ibid., 411.
39. Jonathan Zatlin, *The Currency of Socialism: Money and Political Culture in East Germany* (New York, 2007), 286–88.
40. Betts, *Within Walls*, 188–89.
41. Archivgut des DFV, I/2, Günter Schneider, "Dokumentation über 45 Jahre Fußball in der SBZ/DDR" (unpublished, c. 1996).
42. On sporting tensions between East and West Germany in the context of the 1972 Olympic Games, see Kay Schiller and Christopher Young, *The 1972 Munich Olympics and the Making of Modern Germany* (Berkeley, C.A., 2010), chap. 6.
43. Jutta Braun and René Wiese, "DDR-Fußball und gesamtdeutsche Identität im Kalten Krieg," *Historische Sozialforschung* 30/4 (2005): 192–97.

44. Hinsching, "Der Bereich 'Freizeit- und Erholungssport,'" 16–18; Kluge, *Das Sportbuch*, 178–79.
45. Wilton, "The 'Societalisation' of the State," 110–12, 114–15.
46. Wilton, "Regime versus people?" 119.
47. SAPMO-BArch, DO 101/027/1-2, Analyse, 12 February 1969; Analyse der Eingaben 1976, 23 February 1977; Analyse der Eingaben im Jahr 1977, 7 June 1978.
48. Joachim Staadt, *Eingaben. Die institutionalisierte Meckerkultur in der DDR* (Berlin, 1996).
49. Mark Allison, "1977: The GDR's Most Normal Year?" in *Power and Society*, 256–65.
50. SAPMO-BArch, DY 30/4986, Aktennotiz zur Aussprache mit Sportfreund Roßner am 11. Juli 1985; SAPMO-BArch, DY 30/4963, Protokoll der Videoauswertung des Endspiels im FDGB-Pokal vom 8. Juni 1985 zwischen dem BFC Dynamo und der SG Dynamo Dresden zur Beurteilung der Schiedsrichterleistung, 3 July 1985.
51. SAPMO-BArch, DY 30/4979, petition from the football section at BSG Fortschritt Heubach to Rudi Hellmann, 22 May 1986.
52. SAPMO-BArch, DY 30/4983, petition from Wolfgang K. to Erich Honecker, 28 November 1983.
53. For an overview of the complexities of the GDR's petition culture, see Fulbrook, *The People's State*, chap. 13.
54. Ina Merkel and Felix Mühlberg, "Eingaben und Öffentlichkeit," in *"Wir sind doch nicht die Mecker-Ecke der Nation." Briefe an das DDR-Fernsehen*, ed. Ina Merkel (Cologne, 1998), 11.
55. Doug Gilbert, *The Miracle Machine* (New York, 1980), 92–93.
56. Betts, *Within Walls*, 186.
57. Merkel and Mühlberg, "Eingaben und Öffentlichkeit," 24–27; Betts, *Within Walls*, 186–88.
58. Betts, *Within Walls*, 174; Fulbrook, *The People's State*, 271.
59. Braun, "The People's Sport?" 418. On the provision of running shoes during the jogging boom that began in the late 1970s, see Grix, "The Decline of Mass Sport Provision," 411–15.
60. SAPMO-BArch, DO 101/027/3-4, petition from Werner M. to Konrad Naumann, 14 May 1979.
61. ThHStAW, Bezirkstag und Rat des Bezirkes Erfurt Altregistratur Nr. 46939/1, petition from Traktor Hochstedt to Erfurt district council, 21 April 1989.
62. SAPMO-BArch, DO 101/027/1-2, petition from the football section at SG Dynamo Forst to Erich Mielke, 7 August 1978.
63. SAPMO-BArch, DY 30/4979, petition from the football section at BSG Tiefbau Berlin to Rudi Hellmann, 17 November 1981.
64. SAPMO-BArch, DY 30/4979, petition from Tiefbau Berlin to Hellmann, 17 November 1981.
65. Ibid.; SAPMO-BArch, DO 101/027/1-2, petition from Dynamo Forst to Mielke, 7 August 1978.
66. ThHStAW, Bezirkstag und Rat des Bezirkes Erfurt Altregistratur Nr. 46939/1, petition from Traktor Hochstedt to Erfurt district council, 21 April 1989.
67. SAPMO-BArch, DO 101/027/1-2, petition from Dynamo Forst to Mielke, 7 August 1978.
68. SAPMO-BArch, DY 30/4979, petition from Tiefbau Berlin to Hellmann, 17 November 1981.

69. Ibid., petition from the football section at BSG Tiefbau Berlin to Rudi Hellmann, 2 October 1982.
70. Robert Edelman, *Serious Fun: A History of Spectator Sports in the USSR* (Oxford, 1993), 68.
71. Grix, "The Decline of Mass Sport Provision," 412–13; Wilton, "Regime versus people?" 174.
72. On Chemie Leipzig, see SAPMO-BArch, DY 30/4982, petition from Hans H. to Rudi Hellmann, 22 April 1983; on Sachsenring Zwickau, see SAPMO-BArch, DY 30/4983, petition from Rainer K. to Erich Honecker, 1 August 1984.
73. Wilton, "The 'Societalisation' of the State," 122.
74. SAPMO-BArch, DY 30/4979, petition from BSG Tiefbau Berlin to Hellmann, 17 November 1981; ThHStAW, Bezirkstag und Rat des Bezirkes Erfurt Altregistratur Nr. 46939/1, petition from Traktor Hochstedt to Erfurt district council, 21 April 1989.
75. SAPMO-BArch, DY 30/4979, petition from BSG Tiefbau Berlin to Hellmann, 2 October 1982; Aktennotiz über eine Aussprache zur Klärung einer Eingabe der Sektion Fußball der BSG Tiefbau vom 2.10.1982.
76. ThHStAW, Bezirkstag und Rat des Bezirkes Erfurt Altregistratur Nr. 46939/1, letter from Erfurt district council to the football section at BSG Traktor Hochstedt, 7 June 1989. On official responses to housing shortages in the Saalfeld district in Thuringia, see Andrew I. Port, *Conflict and Stability in the German Democratic Republic* (New York, 2007), 262–69.
77. SAPMO-BArch, DO 101/027/1-2, Stellungnahme zur Eingabe der Sektion Fußball der Sportgemeinschaft Dynamo Forst vom 7.8.78, 29 August 1978.
78. ThHStAW, Bezirkstag und Rat des Bezirkes Erfurt Altregistratur Nr. 46939/1, letter from Erfurt district council to BSG Traktor Hochstedt, 7 June 1989.
79. Johnson, *Training Socialist Citizens*, 109–10.
80. Gilbert, *The Miracle Machine*, 94.
81. ThHStAW, Bezirkstag und Rat des Bezirkes Erfurt Altregistratur Nr. 46939/1, petition from Traktor Hochstedt to Erfurt district council, 21 April 1989; SAPMO-BArch, DO 101/027/1-2, petition from Dynamo Forst to Mielke, 7 August 1978.
82. SAPMO-BArch, DO 101/027/1-2, Stellungnahme zur Eingabe der Sektion Fußball, 29 August 1978.
83. SAPMO-BArch, DY 30/4979, petition from BSG Tiefbau Berlin to Hellmann, 2 October 1982.
84. Braun, "The People's Sport?" 414.
85. See, e.g., Zatlin, *The Currency of Socialism*, chap. 4.
86. Grix, "The Decline of Mass Sport Provision," 414.
87. On *Trendsport* in the late GDR, see Braun, "The People's Sport?" 420–23; Wilton, "The 'Societalisation' of the State," 122–25.
88. Eduardo Galeano, *Soccer in Sun and Shadow* (London, 1998), 209.
89. http://www.fc-nordost-berlin-web.de (Chronik); Beyer, *Rotation Leipzig*, 20–26.

CONCLUSION

Structures and Subjectivities in GDR History

MARY FULBROOK

The GDR was clearly a repressive dictatorship. One need only mention the Berlin Wall and the Stasi to summon a whole field of associations, and the structures of power reflected the lack of any widespread popular support. This much is accepted across a wide variety of historical approaches and interpretations, and underlies many of the attempts at typologizing that accompanied earlier historiographical debates on the GDR.[1] What is far less well explored, however, are the ways in which East German subjectivities changed over time, and the ways in which changing subjectivities and structures were interrelated in processes of historical development that were far from predictable in an uncertain world. The end was not given in the origins.

Narratives of GDR History

Some aspects of the GDR are now widely taken for granted. We know, for example, that, for many Germans, the transition from Nazism to communism was deeply unpopular. The end of the war was for the vast majority of Germans an experience of massive national defeat, not "liberation," with widespread experiences of humiliation, flight and expulsion, and brutal treatment by Red Army soldiers. Once established from these unpromising beginnings, the GDR was widely seen as an imposed dictatorship sustained by Soviet power—unlike its Nazi predecessor, which had been a homegrown dictatorship led by a supposed savior figure whom many had supported with enthusiasm. We also know much about the social, economic, and political transformations that constituted the building of the East German Communist dictatorship on the ruins of Adolf Hitler's state—and the extent to which these transformations were experienced as traumatic and deeply disruptive on the part of those ousted from their livelihoods or separated from friends and family in an already war-torn society. We know a great deal about the experiences of particular social groups who suffered in a myriad of ways during the transition from one socioeconomic and political system to another: large landowners, capitalists, different professional groups among the educated and propertied bourgeoisie.[2] Very few were like those of humble social origins and left-wing inclinations who benefited from the new opportunities offered to them in the "workers' and farmers' state," especially among those born in the later years of the Weimar Republic (the "1929ers").[3] In view of all this, it is indeed impossible to separate the "political" from the "social" in this period of highly intrusive and radical change.

It does not take much, from such a starting point, to place the emphasis of any historical account of the GDR on the power of the Socialist Unity Party (SED) and on the structures and strictures of Communist rule. Moreover, this narrative of GDR history would appear to fit well, at first glance, with a totalitarian portrayal of the SED regime as inherently manipulative and repressive, and of "the people" as essentially innocent victims coerced by and intrinsically opposed to the new, imposed Communist project. But this is precisely where an overwhelming focus on the repressive structures of the regime—at the expense of exploring patterns of subjectivity—is inadequate.

The unequal power relations implied by such a depiction are not far off the mark. Yet, such an account tends to leave out the indigenous origins of many developments in the GDR itself. The new system did not come solely as a result of Soviet domination, and much of what developed over succeeding decades not only had roots in pre-1945 traditions, but was also carried out by Germans whose experiences lay in contesting rather than sustaining the Nazi dictatorship. It also underplays the fundamental question of how, despite this historical legacy, so many people came to terms with and accommodated themselves to the new demands of the SED regime, and how, over forty years, that regime and those who lived within it were transformed through complex processes of historical and generational change. In view of the deep antipathy of so many Germans toward the new Communist dictatorship, it is important also to bear in mind the murderous character of the regime that had preceded it, as well as the fact that many who had helped sustain Nazism feared retribution under the new "Bolshevik" state. Dislike of the Communist dictatorship was not always rooted entirely in any principled support for democracy.

Many people, regardless of whether or not they had previously supported the Third Reich, were deeply critical of significant aspects of the GDR—not least the Wall, the Stasi, and the many restrictions on human rights. They were nevertheless inescapably affected by having lived through this period of history: their assumptions, values, and patterns of behavior developed in the context of particular networks of social and political relations, as well as prevalent, often unexamined cultural frameworks of interpretation. Many individuals who were critical of the SED regime and had held out high hopes for unification with the West registered, after unification, just how different their systems of values and aspirations had become from prevalent norms on the other side of the German-German border.

The multiple transitions from Nazism to communism and then to capitalist democracy left traces in the ways in which people themselves interpreted and gave significance to their world. They became, in short, "East Germans"—a transformation that was often only registered, to its full extent, *after* the fall of the Wall. It was only when the contours and demands of survival in the more competitive West German society, now imported to the East, became clear in practice to East Germans—contrasting with what had, until then, been largely implicit and unspoken assumptions and expectations about constrained and secure life-courses—that key contrasts were explicitly registered and articulated. The initially surprising post-unification development of nostalgia (*Ostalgie*) for East German *society*, not for the widely hated SED state, highlighted differences that had had emerged over time.[4]

Of course the establishment, the relative stability and longevity, as well as the ultimate demise of the GDR had more to do with Soviet domination and the Cold War division of Europe than with any popular consent to Communist rule. Yet, for all the agreement about the coercive and repressive features of the second German dictatorship, major areas of theoretical disagreement remain, particularly over the interpretation of changing subjectivities under dictatorial regimes—and indeed across the transition from Nazism to Communism. This remains a contentious and inadequately explored field—as do, more generally, the ways in which subjectivities are themselves historically constituted and the ways in which they change.

Changing Subjectivities

These theoretical problems are not restricted to analyses of the GDR, but apply to any period of history, as long-running debates over structure, agency, and "structuration" (designating the inextricable linkages between agency and structure) readily attest. From the classics—Karl Marx, Friedrich Nietzsche, Max Weber, and Sigmund Freud—to more recent theoretical developments (structuralism and poststructuralism, hermeneutics, discourse theories, the "cultural turn," the pervasive influence of theorists such as Pierre Bourdieu and Michel Foucault), the issues around self-perceptions, representation, structure, and agency have been repeatedly addressed and assessed from a variety of analytic perspectives.

Moreover, there are serious practical problems involved, irrespective of theoretical starting point. It is not easy to make connections between broad historical changes, on the one hand—generally reconstructed and recounted on the basis of residues found in the archives and public records—with, on the other, inner processes of thinking, feeling, and reflection on questions of morality in the subjective perceptions of historical actors. Only rarely can we compare personal sources and self-representations, both from the time and later, with external records of behavior and action—and even then, there remain many areas beyond the reach of the historian.[5] A further twist is added in the case of recent German history by the fact that one dictatorship was succeeded by another with a radically different political ideology, constraining and shaping people's self-representations in ways that are extremely hard to capture and interpret. Yet, for all the difficulties, analysis of the transitions across regime boundaries in recent German history provides a particularly fertile ground for exploration.

There are major methodological pitfalls to be navigated in this area. An uncritical reproduction of popular perceptions and memories runs the risk of (mis)taking the worm's-eye view as an adequate guide to the shape of the forest as a whole, and of reproducing partisan accounts from perspectives that are necessarily partial (in both senses of the word). Particularly if the focus is on people who were not targeted by the Stasi, who were not knowingly victims of surveillance and intimidation, who were not politically active and thus exposed to the difficulties resulting from such activities, who were relatively happy to lead a quiet life and accept constraints they could not challenge or change, there is the risk that any "thick description" will be misinterpreted as an attempted exoneration of the regime rather than as a contribution to understanding its stability over forty years—more than three times as long as the Third Reich. Leaving aside simplistic misunderstandings of this sort, it is clear that any account that uncritically reproduces the highly variable and often mutually contradictory subjective perceptions of the time runs the risk of simply recording the conflicting interpretations, prejudices, priorities, and partial misconceptions that obtain in any society. As far as professional history is concerned, mapping subjectivities without some critical distance and interpretive framework is, in principle, both impracticable and theoretically unsustainable. There needs to be, then, an explicit engagement with the question of recouping but, at the same time, also of interpreting patterns of subjectivity across the range: this involves investigating and enabling voices "to be heard," but also engaging in critical interpretation of those voices.

To take a simple example: following the opening of the archives in the early 1990s, a great deal was suddenly learned about the sheer extent of Stasi surveillance and infiltration of society. Media revelations and historical research on the Stasi provoked a widespread sense of shock. We therefore have to confront the now known facts about the structures and practices of the Stasi with prevalent claims among East Germans to the effect that they were able to lead what many called "perfectly normal lives," relatively untroubled by coexistence with the Stasi. One way of addressing this is to explore the disjuncture between the actual extent of Stasi activity and prevalent perceptions or knowledge of Stasi structures and practices. This requires a differentiated approach. We can map relative ignorance about the Stasi in relation to, for example, social location, political relevance, age, and generation: those born in the 1970s and 1980s were far less likely to have been aware of or troubled by the Stasi than those who were older. Conversely, those active in the churches or oppositional movements, or who worked in key areas of industry and politically sensitive areas for the state, had a far greater awareness of the Stasi than those at a greater distance from power struggles. The different subjective perceptions and associated anxieties are themselves part of East German history, to be explored against what is now known of the actual structures of power. This disjuncture between subjective perceptions and structural realities is itself important: ignorance itself has a history, a discourse, and its character and significance requires historical exploration. Although the subject matter and the implications of "ignorance" are very different, the question is not dissimilar in principle from that of the post-Nazi claim to have "known nothing" about the extermination of the Jews—a claim that has now been subjected to extensive historical investigation.[6] Analysis of prevalent discourses can, on its own, be no substitute for analysis of structures of power and historical developments; but discourses certainly play a key role both in how people are involved in particular regimes, permitting certain developments to take place, and how they later reflect upon particular periods of history and participate in a later present.

By contrast, an overly critical approach to what people themselves said about their lives under dictatorial conditions—before and after 1945 (for those who were old enough), as well as before and after 1989—runs the risk of becoming reductive, effectively interpreting away all residues of individual autonomy. Totalitarian theorists, for example, tend to read Western responses into the situation, prioritizing a certain description and critique of the political system and assuming that no apparent support could actually have been authentic. It is easy, from this perspective, to discount evidence of conformity as having arisen from coercion, pressure, fear, regime propaganda, and ideological indoctrination. Even where the authenticity of subjective perceptions is conceded, or the personal benefits of particular policies or actions are recognized, a functionalist argument is often adduced to show that, whatever the perceived benefits or individual motives for support, people who conformed were effectively "collaborators" who ensured the smooth functioning of an unjust regime, thus contributing to their own subjugation and to the stabilization of power structures.[7] Apparent agency can, in this way, be dismissed in terms of its functional consequences for the regime; subjectivities can be written off as essentially irrelevant. Frequently, the only real agency to appear in totalitarian accounts is that of the dominant political forces (the SED, the Stasi, "Moscow," and so on), on the one hand, and those who challenged Communist domination, on the other; the vast majority of the people "in between" are represented as more or less passive dupes or as the "victims of history." Any attempt to explore the ways in which they perceived their own situation and actively sought to lead their lives in circumstances not necessarily of their own choosing, which brings to attention the ways in which they made sense of their lives, can, from this perspective, be dismissed as political "whitewashing" of a repressive regime; in extreme cases, political diatribe takes the place of scholarly engagement with the issues at hand.[8]

"Mentalities" and cultural traditions are thus given short shrift by totalitarian theorists: in an ironic reversal of Marxist conceptions of "false consciousness," totalitarian theorists tend to discount expressions of subjective perceptions, often interpreting pre-1989 records of opinion as the result of propaganda, ideology, or fear, while discounting post-1990 memories as nostalgic distortions born of difficult post-unification conditions. There is, of course, an element of truth to this skepticism, but it runs the risk of leading to the wholesale dismissal of this entire area of investigation. There are innumerable sources for changing patterns of mentality and subjectivity prior to 1989 that have barely been explored and that potentially allow for a discerning and critical evaluation, especially with respect to change over time. As for any period and any regime, due attention has to be paid to the provenance, conditions, and purposes of the sources. As far as post-unification representations are concerned, a longing for "the good old days" is a well-known historical and psychological phenomenon: in startling contrast to Whig theories of history, disappointed contemporaries tend to view the past as having been somehow better. But here again it is possible to engage in critical exploration and interpretation of assumptions, ways of thinking, patterns of discourse, and remembered experiences. Oral history practitioners have been especially careful to develop a method for *understanding* without necessarily *believing* what their respondents say. A simple dismissal of such sources is shortsighted.

Disagreements over interpretations of subjectivities in the GDR are rather different from comparable controversies in relation to the Third Reich. While there has been much scholarly debate about the balance between apparently widespread popular enthusiasm for Hitler as a charismatic leader, on the one hand, and the massive forces of repression and violence in the genocidal Third Reich, on the other, similar debates over the drab, constrained domestic dictatorship led by East German Communists under Soviet domination are only really beginning as a serious scholarly endeavor, and are still on occasion plagued by unwarranted politicization of differing theoretical approaches. Perhaps condemnation of the Third Reich is so taken for granted that historians exploring popular support for Hitler need not repeatedly avow their personal antipathy for Nazism. Whatever the reason, historians exploring support for Hitler are in little danger of being accused of personally harboring Nazi sympathies—in contrast to historians of the GDR who face accusations of "whitewashing" the dictatorship when exploring how some East Germans managed to come to terms with the state in which they had to lead their lives.[9]

There is a closely related distinction with respect to the styles of history writing about the two dictatorships. It was more than forty years after the end of the war when, in the 1980s, Martin Broszat and Saul Friedländer engaged in their now well-known debate about ways of "normalizing" the writing of Third Reich history. This debate signaled a key stage in Western writing about the Nazi period, but raised issues that have not yet been fully resolved: in particular, the question of whether a supposedly objective or "neutral" writing of Third Reich history, as if it were a period like any other, distorts or downplays the traumatic and seismic break that this period signified for its victims; and how the subjectivities of those living through this period, "witnesses" whose voices were often seen as purely "illustrative," should be incorporated into scholarly accounts that primarily focused on policies and political structures. Friedländer's two-volume narrative of the Nazi persecution and attempted extermination of European Jews stimulated further questions about subjectivities and scholarly history writing, although again without resolution.[10] While there has not yet been a comparable debate over the style and tone of GDR history writing, it is notable that two key variants have vied with each other: the lightly ironic, and the critical verging on hostile.[11] In different ways, both have downplayed the perceptions and subjectivities of people living at the time.

Intertwining Patterns

One way forward is to explore in more detail the character of subjective perceptions in historical context, exploring variations in patterns of subjectivity—constrained and enabled by changing structural circumstances and sociopolitical conditions—across individuals and generations, and among different groups, within the context of changing structural circumstances and wider historical conditions. The chapters in this book suggest some productive ways out of what has increasingly become sterile theoretical terrain. In particular, by considering the history of East Germans from a variety of perspectives, the essays point to interesting areas of continuity, convergence, and divergence.

The future was constantly contested, as demonstrated by the variety of debates over ways of overcoming fascism and creating a new future, while differentially interpreting the recent past. "Memory cultures" were never as simple as critiques of the allegedly monolithic "anti-fascist myth"—as opposed to "private views" or "popular opinion"—would suggest. There were complex interrelations between dominant or official narratives and prevalent or marginalized personal narratives, with negotiations around what could be said and the forms in which subjectivities could be expressed and identities developed. Moreover, East Germans themselves changed over time as they negotiated their way through new post-Nazi circumstances and sought to build new lives, partially disavowing or amending their own biographical pasts—or, less often, stubbornly sticking to some notion of "how it really was" in the hope that their voice would eventually be heard. The interactions among different scripts—dominant, salient, marginalized, suppressed—within East German negotiations of the fascist past need to be explored more fully, and in more subtle ways than a concentration primarily on official "propaganda" and "ideology" allows.

Changing views and contested narratives among the cultural intelligentsia, former prisoners of war, members of the left-wing resistance against Nazism, as well as among wider groups of perpetrators, victims, and "ordinary Germans"— selectively sampled in Part I, on "Memory and Identity after Nazism"—not only suggest some of the ways in which to pursue such an undertaking, but also serve to open up new areas of inquiry. Andreas Agocs's contribution reveals how intellectual and cultural history cannot be separated from political history, and how indigenous divisions were far more complex than notions of the imposition of a Stalinist dictatorship suggest. Joanne Sayner's analysis of memories of the "Red Orchestra" breaks down the model according to which the official anti-fascist narrative is either presented as being simply at odds with personal memories, or is gratefully accepted as a means of evading any sense of guilt or engaging in confrontations with the Nazi past. Her approach nevertheless leaves open questions about the wider resonance of contested and partial official narratives. Sayner's analysis of Greta Kuckhoff's attempts to influence a more accurate representation of the "Red Orchestra" opposition movement during the Third Reich makes very clear which discursive frameworks were dominant where and when, and just how difficult it was even for a woman as intelligent, politically experienced, and tenacious as Kuckhoff to correct or amend views articulated by more powerful voices.

Yet, even within a context of official discourses backed by power, personal interests could still play a role and allow distinctive individual inflections of an account. Christiane Wienand's focus on the shifting self-representation of Bernt von Kügelgen raises questions about degrees of personal authenticity as well as the instrumentalization of dominant views under changing circumstances, tracing how a personal narrative of anti-fascist conversion could be adapted while remaining constrained within the broader framework of changing official discourses. My own chapter raises questions about the ways in which different communities of experience are affected by the later contexts in which they form new lives, and the longer-term significance of post-rupture circumstances for later communities of connection and identification. A people-oriented focus on the continuing significance of a salient past can, in this way, suggest rather different interpretations from those prevalent in the kinds of "collective memory" studies that remain primarily at the level of official representations, rituals of remembrance, political debates, and public memorialization.

Part II, on "Health, Food, and Embodied Citizens," continues the people-oriented focus, now paying greater attention to physical aspects of "becoming East German" in an ever-changing international context. Many individuals in positions of influence, including not only SED politicians and left-leaning intellectuals but also, for example, health professionals, continued to develop traditions that had existed in Germany prior to 1945 (or 1933) and that remained influential, in a different political context, in West Germany. Moreover, Cold War competition could lead not only to explicit divergence but also eventually to convergence in terms of aims, policies, and practices, albeit often by somewhat meandering routes. Donna Harsch and Jeannette Madarász-Lebenhagen, for example, show how health policies and particular strategies of disease containment and prevention—while distinctive in many respects, especially in regard to the roles and responsibilities allotted to the state versus the individual, and despite different philosophies and structures for the delivery of health care—eventually converged in East and West Germany. While Madarász-Lebenhagen's careful analysis shows how a period of divergence in competition for common goals eventually led to the adoption of the same model of risk factor analysis, Harsch draws attention to generational shifts in the medical profession, as well as changing views of parents (in terms of their willingness to present their children for vaccination) and patients (with respect to voluntary submission to forms of treatment, including isolation).

Convergence between East and West across later postwar generations is also evident in Neula Kerr-Boyle's work on eating habits and dieting in the GDR. Kerr-Boyle's analysis of dieting discourses and practices makes clear that wider political and cultural influences—including cultural currents shared across the Western world—played a role in the efforts of women, in particular, to lose weight even when they were already of average or less than medically ideal weight. But there were many factors involved in women's efforts to slim, including the continuation of a still gender-unequal society in which it was considered more important for women than for men to care for their appearance, and in which dieting concerns were more prevalent among educated and professional women than among their blue-collar, less well-educated counterparts. Why this was the case remains a matter of speculation, both among historians and historical actors themselves.

There were often discrepancies between an individual's behavioral practices and his or her own capacity to articulate and account for such behaviors. But there are clear parallels with developments in contemporary capitalist societies, where professional success has been linked to body image, and where there is no direct or obvious link between women's subjective perceptions of their eating behaviors and official propaganda. Both the explicit adoption of the risk factor model of disease and the often subconscious processes of pursuing bodily ideals of slenderness crossed the boundaries between East and West, between democratic and dictatorial political systems, and between Communist and capitalist socioeconomic systems. Even the area of luxury dining can be viewed in light of changing patterns of cultural diplomacy and a partially shared international and domestic language of embodied status distinctions, as Paul Freedman demonstrates. These are a few examples of areas where the GDR needs to be examined not only in terms of its own pre-1945 Nazi past and its Communist present, but also in the wider context of modern industrial societies, with an increasingly transnational media presence, individualist goals, and faith in science.

These essays also have relevance for questions about constraint and conformity. Not all discipline is the obvious *repressive* kind, and power is not only about the political structures and institutions of a "walled-in" state, as important as these are. Norms are integrally related to the self: "discipline" is not merely imposed from without, but is also a matter of self-discipline, regardless of whether those practicing self-discipline are consciously aware of what they are doing, in spheres as apparently divergent as individual eating habits, self-narratives, political challenges, or behavioral conformity.

Part III, on "Constraints and Conformity: Friends, Foes, and Disciplinary Practices," seeks to shed new light on contested political terrain over time, exploring unfolding processes in the sphere of subjectivities as well as of structures. Not only the shifting character of power and repression and the (class) character of ideology, but also processes of learning from the past in ever-changing later contexts—again, both national and international—were highly important. As Andrew Port shows in his comparative exploration of practices of terrorizing and enthusing workers, and of suppressing workers' unrest, in the Third Reich and the GDR—the self-professed workers' and farmer's state—analysis of systems of repression needs to be augmented by exploration of changing "sensibilities" over time; people learned from past experiences and adjusted their aspirations and expectations accordingly. David Tompkins's analysis of the shift in official views of Israel, from friend to foe, reveals continuing undercurrents of anti-Semitism emerging in new forms, with early widespread support for the Jews' right to a homeland later tempered by criticism of Israeli policies in the Middle East. Again, there was a process in which policies and attitudes changed under different circumstances, with a particular role played in this case by wider international considerations. Phil Leask's analysis of accounts of inner-party humiliation explicitly highlights the ways in which discipline may be imposed through strongly emotional experiences of humiliation. It is striking how frequently both real individuals and fictional characters experienced humiliating rituals of initiation and were subjected to humiliating incidents at an early stage of their career, before later holding positions from which they imposed humiliating experiences on others. This was a widespread disciplinary practice in a Marxist-Leninist party—and it was a discipline of a very different order from that explored in other chapters, where less obvious normative constraints played a significant role. These too, however, are highly significant for our understanding of East German history.

The willingness and capacity of people to express their frustrations and agitate for improvement may change, even when the grounds for discontent have not deteriorated significantly. Looking at lower-level sports functionaries and ordinary football players, Alan McDougall reveals how increasing "individualization" during the Honecker period—along with enhanced avenues for voicing discontent (such as *Eingaben,* or citizens' complaints and petitions) and heightened expectations of improvement in the near future—played a role in the expression of grassroots discontent in the 1970s and 1980s.[12] An analysis of such an everyday field (both literally and metaphorically) can demonstrate the extent to which people had adapted to, and knew how to play by, the rules of the Socialist game, actively participating in the microstructures of what I have elsewhere called the "honeycomb state" while at the same time pursuing their own individual ends.[13]

The chapters also interrelate, of course, with the overriding themes relating to structures and subjectivities having relevance in different ways across diverse areas at different times. There is no sense in which we would wish to suggest any new master narrative, but it is worth registering just how much changed across the forty years of the East German dictatorship, and reflecting on how shifting subjectivities can be reconceptualized in light of broader structural and historical changes. The notion of "trauma" has been widely used in recent decades to understand better the long-term reverberations of massive ruptures in individual and collective lives.[14] There is no doubt that the consequences at a personal level of war and the postwar upheavals, which have been intensively explored for areas of Western Europe, also played a major and still inadequately explored role in the GDR (as in other postwar Communist states).[15] An overriding concern with issues of dictatorship and socioeconomic transformation has perhaps occluded our view of the lingering consequences of experiences of war and Nazism for East Germans at a personal level. This focus has also, arguably, occluded our perceptions of key shifts over time. Even though it came later, and in different ways than in the West, a fragile stabilization eventually set in in the GDR as well, at not only the political but also the personal level.

The concept of "normalization" may help us to understand this process better. It raises explicitly the question of links between broader social and political stabilization—on both the national and international levels—and aspects of the routinization of everyday life, including some sense of a "return to normality" in everyday life, if only as an absence of existential fears about hunger, bombing, or the loss of loved ones—however tempered this "absence" may have been by newer Cold War anxieties. It also points to the significance, under new conditions, of learning new "rules of the game" and, in some cases, the internalization of new norms or adaptation to new codes of conduct.[16] In periods of massive upheaval and rapid social transformation, people often grope their way forward, dealing with often horrendous personal legacies of the recent past and unstable present, and not knowing the best course of action in the face of an uncertain future. Once matters have settled down into some kind of routine—however disagreeable—people are better able to adapt their behavior in the light of expectations about the likely consequences of different kinds of conduct. They know about and can orient themselves toward the likely responses of those in dominant positions; they are aware of the explicit and implicit rules governing social processes, and can assess the probable outcomes of different courses of action—including likely sanctions and penalties for nonconformity, as well as, ironically, the very terrifying unpredictability itself of official responses. Material and personal self-interest, family considerations, as well as political, religious, or moral views, all play a role in affecting how different individuals perceive and respond to changing "regimes"—in the moral and social, as well as the political sense—and how they adapt their behavior, and often also their self-perceptions, accordingly. This does not necessarily mean people will choose to conform; but it does mean that they are aware of the likely consequences of transgressing the normative as well as physical boundaries of the regime. They may, over time, also change their personal views and professed values so that they need not live in a constant state of dissonance between "inner" and "outer," between beliefs and behavior, but can find ways of "living with themselves" with a sense of internal consistency. Or they may simply joke about *Doppelzüngigkeit*, living with two tongues, one for "officialspeak" in public places and the other for where they feel "at home," with trusted friends and family. Command over multiple discourses, with deployment as relevant in different situations, was not unique to people living in the GDR.[17]

Many East Germans were—both at the time and in retrospect—highly critical of the SED regime, angry or bitter about ways in which the constraints of the system had, in some sense, constrained or even "deformed" the paths they felt their lives should or could have taken under different circumstances. They could also be very critical of the impact their own status had on their children's chances of education and career advancement—without necessarily making any direct connection between the Communist project of societal transformation and the legacies of the Nazi past. Nevertheless, a particularly striking feature of many East Germans' accounts of their lives is the emphasis on personal agency and choice, even when the consequences of such choices were not always easy to live with. This was evident in letters and diary writing at the time, where people thought about what choices to make, or reflected on the consequences of earlier choices. It was evident, too, in accounts of their lives after unification. Even when oral history interviewees were highly critical of the building of the Berlin Wall in 1961, for example, they tended to emphasize the reasons why they had "chosen" to stay in the GDR rather than flee to the West while the possibility had still existed. Equally striking is the widespread sense of pride in what they had managed to achieve as individuals in the GDR—with or without the assistance of the state, and despite the constraints of the regime and its policies. On a different plane, as Freedman points out, the tastes and culinary memories of the GDR have provided a key source of nostalgia.

An examination of variations not only in the ways in which people represent and interpret their own past under changing circumstances, but also the ways in which the new circumstances affect the very constitution of the people themselves, can provide a way to analyze the relations between structures and subjectivities. Such has been, in part, the project of this book. Looking at patterns of negotiation and compromise, the chapters have examined how people helped shape the worlds in which they lived, even as they were themselves formed by the circumstances and periods into which they were born. The chapters have also depicted the character and negotiation of power relations by demonstrating the sundry possibilities for individual agency in the GDR, as well as the often unintended consequences of regime policy. Going beyond an analysis purely of power relations, the authors have explored the ways in which East Germans conceptualized, sought to control, and were simultaneously constituted by the regimes and periods through which they lived—even at the most physical, bodily level. Not only political, economic, and social relations, but also aspects of health and illness, food and dieting, leisure activities, and the ways in which people reflected on their past and their present: all of this helped to shape—often literally—distinctively new kinds of people, with experiences, outlooks, and ways of being that were both like and unlike those of their European neighbors to the East and West. In this way, analyses of the ways in which people "became" East Germans, and at the same time contributed to and transformed the state in which they lived, may help us develop new and fruitful approaches to understanding wider patterns of change in modern Europe.

Notes

1. See further Andrew I. Port's Introduction and his chapter in this volume.
2. The literature in these areas is now substantial. For further references see Andrew I. Port's Introduction to this volume.
3. On the 1929ers, see further Mary Fulbrook, *Dissonant Lives: Generations and Violence through the German Dictatorships* (Oxford, 2011).
4. See, e.g., Caroline Pearce and Nick Hodgin, eds., *The GDR Remembered: Representations of the East German State since 1989* (Rochester, N.Y., 2011); David Clarke and

Ute Wölfel, eds., *Remembering the German Democratic Republic: Divided Memory in a United Germany* (New York, 2011).
5. I became acutely aware of this problem when confronting the picture presented in the archival legacies with the conflicting evidence of contemporary letters, later statements of self-defense, and private memoirs of a former Nazi *Landrat*; see Mary Fulbrook, *A Small Town Near Auschwitz: Ordinary Nazis and the Holocaust* (Oxford, 2012).
6. See, e.g., Frank Bajohr and Dieter Pohl, *Der Holocaust als offenes Geheimnis: Die Deutschen, die NS-Führung und die Alliierten* (Munich, 2006); Bernward Dörner, *Die Deutschen und der Holocaust. Was niemand wissen wollte, aber jeder wissen konnte* (Berlin, 2007); Peter Longerich, *"Davon haben wir nichts gewusst!" Die Deutschen und die Judenverfolgung 1933-1945* (Munich, 2006).
7. See, e.g., Peter Grieder, "In Defence of Totalitarian Theory as a Tool of Historical Scholarship," *Totalitarian Movements and Political Religions* 8/3 (2007): 562–89.
8. These points are developed in Mary Fulbrook, "The State of GDR History," *Francia. Forschungen zur westeuropäischen Geschichte* 38 (2011): 259–70. See also Andrew I. Port's Introduction and his chapter in this volume.
9. This is something I have experienced personally in reviews of my own work: see, e.g., Ilko-Sascha Kowalczuk's review of *Power and Society in the GDR, 1961-1979: The "Normalisation of Rule"?* (New York, 2010) in *Historische Zeitschrift* 291 (2010): 278–79; and Klaus Schroeder's review of *Ein ganz normales Leben: Alltag und Gesellschaft in der DDR* (Darmstadt, 2008), in *Zeitschrift des Forschungsverbundes SED-Staat* 26 (2009):177–80.
10. See, e.g., the third chapter of Alon Confino, "Narrative Forms and Historical Sensation," *Foundational Pasts: The Holocaust as Historical Understanding* (Cambridge, 2012).
11. Two examples must stand for many: Stefan Wolle, *Die heile Welt der Diktatur. Alltag und Herrschaft in der DDR 1971-1989* (Berlin, 1998), adopts the ironic mode, while Klaus Schroeder, *Der SED-Staat. Partei, Staat und Gesellschaft, 1949-1990* (Munich, 1998) adopts the castigatory stance. Despite their differences in tone and narrative style, both are critical of the dictatorial conditions and largely downplay (and thus effectively belittle) the authenticity of subjective responses.
12. On the idea of increasing "individualization" in the GDR in the 1970s and 1980s, see Mary Fulbrook, *The People's State: East German Society from Hitler to Honecker* (London, 2005).
13. Fulbrook, *People's State*.
14. See, e.g., the discussion in Ido de Haan, "Paths of Normalization after the Persecution of the Jews: The Netherlands, France and West Germany in the 1950s," in *Life after Death: Approaches to a Cultural History of Europe during the 1940s and 1950s*, ed. Richard Bessel and Dirk Schumann (Cambridge, 2003), 65–92.
15. There are explorations of the reverberations of both the Holocaust and war at a political level: see, e.g., Jeffrey Herf, *Divided Memory: The Nazi Past in the Two Germanys* (Cambridge, M.A., 1997); Christina Morina, *Legacies of Stalingrad: Remembering the Eastern Front in Germany since 1945* (Cambridge, 2011). But there remains much to be done at a personal level, beyond the actors on the public stage.
16. See the Introduction in Fulbrook, *Power and Society*; also discussed in idem, *Dissonant Lives*.
17. See, e.g., Alexei Yurchak, *Everything Was Forever, Until It Was No More: The Last Soviet Generation* (Princeton, 2006).

CONTRIBUTORS

Andreas Agocs is visiting assistant professor for modern European history at the University of the Pacific in California. He received his Ph.D. from the University of California, Davis, and his master's degree from the Heinrich-Heine University in Düsseldorf, Germany. His article "Restrained Revolution: Antifascist Committees and the End of Mass Politics in East and West, 1944-1947" was published in 2009 in *Témoigner: Entre Histoire et Mémoire. Revue pluridisciplinaire de la Fondation Auschwitz Bruxelles*. Agocs's book manuscript "Other Germanys: Politics and Cultural Renewal from Antifascism to Cold War, 1935–1953" is currently under review with an academic press.

Paul Freedman is Chester D. Tripp Professor of Medieval History at Yale University, where he has taught since 1997. From 1979 until 1997 he was in the History Department at Vanderbilt University. He has written on the peasantry and church, as well as the society and culture of the Middle Ages, especially in Catalonia from the eleventh to fifteenth centuries. His 1999 book *Images of the Medieval Peasant* was awarded the Haskins Medal by the Medieval Academy of America. He has also worked on the history of food and cuisine and, in 2008, published *Out of the East: Spices and the Medieval Imagination*. Freedman was the editor of *Food: The History of Taste* (2007), which has been translated into nine languages. Among his current projects is a book on changes in American restaurants from 1830 to the present.

Mary Fulbrook, FBA, is professor of German history at University College London. Her most recent books are *A Small Town near Auschwitz: Ordinary Nazis and the Holocaust* (2012) and *Dissonant Lives: Generations and Violence through the German Dictatorships* (2011). She is currently directing an AHRC-funded collaborative project on *Reverberations of War in Germany and Europe: Communities of Experience and Identification since 1945*. A former chair of the German History Society, and chair of the Modern History Section of the British Academy, Fulbrook has written widely on the GDR, including *Anatomy of a Dictatorship: Inside the GDR* (1995) and *The People's State: East German Society from Hitler to Honecker* (2005), as well as writing and editing many other books.

Donna Harsch is professor in the Department of History at Carnegie Mellon University in Pittsburgh. Her field of research is modern Germany. She has published numerous articles as well as two books: *Revenge of the Domestic: Women, the Family, and Communism in the German Democratic Republic, 1945-1970* (2007) and *German Social Democracy and the Rise of Nazism, 1928-1933* (1993). She is currently working on a comparative history of health cultures in the Federal Republic of Germany and the German Democratic Republic.

Neula Kerr-Boyle studied history at the University of Glasgow and the University of Mainz before continuing on to the University of Warwick, where she completed an M.A. in the Social History of Medicine. Her Ph.D. thesis (University College London, 2012) is a historical study of anorexia nervosa in the German Democratic Republic. Through an investigation of the material conditions, cultural discourses, and social practices surrounding eating and the body, the thesis analyses the interconnectedness of body, self, and society in East Germany between 1949 and 1990.

Phil Leask is a writer and researcher with a Ph.D. from University College London. His doctoral dissertation considers the concept of humiliation and its significance in representations of the GDR. He is currently working on a research project on narratives of identity across generations and across borders, drawing on personal accounts of people in or from East Germany.

Jeannette Madarász-Lebenhagen read history at Cambridge University and then went on to do her Ph.D. at University College London. She published her dissertation in 2002 under the title *Conflict and Compromise in East Germany, 1971-1989: A Precarious Stability*. She published a second monograph, *Working in East Germany: Normality in a Socialist Dictatorship, 1961 to 1979* in 2006, and then, in 2010 (with Martin Lengwiler), *Das präventive Selbst. Eine Kulturgeschichte moderner Gesundheitspolitik*. Since 2011, Madarász-Lebenhagen is working at the Institute for the History, Philosophy, and Ethics of Medicine in Mainz, researching gender representations and prevention in a German-German comparison.

Alan McDougall was educated at Oxford University and is associate professor in modern European history at the University of Guelph in Canada. His first monograph was *Youth Politics in East Germany: The Free German Youth Movement 1946-1968* (2004). He is currently writing a social and political history of football under East German communism.

Andrew I. Port is associate professor of history at Wayne State University in Detroit, Review Editor of the *German Studies Review*, and, beginning in 2014, editor of *Central European History*. He received a Ph.D. in modern European history from Harvard University, a B.A. in history from Yale University, and a certificate in political science from the Institut d'Etudes Politiques in Paris. His research focuses on modern Germany, communism and state socialism, labor history, social protest, and comparative genocide. His first book, *Conflict and Stability in the German Democratic Republic* (2007), appeared in German translation as *Die Rätselhafte Stabilität der DDR* (2010), and his current project looks at German reactions to genocide in other parts of the world since 1945.

Joanne Sayner is senior lecturer in cultural theory and German studies in the Department of Modern Languages at the University of Birmingham in the United Kingdom. She specializes in the politics of remembrance, women's literature, and autobiography. Her first book, *Women without a Past? German Autobiographical Writings and Fascism*, appeared in 2007. Her second book, a project about memory and the GDR, is entitled *Reframing Antifascism: Memory, Genre and the Life Writings of Greta Kuckhoff* (2013).

David G. Tompkins is assistant professor of history at Carleton College in Minnesota. He specializes in the history of modern Central Europe, and is particularly interested in the relationship between culture and politics. His book *Composing the Party Line: Music and Politics in Early Cold War Poland and East Germany* will appear in 2013; he has published articles in *German History*, *The Polish Review*, and several edited volumes. His current project examines images of the "Other" in the Soviet bloc.

Christiane Wienand is research fellow in the Department of German at University College London, working in the AHRC-funded interdisciplinary research project *Reverberations of War in Germany and Europe: Communities of Experience and Identification since 1945*. Her research focuses on the history of memory in Germany and Europe after World War II, and her current project looks at youths as "reconciliation activists" in Europe and Israel since 1945. She is currently preparing for publication her Ph.D. thesis, which is entitled "Performing Memory: Returned German Prisoners of War in Divided and Reunited Germany."

❦ INDEX ❧

Abusch, Alexander, 58–59, 62, 65, 68, 70, 73, 99–112
Academy for Medical Training and Education (*Akademie für Ärztliche Fortbildung*), 132
Ackermann, Anton, 69
Adenauer, Konrad, 36
Advice Bureau for Children and Young People's Health Protection (*Beratungsstelle für Kinder- und Jugendgesundheitsschutz*),176n34
African Americans, 13, 22, 23
agency, 2, 3, 5–7, 17, 38, 81, 112, 173, 279, 281, 288–89
agricultural cooperatives (LPG), 44, 246
Albania, 191
Algeria, 187
Aly, Götz, 209
Andersch, Alfred, 68
Anschluß, (1938) 209
Anschütz, Rolf, 189
anti-fascism (anti-fascist), 17, 57–59, 62–64, 66–73, 79–94, 99–112, 185, 210, 222, 226, 241
anti-formalist campaign, 66, 71
Anti-Radical Decree (1972), 21
anti-Semitism, 19, 27n29, 61–62, 220, 222–24, 226, 229, 230, 232
Arab countries, 220–22, 224–25, 227–30
Arab Legion, 221
Arafat, Yasser, 184
Arendt, Hannah, 26n29
Arndt, Melanie, 142
Aronowitz, Robert, 123
"asocials," 21, 143–47, 151
Association for the Protection of German Writers (*Schutzverband deutscher Autoren*), 59–60

Association of Returnees, POWs, and Family Members of MIAs (*Verband der Heimkehrer, Kriegsgefangenen und Vermisstenangehörigen e.V.*), 107, 110
Aufbau (journal), 64, 66
Aufbau (publishing house), 65
Augustine, Dolores, 21
Auschwitz, 39, 41
Auschwitz trial, 50
Austria, 40, 142, 145, 209
Aziz, Tariq, 185

Babelsberg, 228
Bacillus Calmette-Guérin (vaccination), 142–43, 147–51
Baldwin, Peter, 121
Baltic Sea, 187
Barnard, Christiaan, 128
Basic Law, 21
Bavaria, 204
Becher, Johannes R., 62, 70–71, 75n28
Becker, Jurek, 49
Berlin, 40, 47, 79–80, 191, 225, 228–29
Berlin Children's Hospital, 176n34
Berlin Wall, 10–12, 16, 18–21, 28n42, 47–48, 150, 185, 188, 203, 210, 278, 284
Berliner Zeitung (newspaper), 158, 166
Besymenski, Lew, 87
Biermann, Wolf, 242
Biernat, Karl Heinz, 91
Biess, Frank, 100
Birkenfeld, Günther, 56, 59–60, 69
Bitburg, 50
Bitterfeld, 243, 246
Bizone, 58
Black Sea, 187
Black, Monica, 15
Blackbourn, David, 5

Blitzkrieg, 207
Boder, David, 39
Body Mass Index (BMI), 169–70
Böll, Heinrich, 68
Bolshevism (Bolsheviks), 40, 244
Bonn, 226
Bourdieu, Pierre, 279
Brandenburg prison, 40
Brandt, Willy, 132, 184
Bredel, Willi, 244
Brigitte (journal), 162
Broca-Index, 174n10
Brockdorff, Erika von, 89
Broszat, Martin, 13, 283
Bruce, Gary, 4, 14, 26n29, 27n34
Buchenwald, 36, 39
Bulgaria, 185
Butler, Judith, 23

Cairo, 225
Camus, Albert, 66
Carville, James, 217n31
Castro, Fidel, 185
Ceaușescu, Nicolae, 184
censorship, 60–61, 129, 238
Central Institute for Cardiovascular Research (*Zentralinstitut für Herz-Kreislaufforschung*), 132
Central Institute for Nutrition (*Zentralinstitut für Ernährung*), 162, 164–66, 168, 175n14, 176n38. *See also* Institute for Nutrition
Central Institute for Youth Research (*Zentralinstitut für Jugendforschung*) (ZIJ), 164, 166, 168, 171, 259
Central Office of the State Justice Administrations for the Investigation of National Socialist Crimes (Ludwigsburg) (*Zentral Stelle*), 50
Checkup 35 program, 131
childcare, 12, 16, 171, 208
children, 34, 42–45, 47, 50, 148–50, 156n39, 164–65, 168, 176n34, 176n38, 202, 227, 266, 285, 288
Christian Democratic Union (*Christlich Demokratische Union*, CDU), 64
churches, 1, 5, 50, 281
civil society, 8, 23, 263

class, 13, 79, 86, 88, 158, 169–71, 240, 243, 246
Clinton, Bill, 217n31
Cold War, 4, 18–19, 56–57, 68, 87, 93, 107–8, 142, 151, 173, 175n24, 190, 222–23, 228, 231
Cominform (Communist Information Bureau), 58
Comintern school, 244–45
Committee of Antifascist Resistance Fighters (*Komitee der antifaschistischen Widerstandskämpfer*), 37, 103
Communist Party of Germany (KPD), 86, 89, 103, 248
Communist Party of Israel, 225, 233
Communist Party of the USSR, 247
Confessing Church, 71
Congo, Democratic Republic of, 185
Congress of Cultural Freedom (West Berlin, 1950), 70
Constanta, 187
Constitution (1949), 102
   Article 6, 240
Constitution (1968), 240
Constitution (1974), 262
Coppi, Hans, 90, 92
Council of Peace, 80
Counter Intelligence Program (COINTEL), 21
Countrywide Integrated Noncommunicable Diseases Intervention (CANON/CINDI), 130
Craxi, Bettino, 185
"Crystal Night" (*Kristallnacht*), 104
Cuba, 185, 187–88
Cultural League for the Democratic Renewal of Germany (*Kulturbund zur demokratischen Erneuerung Deutschlands*), 56, 58–62, 64–71, 74n2, 74n10
Czechoslovakia, 23, 220, 222–23

Dahlem, Franz, 84
Dallin, David, 85
Davis, Natalie Zemon, 15
Dayan, Moshe, 227
DEFA. *See* East German Film Studios

Deine Gesundheit (journal), 126, 164, 166
Delikat shops, 181
democratic centralism, 246, 251–52
denazification, 1, 35–36, 143
destalinization, 147, 151, 203
détente, 20, 84. See also Ostpolitik
Detroit, 23
Deutsches Ärzteblatt (journal), 126, 131
dieting, 17–18, 20, 158–77
    Hungerkuren (starvation diets) 161, 169
dining, 17–20, 179–93, 286
discourse analysis, 79–94
diseases
    anorexia nervosa, 169, 176n38
    arteriosclerosis, 121, 123
    bulimia nervosa, 169
    chronic disease, 121, 126, 130
    heart disease, 17–18, 121, 123–24, 129–30
    hypertension, 121
    infectious disease, 121, 123, 126
    "manager's disease," 124
    tuberculosis (TB), 17–19, 141–52, 159
dispensary system, 129–30
Displaced Persons (DP) camps, 39, 141
Döblin, Alfred, 59
"Doctors' Plot," 222–23
Dresden, 41, 185, 226, 228, 230
Drewitz, Ingeborg, 91
Drummer, Kurt, 182
Dulles, Allen Welsh, 84
Duncker, Hermann, 61–62
Dymshits, Alexander, 61

East German Film Studios (*Deutsche Film-Aktiengesellschaft*, DEFA), 87, 91
Eastern Bureau (*Ostbüro*), 215n11
Eastern Policy (*Ostpolitik*), 132, 184. See also détente
Egypt, 223–24
Eichmann, Adolf, 225
    Eichmann trial, 50
Eigen-Sinn, 5, 205, 258–59, 265, 271–72
Eile mit Meile (jogging campaign), 263, 266

Engels, Friedrich, 247, 253
Engholm, Björn, 185
England, 190
epidemiological research, 129–32
"euthanasia" program, 38
exile, 86, 101, 109, 125, 127, 210
exiles, 59, 61–68, 71–72, 86, 105, 215n11, 245
existentialism, 66, 71, 76n48
expellees, 43, 141
Exquisit shops, 181

factories (*Volkseigene Betriebe*, VEB), 9, 47, 158, 202, 204, 209, 223–24, 228, 230, 259–60, 262, 265, 267–68
    Berliner Werkzeugmaschinenfabrik Marzahn, 271
    Karl-Marx-Werk, 228
    Tiefbau Berlin, 266–70
    VEB Grubenlampe, 229
    VEB Thüringer Kugellagerfabrik, 229
    VEB Werkzeugfabrik, 229
Fainsod, Merle, 6
Fallada, Hans, 62
farmers, 12, 29n65, 64, 79n80, 261
fascism, 4, 20, 59, 66–67, 86, 92, 283
Federal Office of Health Education (*Bundeszentrale für gesundheitliche Aufklärung*), 131–32
Federal Republic of Germany (West Germany), 4, 6, 10, 20–21, 80, 82, 84–85, 89–91, 99, 107–8, 142, 145–47, 149–51, 159–60, 174n12, 182–85, 190–91, 222, 225–28, 231, 233
Finkelstein, Norman, 49
First German Writers' Congress (1947), 17–18, 56–70
Flicke, Wilhelm, 83–84, 86, 88, 90
football (soccer), 20, 257–76, 287
football teams
    Bayern München, 259
    Berliner FC Dynamo (BFC), 264–65, 271
    Chemie Leipzig, 268
    Dynamo Cottbus, 267, 269
    Dynamo Dresden, 259, 264

Dynamo Forst, 266–69
Eintracht Mahlsdorf, 261
FC Nordost Berlin, 271
Fortschritt Heubach, 264
Lokomotive Weißenfels, 262
Rotation Leipzig 1950, 261, 271
Traktor Bürgwerben, 262
Traktor Gusow, 260
Traktor Hochstedt, 257, 266–69
Traktor Letschin, 260
Union Berlin, 259
Fortschritt, Der (journal), 85
Foucault, Michel, 21, 79–94, 95n9, 279
Four Year Plan (1936), 206
Fourth German Writers' Congress (1955), 70
Framingham Study, 123
France, 11, 37, 46, 49, 147, 209, 223, 226
Frau von heute, Die (journal), 159, 161, 175n26
Free German Trade Union Federation (*Freier Deutscher Gewerkschaftsbund*, FDGB), 40, 179, 187, 207, 228, 260, 263
Free German Youth (*Freie Deutsche Jugend*, FDJ), 228, 260, 263
Freud, Sigmund, 279
Freyburg, 185
Friedensburg, Ferdinand, 64
Friedländer, Saul, 13, 283
Fühmann, Franz, 102, 114n19
Fulbrook, Mary, 12, 167, 173–75, 177–78
funerals, 214n6
Für Dich (journal), 90, 162–63, 166–67, 175n26

Galeano, Eduardo, 271
Gaus, Günter, 259, 177n50
Gaza, 227
Gdansk, 187
gender, 20, 158, 162–63, 168–71, 202, 216n21
gender relations, 10, 18, 20, 158, 162–63, 171, 285
genocide, 4, 9, 13, 20, 27n29, 33–34, 39, 49, 80, 209
Gera, 227

German Cardiovascular Prevention Study (*Deutsche Herz-Kreislauf-Präventionsstudie*), 131
German Football Association (*Deutscher Fußball-Verband der DDR*, DFV), 259, 264
German Gymnastics and Sports Federation (*Deutscher Turn- und Sportbund*, DTSB), 268, 271
German Hygiene Museum (*Deutsches Hygiene-Museum*), 125, 132, 160, 164
German Resistance Memorial (*Gedenkstätte Deutscher Widerstand*), 108, 111
German-Soviet Friendship, 100, 106, 109
German Writers' Association (*Deutscher Schriftstellerverband*, DSV), 70
Gestapo, 39–41, 201, 210
"Gewissen in Aufruhr" (film), 101
Gilbert, Doug, 265, 269
Ginzburg, Carlo, 15
Gleichberechtigung. *See* gender relations
Globke, Hans, 46
Goellner, Joachim, 248–50
Goethe Communities (*Goethegemeinden*), 66
Goldbroiler, 181
Goldhagen, Daniel J., 27n29
"Good Bye Lenin!" (film), 18, 181
Gorbachev, Mikhail, 184, 250, 252
Götting, Gerald, 72
Great Britain. *See* United Kingdom
Great Depression, 23
Greece, 185, 187
Grieder, Peter, 3–4, 6, 24
Grix, Jonathan, 262
Gromyko, Andrei, 184
Grotjahn, Alfred, 124, 141, 144
Group 47 (*Gruppe 47*), 68
Guddorf, Wihelm, 88

Haenel, Helmut, 162, 165, 177n57
Haffner, Sebastian, 14
Hager, Kurt, 180–81
Halbwachs, Maurice, 33
Halle, 229
Halle, Günther, 87
Hallstein Doctrine, 225

Hamburg, 47
Harich, Wolfgang, 64, 66–67, 70, 73
Harnack, Arvid, 84, 88–89
Harsch, Donna, 10
Hauptmann, Gerhart, 62
Havana, 188
health (health-care), 5, 20, 37, 40, 121–34, 141–52, 159–73, 183, 260, 270, 285, 289
    health education, 125–26, 132
    health policy, 17, 124–25, 133–34
heart surgery, 128
Heidegger, Martin, 66
"Heimkehr in ein fremdes Land" (film), 101–2
Hein, Christoph, 242
Heinemann, Lothar, 129
Hellmann, Rudi, 266–67, 270
Hensel, Helmut, 41
Herbert, Ulrich, 208
Heym, Stefan, 10, 241, 245
"Historians' controversy" (*Historikerstreit*), 49
Hitler, Adolf, 22, 27n29, 35, 40, 44, 79, 212, 213n2, 224, 227, 229
"Hitler Myth," 209, 282–83
Hitler Youth (*Hitler Jugend*, HJ), 44
Hitler Youth generation, 261
HO stores, 191
Hobsbawm, Eric, 22
Höhne, Heinz, 89–91
Holocaust. *See* genocide
Holocaust (TV miniseries), 48
homosexuals (homosexuality), 21–22, 38
Honecker, Erich, 2, 12, 18–19, 87, 92, 102, 104, 128, 132, 167, 173, 174n3, 183–84, 242, 257–58, 262–71
hooliganism, 258, 271
Horizonte (journal), 59, 69
hotels
    Astoria, 186–87
    Chemnitzer Hof, 182
    Neptun, 187
House Un-American Activities Committee (HUAC), 21
Huch, Ricarda, 61
Humanitas (journal), 176n38
humiliation, 237–53

Hungarian Revolution (1956), 206, 223
Hungary, 185
Hunt, Michael, 29n70

Iceland, 188
identity 2, 35, 39, 41, 63–64, 68, 71, 77n72, 80, 106, 109–12, 118n82, 167–68, 183, 191, 226, 261, 284
individualism, 12, 167–68, 177n48
inner émigrés, 62–63, 67, 72
Inquisition, 245
Institute for Marxism-Leninism (*Institut für Marxismus-Leninismus*), 88
Institute for Nutrition (*Institut für Ernährung*), 161. *See also* Central Institute for Nutrition
intellectuals, 18, 56–59, 61–68, 72–73, 78n80, 252, 285
Intelligentsia, 102, 169, 171, 204, 223, 230, 284
Intershops, 181
Iraq, 185
Iron Curtain, 6, 15, 165, 170, 172, 174n8
Israel, 18, 46, 219–31
Iwanow, Konstantin, 225

Jaspers, Karl, 59, 66
Jerusalem, 227
Jesus, 226
Jewish Historical Institute (Warsaw), 39
Jews, 22, 27n29, 35, 39, 46, 48–50, 209, 286
Jim Crow Laws, 13, 22
Johnson, Molly Wilkinson, 261
June 17, 1953 uprising, 1, 18–19, 47, 202, 204–8, 210–12, 216n23, 261
Junge Welt (newspaper), 90
Jünger, Ernst, 64

Kadar, Janos, 185
Kahan, Anette, 47
Kant, Hermann, 102, 110
Kantorowicz, Alfred, 62, 68–70
Kasslerrollen, 180, 183, 190
Kataïev, Valentin, 57, 61
Kaul, Friedrich Karl, 225
Kennedy, John F., 22
Kershaw, Ian, 13, 204, 215n11

Khrushchev, Nikita, 206
kibbutzim, 219, 227
Klemperer, Victor, 224
Kleßmann, Christoph, 122
Kocka, Jürgen, 10
Königsee, 229
Kopstein, Jeff, 213n2
KPD. See Communist Party of Germany
Krause, Jürgen, 183
Kraushaar, Luise, 91
Kroboth, Rudolf, 182
Küchenmeister, Claus, 91
Küchenmeister, Wera, 91
Kuckhoff, Adam, 63, 91
Kuckhoff, Greta, 63, 79–94, 284
Kügelgen, Bernt von, 103–12, 284
Kurella, Alfred, 71

Lafontaine, Oskar, 185–86
Langgässer, Elisabeth, 62
Lanzmann, Claude, 50
Laos, 185
Lasky, Melvin J., 57, 60–62, 70, 73
League of German Girls (*Bund deutscher Mädel*, BdM), 44
League of German Officers (*Bund deutscher Offiziere*), 102
Lebanon, 230
Lehmann, Klaus, 85
Leipzig, 202, 230
Lengsfeld, Vera (Wollenberger), 47
Lenin, Vladimir, 105, 232, 237, 240, 244–45, 247, 249, 251
Leningrad, 187
Leninism. See Marxism-Leninism
Leonhard, Wolfgang, 58, 244–45
liminality, 258, 271
Lindner, Ulrike, 151
LPG. See agricultural cooperatives
Lübeck, 29n63, 147–49, 151
Lübke, Heinrich, 46
Lüdtke, Alf, 3, 5, 206, 209

Magazin, Das (journal), 159, 162
Magdeburg, 227
Mann, Thomas, 59
Mannheim, Karl, 79
Marcusson, Erwin, 125, 132, 145

Maron, Monika, 47, 241, 245
marriage ceremonies, 214n6
Marshall Plan, 58
Martini, Winfried, 89–90
Marx, Karl, 212, 247, 249, 252, 279
Marxism-Leninism (Marxist-Leninist), 48, 220, 237, 240, 244–45, 248–52, 282, 287
Marxism. See Marxism-Leninism
Mason, Timothy, 13, 201, 203, 206, 213n2
McCarthyism, 29n70
McLellan, Josie, 19, 167, 173, 177n52–53
Medical Commission of the SED Central Committee (*Medizinische Kommission des ZK*), 174n11
Mein Kampf, 79
Meinecke, Friedrich, 65, 73
Meiningen, 223
Meir, Golda, 222
Meissen, 185
Memorial to the Murdered Jews of Europe, 51
memory, 5, 17, 20, 23, 33–36, 40, 42–43, 51, 52n5, 79–94, 99–100, 103, 105, 108–12, 118n82, 147, 149, 151, 179–83, 189–93, 207, 280, 282, 284, 289
    memory culture, 72, 99, 100, 104, 283
    memory literature, 105
mentalities, 6, 9, 20, 24, 282
Merker, Paul, 221
Meuschel, Sigrid, 22
Mexico, 188
Meyer, Hans, 62
middle classes, 2, 79, 102, 123–24, 169
Middle East, 221, 225
Mielec, 41
Mielke, Erich, 87–88, 91, 240, 266
militarism, 216n15
military service, 19, 47
Ministry for State Security (MfS, or Stasi), 1, 3, 9, 12, 14, 45, 87, 91, 103, 204, 210, 237, 240–41, 250, 258, 264, 266, 278, 280–82
    informants (*Inoffizielle Mitarbeiter*, IM's), 1, 14, 104

Ministry of Health
(*Gesundheitsministerium*), 124,
144–49, 159–60
"modern dictatorship," 10, 28n60
MONICA (Multinational MONItoring
of trends and determinants in
CArdiovascular disease), 129
Moscow, 4, 14, 62, 80, 87, 91–92, 222,
250, 282
MRFIT (Multiple Risk Factor
Intervention Trial), 131
Munich Olympics (1972), 22, 263

Nantucket, 187
Nasser, Gamal Abdel, 224
National Committee for a Free Germany
(*Nationalkomitee Freies Deutschland*),
101–5, 107–8, 111
National Committee for Health
Education (*Nationales Komitee für
Gesundheitserziehung*), 126, 159–60,
169
National Democratic Party of Germany
(*National-Demokratische Partei
Deutschlands*, NDPD), 36, 102–3
National Front (*Nationale Front*, NF),
36
National People's Army (*Nationale
Volksarmee*, NVA), 47, 101
National Research and Memorial Sites of
Classical German Literature (*Nationale
Forschungs- und Gedenkstätten der
klassischen deutschen Literatur*), 72
National Socialism (National Socialists,
NSDAP), 6–7, 13, 17, 19–23,
30n79, 33–51, 59–68, 78n80, 79–85,
89–90, 92–93, 99–104, 100, 102,
107–8, 112, 114n19, 122, 124, 126,
133–34, 143–46, 151, 171–73,
174n5, 174n12, 201–12, 213n3, 222,
224, 227, 229–31, 236, 241–42, 261,
277–80, 282–84, 286–88
Naumann, Konrad, 266
Nazism. *See* National Socialism
Neue Menschen (journal), 100
Neues Deutschland (newspaper), 40, 90,
221, 226–27, 250
Neutsch, Erik, 243

New Course, 207
"new cultural history," 2
New Forum, 270
New York Left, 61
Nicaragua, 185
Niethammer, Lutz, 27n39
Nietzsche, Friedrich, 279
Nora, Pierre, 33
Norden, Albert, 183, 225, 227
"normalization," 11–14, 173, 174n2,
287–88
Norway, 188
nouvelle cuisine, 191
November Revolution (1918), 204, 207,
213n2
Novyj Mir (journal), 87
NSDAP. *See* National Socialism
Nuremberg Laws, 13, 22

Oberländer, Theodor, 46
Oberliga (domestic football league),
258–59, 264
obesity, 160, 163, 165, 172, 174, 174n8
Office for Human Research Protection,
22
Office of the Military Government in
Germany (OMGUS), 60
Ophüls, Marcel, 49
Ortega, Daniel, 184–86
Ost und West (journal), 68, 76n55
Ostalgie, 7, 12, 18, 30n79, 190–92, 279
Ostbüro. *See* Eastern Bureau
Ostpolitik. *See* Eastern Policy
Ould, Herman, 68

Palace of the Republic, 181, 189
Palais Unter den Linden, 184–185
Palestine, 221
Papandreou, Andreas, 185
"participatory dictatorship," 9
Partisan Review (journal), 60
Pätzold, Kurt, 48, 50
Paulus Church (Halle), 229
Paxton, Robert, 49
Peitsch, Helmut, 93
"people's community" (*Volksgemeinschaft*),
42, 207
Pérez de Cuéllar, Javier, 185

Perrault, Giles, 89
Petershagen, Rudolf, 101–2
petitions (*Eingaben*), 9, 204, 257–58, 262–68, 270–71, 287
Peukert, Detlev, 206
physicians, 143, 146–50, 152
Pieck, Wilhelm, 187, 221
Piscator Theater, 40
Plötzensee, 40
Poland, 35, 50, 206, 211, 224
Politburo (SED), 184, 189, 225, 227
polyclinic, 148
Popovič, Jovan, 67
Port, Andrew, 177n48, 248
Prague Spring, 45
PRISMA (television show), 265
production quotas, 19, 210
Protestant Reformation, 67, 71
Protestantism, 224

racial hygiene, 145, 151
racism, 13, 22–23, 35–37, 45, 63, 79, 92, 124, 209, 212
Ravensbrück, 41
Rawls, John, 240–41
"real existing socialism," 8, 189, 263
rearmament, 205–7
Red Army, 35, 204, 212, 239, 277
Red Orchestra, 79–94
Redetzky, Hermann, 125, 132
refugees, 43, 141
Resistenz, 6
restaurants
    Jägerhütte, 187
    Tampico, 182
    Thüringer Hof, 186
    Trader Vic's, 190
    Waffenschmied, 189
returnees, 99–112
Rhineland, 209
Ribnitz, 229
Richter-Schnog, Eva, 63
Riedel, Otto, 71
Riga, 187
"risk factor model," 122–23, 127–28, 130–32, 165–66, 172
Ritter, Gerhard, 85, 90
Roeder, Manfred, 83, 85, 89–90

"Röhm Putsch," 44
Romania, 191
Roosevelt, Franklin Delano, 4
Rose, Geoffrey, 130
Rostock, 187, 223
Rotkäppchen (sparkling wine), 185–86

Saalfeld, 214n6
Saar, 185
Saarland Referendum (1935), 209
Sabrow, Martin, 93
Sachsenhausen, 36
Sachsenring Zwickau, 268
Samrin, Heng, 184
sanatorium, 142, 144, 146–47
Sartre, Jean-Paul, 66
Sartzetakis, Christos, 185
Scheel, Heinrich, 89
Scheinis, Zinovii, 225
Schleswig-Holstein, 185
Schmidt, Henry, 41
Schneider, Michael, 202
Schnog, Karl, 63
Schroeder, Klaus, 6
Schulze-Boysen, Harro, 84, 88–89
Schutzstaffel (SS), 39–42, 44
Schwerin, 230
"secret speech" (1956), 206
Seghers, Anna, 71, 244
self-censorship, 238
self-criticism, 245, 251
shame, 239, 241, 249
ships
    Andrea Doria, 187
    Arkona, 188
    Fritz Heckert, 187–88
    Stockholm, 187
    Völkerfreundschaft, 187–88, 192
Shoah (documentary), 50
Sieg, John, 88
Six-Day War (1967), 220, 226, 230
Slánský trial (1952), 30n78, 222–23
Slow Food movement, 191
Smolensk, 6
soccer. *See* football
Social Democrats, 40, 44, 141–45, 210–11, 213n1, 215n11
social divisions, 211

social hygiene (social hygienists), 122–25, 141, 143, 145, 166
social mobility, 10, 208
socialist humanism, 65
socialist realism, 70, 73, 237
Sochi, 187
"Sonderweg thesis," 11, 14
Sopade reports, 215
Soviet bloc, 18–20, 22–23, 176n40
Soviet Military Administration in Germany (SMAD), 58, 141, 144
Soviet Union (USSR), 1–2, 6, 10, 23, 29n70, 100, 110, 141, 147–48, 188, 191, 204, 209, 225, 227, 244–45, 247, 252
Soviet Zone of Occupation (SBZ), 57, 80, 83, 85, 99, 159
Spain, 188
Spanish Civil War, 63
Spartakiad, 260, 274n23
Spiegel, Der (journal), 89–90
sports clubs (*Sportvereinigungen*, SV)
    SV Chemie, 261
    SV Dynamo, 264, 267
    SV Lokomotive, 259
    SV Stahl, 260
    SV Vorwärts, 259
Sports Department of the SED Central Committee (*Sportabteilung des ZK*), 261–62, 266
Spreewaldgurken, 17, 181
Sputnik (journal), 250
SS. *See* Schutzstaffel
stability, 9, 11–12, 14, 16, 22–24, 73, 132, 181, 201, 279–80
Stadtroda, 145
Stakhanovism, 211
Stalin, Josef, 4, 105, 109, 223, 232, 244–45, 248
Stalingrad, 101, 209
Stalinism (Stalinization), 17, 35, 57, 69, 73, 210, 237, 244, 248, 251
Stamler, Jeremiah, 130
Stasi. *See* Ministry for State Security (MfS)
Steidle, Luitpold, 102, 146
Steinbeck, John, 59–60
Stern (journal), 85, 90
Stöbe, Ilse, 89
Strength through Joy (*Kraft durch Freude*), 206
Strittmatter, Erwin, 246
Strüwe, Kurt, 228
Suez Canal crisis (1956), 223–24, 228
Suhl, 189
Sweden, 147–48

Tallinn, 187
Tat, Die (journal), 89
TB (tuberculosis). *See* diseases, tuberculosis
Tempolinsen, 181
Thälmann, Ernst, 36, 101
Theresienstadt, 39, 41
Third Reich. *See* National Socialism
Thompson, Edward P., 5, 16
Thormeyer, Walter, 41
Thuringia, 144, 203
Timmermann, Carsten, 123
totalitarianism (totalitarian theory), 1–9, 14–16, 20, 22, 24, 26n28, 60, 79, 93, 258–59, 271, 281–82
Trabant (automobile), 192
Truman Doctrine, 58
Tuchel, Johannes, 87, 91, 95n24
Tunisia, 187
Turkey, 188
Tuskegee Syphilis Study, 22

Uhse, Bodo, 244
Ulbricht, Walter, 2, 19, 22, 86–88, 102, 108, 128, 132, 208, 210, 225–26, 229, 242, 248, 258, 260–61, 263
Union of those Persecuted by the Nazi Regime (*Vereinigung der Verfolgten des Naziregimes*, VVN), 37–40, 85
United Kingdom, 2, 11, 15, 147, 169, 178n67, 190, 220–21, 223, 226
United Nations, 220
United States, 13, 21–23, 29n70, 142, 145, 151, 160, 166, 169, 178n67, 190, 220–24, 226–38, 231
USSR. *See* Soviet Union

Verlag der Nation (publishing house), 102–3

Versailles Treaty (1919), 209, 212
Victims of Fascism (*Opfer des Faschismus*, OdF), 37
Vietnam, 226
Vishnevski, Vsevolod, 57
Voigt, Jutta, 180
Volkseigene Betriebe (VEB). *See* factories

Wandlitz, 184, 189
Warnemünde, 187–89
Warsaw Pact, 189–90
Wartburg Congress (1954), 71
Washington, D.C., 4
Weber, Max, 23, 279
Wehler, Hans-Ulrich, 10
Wehrmacht, 99–105, 108
Wehrmacht exhibition, 50–51
Weimar (city), 72
Weimar Republic, 17, 174n5, 211, 277
Weisenborn, Günther, 58–59, 62, 67–69, 72–73, 85, 89–90
"welfare dictatorship," 9
Welt, Die (newspaper), 89
Weltbühne, Die (journal), 221
Wende Museum, 184
West Germany. *See* Federal Republic of Germany
Westmoreland, William, 184
Willmann, Heinz, 69
Wilthen, 185–86
Wilton, Dan, 263–64
Windisch, Hubert, 227
Winter, Kurt, 125, 127
Winterhilfe, 205
Wismar, 224
Wolf, Christa, 49
Wolf, Friedrich, 239

Wolle, Stefan, 191–92
Wollenberger, Albert, 127, 132
women, 2, 7, 10, 16–18, 20, 47, 80, 89, 91, 125–26, 149, 157n59, 159, 161–65, 168–73, 176n38, 178n70–72, 182, 190, 211, 260, 285–86
workers
    industrial, 2, 5, 12, 19–20, 160, 169, 171–72, 201–12
    white-collar, 169–71, 249
Working Group of Former Officers (*Arbeitsgemeinschaft ehemaliger Offiziere*), 102–3
World Health Organization (WHO), 129–32
World War II, 22, 87, 99–101, 111, 122, 124, 141, 147, 224, 229–31

Yalta, 187
Yemen, 185
Yom Kippur War (1973), 230
youth confirmation (*Jugendweihe*), 203
youths, 2, 17, 23, 29n65, 36, 44–48, 51, 68, 92, 101, 105, 151–52, 164–65, 168–69, 176n34, 190, 203, 223, 228–29, 245, 259–60, 263–64, 267, 269, 274n23
Yugoslavia, 244

Zella-Mehlis, 229
"Zero Hour" (*Stunde Null*), 18, 51
Zhikov, Todor, 185
Zimmermann, Rudolf, 41, 43
Zionism, 220, 222–25, 232
Zwahr, Hartmut, 202
Zwerenz, Gerhard, 110
Zwickau, 229

www.ingramcontent.com/pod-product-compliance
Lightning Source LLC
Chambersburg PA
CBHW072145100526
44589CB00015B/2097